American [W9-AVC-119] Association

Physicians dedicated to the health of America

Evidence-Based to Value-Based Medicine

AMA Press
Vice President, Business Products: Anthony J. Frankos
Publisher: Michael Desposito
Director, Production and Manufacturing: Jean Roberts
Senior Acquisitions Editor: Barry Bowlus
Developmental Editor: Katharine Dvorak
Copy Editor: Kathleen Richmond
Director, Marketing: J. D. Kinney
Marketing Manager: Amy Postlewait
Senior Production Coordinator: Rosalyn Carlton
Senior Print Coordinator: Ronnie Summers

Internet address: www.ama-assn.org

Additional copies of this book may be ordered by calling 800 621-8335 or from the secure AMA Press Web site at www.amapress.org. Refer to product number OP841905.

ISBN 1-57947-625-2

Library of Congress Cataloging-in-Publication

Brown, Melissa M.
  Evidence-based to value-based medicine / Melissa M. Brown, Gary C. Brown, Sanjay Sharma.
    p. ; cm.
  Summary: "An introduction to the principles behind value-based medicine and its role in improving the quality of healthcare in the U.S. and maximizing the use of healthcare resources" —Provided by publisher.
  Includes bibliographical references.
  ISBN 1-57947-625-2
  1. Medical care—United States—Cost effectiveness. 2. Medical care—United States—Cost control. 3. Medical care—United States—Finance. 4. Evidence-based medicine—United States. 5. Medical economics—United States. [DNLM: 1. Quality of Health Care—economics—United States. 2. Cost-Benefit Analysis—United States. 3. Evidence-Based Medicine—United States. 4. Health, Resources—economics—United States. W 84 AALB8785e 2005] I. Brown, Gary C., 1949-II. Sharma, Sanjay, M.D. III. Title.
  RA410.53.B776 2005
  362.1'0973—dc22   2004021494

BP86:04-P-021:01/05

To our children, Heather, Heidi, Katie, Neel, and Evan, the very reasons behind our passion.

To the men and women in the arena who will make value-based medicine a reality to improve the quality of care and provide access to care for all.

"It is not the critic who counts. . . . The credit belongs to the man [or woman] who is actually in the arena . . . who strives valiantly; who errs, who comes short again and again . . . but who does actually strive to do the deeds; who knows great enthusiasms, the great devotions; who spends himself in a worthy cause; who at the best knows in the end the triumph of high achievement, and who at the worst, if he fails, at least fails while daring greatly, so that his place shall never be with those cold and timid souls who neither know victory nor defeat."

Theodore Roosevelt
"The Man in the Arena"
Speech at the Sorbonne
Paris, France
April 23, 1910

CONTENTS

FOREWORD

(The delivery of healthcare services is critically important for all citizens, no matter a person's age, gender, ethnicity, level of income, level of education, or place of dwelling. One measure of the effectiveness of a government is its ability to facilitate the delivery of high-quality healthcare services to its citizens. This can be done primarily through a private system, a public system, or though a combination of both, which is currently the situation in the Untied States.)

By most accounts, certainly mine, (the health delivery system is a mess. For those over 65 years of age we have a wonderful universal coverage system—Medicare—that is horribly inefficient, largely because it pays every provider the same price regardless of quality. For those under 65 we have a dynamic market that offers many different health plans—assuming you are healthy and wealthy. If you are sick or middle income, and don't work for a large employer you are likely to be one of the 40 million who are out of luck.)

(We have two totally different health finance systems in the US, a single payer system if you are over 65, and a very unstructured market system if you are under 65. The long-term answer to our healthcare and health spending dilemma, for me, is to merge the best of both systems—to come up with one well-structured and well-regulated system for all Americans, regardless of age, delivered by private payers, making rational coverage and payment decisions, with private capital, not taxpayer dollars, at risk.)

⁎The 2003 Medicare reform bill is a first step in that direction—more people getting Medicare through PPOs and other private health plans. Hopefully the next step—reform of the commercial system—will come once the dust settles from Medicare reform.

· (What is the missing ingredient to make the needed changes in the health system—information.) Information for consumers, for health plans, and even for providers to drive internal change. (Doctors, nurses, hospital administrators—they all want to do the right thing for patients. But there is no objective measure of what works? What adds value?)

Back in 1989, as part of the adoption of RBRVS, the White House (in the person of Dr Bill Roper and me), and Representative Henry Waxman, among others, pushed for a huge expansion of the Agency for Healthcare Research and Quality (AHRQ) to do precisely this—set up practice guidelines, evaluate drugs and devices, and set the standard for what works! AHRQ had a $10 million budget that was increased to $150 million a year. It is now over $300 million. Still the first time they tried to actually establish practice guidelines (for back surgery in 1993), they were attacked by the back surgeons—and Congress tried to abolish the agency! If this "objective evaluation" stuff was easy, it would have happened long ago.

As a result, the agency was forced to retreat from that core mission, and it became a research arm of the Department of Health and Human Services. Dr Clancy has done a terrific job at AHRQ, but I bet she also yearns to venture back into the biggest void in health policy—looking at what works and adds value.

As CMS Administrator I would love to have had objective value-based input on thousands of decisions I had to make, on both coverage and payment policy: What is the added value of the $27,000 insertible defibulator vs the $10,000 product? Do drug-eluting stents really add value, and deserve extra payment? (We decided they did—on very limited data). Is Arenesp in fact preferable to Procrit and does it add value? How about Enbril or Remicade? Are all PET scanners the same (they aren't, but Medicare pays as if they are). Does PET add value to an Alzheimer patient's treatment? Does Taxotere add value over Taxol?

I can assure you that, on January 1, 2006, when CMS starts pumping out $60 billion per year in new outpatient drug payments, they would love have objective answers to unending drug questions: Does Celebrex have the same issues as Vioxx? Does it add value over Motrin? Should the Medicare formularies be allowed to discourage Celebrex in favor of naprosin or Motrin, or Nexium in favor of Prilosec? Does Nexium add value?

(The questions are unending, the answers objective have been sparse. Lacking data on outcomes and quality, or information on added value, the US system pays for everything. And in traditional Medicare, even worse, they pay the same price for any variation on a product or physician or hospital service, regardless of quality. With no connection between payment and quality or outcomes, what to you get? No surprise—just what you created the incentive for—intense competition to churn volume of all goods and services and rapid volume inflation across the board.)

(The only way to change the system is to inject some competition over price and quality. And the only way to do that is to evaluate all health products and services objectively and give that information to everyone—consumers and providers. The debate and the process are 35 years overdue. The sooner it starts, the better.)

Drs Brown visited me at CMS in 2002. I liked their work then, and I like it now. I am not sure that Medicare, or private insurers, are ready to make yes or no coverage decisions based on this type of evaluation now—and I'm not sure I would advocate it. But Medicare, Medicaid, and private insurers would be far better to have access to this type of value-based research when making coverage and payment decisions. And doctors and patients would be far better off having it when they make care decisions.)

(No matter the system of healthcare delivery, value-based medicine provides an extraordinary return on investment. In essence, it gives us an information system that identifies healthcare interventions of the highest quality for the most reasonable cost. By doing so, value-based medicine allows healthcare dollars to be directed to services that return the greatest value.)

Patients will applaud value-based medicine because it empowers them with information to make more informed decisions and affords the opportunity to exercise greater control over their healthcare futures. Physicians and other providers instantly realize that value-based medicine allows them to deliver the highest quality care since it integrates the quality of life variables that the primary outcomes of evidence-based clinical trials often ignore. And policy makers and payers will favor value-based medicine because it enables them to secure the highest quality care and the greatest return on the resources expended for those who depend upon them to make the best decisions.

(In an era in which the annual healthcare budget in the US exceeds the Department of Defense budget by a factor of four, and CMS alone is almost double the budget of the DOD, it is imperative that the American public receives the greatest value for its hard-earned dollars. Value-based medicine will do just that, maximize both the quality of care and the volume of services delivered for the dollars expended. It will allow the healthcare system in the US to be all that it can be for those who depend upon it. The public deserves no less.)

In *Evidence-Based to Value-Based Medicine,* the authors have done a remarkable job detailing the exceedingly important concept of value in healthcare and have shown us the mechanism to use quality-of-life measurements in association with evidence-based medicine and relevant costs. They are to be commended on their superb efforts in seeking appropriate opportunities to quantify the care that is valued and efficacious—meeting the single most critical challenge toward making healthcare accessible and affordable for all Americans.

Tom Scully
Senior Counsel, Alston & Bird, LLP
Former Administrator, Centers for Medicare and Medicaid Services

PREFACE

The need for standardization of quality-of-life measurement instruments and cost-utility analysis has been previously recognized.[1-3] We believe this lack of standardization is the greatest impediment to the establishment of value-based medicine standards, which could improve the quality of healthcare and enhance the efficient utilization of healthcare resources in the United States and other countries. and by it decrease the health care costs.

It is our objective to present a template for standardization of the variables associated with cost-utility analysis to facilitate the creation of subsequent value-based medicine quality standards. Throughout *Evidence-Based to Value-Based Medicine* we make specific recommendations about how to effectively deal with the standardization issue. With time and further refinement, it is very likely, if not certain, that additional refinements will occur. While the methods we suggest may not be perfect—and some may disagree with them—they are far better than the chaotic system that currently exists in the arena of cost-utility analysis. In fact, many different methodologies to standardize input and output variables would be more acceptable than what exists today—a chaotic collection of incomparable analyses that are of minimal help to the clinician and patient. Let's just get it done!

It is our intent to demonstrate the best practices necessary for the performance of the most robust cost-utility analyses, and thus the most valid, value-based medicine database standards. In doing so, we will purposely repeat important concepts throughout the text, a format not typically used in many medical writings. We believe, however, that repetition is merited considering the importance of select concepts and the difficulty of segments of the material.

In regard to the goal of creating value-based medicine quality standards, the major goals of this text are to:

1. provide the reader with a working knowledge of the theory and the variables that go into cost-utility analysis and value-based medicine, and

---

[1]Gold MR, Patrick DL, Torrance GW, et al. Identifying and valuing outcomes. In: Gold MR, Siegel JE, Russell LB, Weinstein MC, eds. *Cost-Effectiveness in Health and Medicine.* New York, NY: Oxford University Press; 1996:82–134.
[2]Gold MR, Franks P, McCoy KI, Fryback DG. Toward consistency in cost-utility analyses: using national measures to create condition-specific values. *Med Care.* 1998;36: 778–792.
[3]Weinstein MC, Siegel JE, Gold MR, Kamlet MS, Russell LB. Recommendations of the Panel on Cost-Effectiveness in Health and Medicine. *JAMA.* 1996;276:1253–1258.

2.   present a coherent method to standardize the variables associated with cost-utility analysis to allow the establishment of a valid and clinically useful value-based medicine database.

Once these goals are accomplished, the incorporation of value-based medical standards and higher-quality care for all is close behind.

ABOUT THE AUTHORS

Melissa M. Brown, MD, MN, MBA   is Director of the Center for Value-Based Medicine, a medical faculty member at the University of Pennsylvania, and an Adjunct Senior Fellow at the Leonard Davis Institute of Health Economics at the University of Pennsylvania. A former nursing instructor at the same institution, she has a broad-based healthcare focus and has authored more than 125 healthcare writings. A nominee for US Congress and a member of the Advisory Council of the National Institute of Aging, Melissa brings a unique public-policy perspective combined with healthcare research and business principles to the value-based medicine arena.

Gary C. Brown, MD, MBA   is Co-Director of the Center for Value-Based Medicine, a professor at Jefferson Medical College, and Director of the Retina Service at Wills Eye Hospital. An Adjunct Senior Fellow at the Leonard Davis Institute of Health Economics at the University of Pennsylvania, he also served as Chairman of the Board of a managed care organization and is the author or coauthor of over 400 medical writings and eight books. Gary brings a unique managed care/health insurer perspective combined with medical research and business principles to the value-based medicine arena.

Sanjay Sharma, MD, MSc (Epid), MBA   is Director of the Cost-Effective Ocular Health Policy Unit at Queens University. An Associate Professor of Ophthalmology and Assistant Professor of Epidemiology at Queens, he is the recipient of multiple awards, including the prestigious Premier's Research Excellence Award. The author of over 200 medical writings, Sanjay brings a valuable blend of epidemiological and biostatistical medical research principles combined with a business perspective to the value-based medicine arena.

1

Background

Introduction to Evidence-Based and Value-Based Medicine

The term *evidence-based medicine* (EBM) has appeared increasingly in the healthcare literature over the past decade.[1–5] While the majority of healthcare professionals are familiar with the term, there are few who are familiar with the next level of healthcare to which EBM naturally transitions—*value-based medicine* (VBM). The purpose of this book is to provide healthcare stakeholders with a working knowledge of VBM, or the practice of medicine based upon the patient-perceived value conferred by interventions for the resources expended. In this book we address EBM, but comprehensively describe VBM and its critical role in improving the quality of healthcare in the United States while concomitantly maximizing the use of healthcare resources.

EVIDENCE-BASED MEDICINE

Evidence-based medicine is the practice of medicine based upon the best scientific data available. It forms the basis for the problem-solving approach—a conceptual framework that professionals and students in the healthcare sciences have used for centuries in gathering information, processing it, and attempting to utilize that which is most important, relevant, and useful.

Definition

> Evidence-based medicine is the practice of medicine based upon the best scientific data available.

Since the introduction of the term *evidence-based medicine* by Guyatt and colleagues in 1992,[2] the concept has become increasingly popular.[4] Yet, when speaking to healthcare professionals, one senses a frustration at the inability to decipher clinical research studies adequately and apply the evidence to practice. Professionals can recite the symptoms and signs of a multitude of diseases, but many have difficulty properly evaluating and critiquing an article written in the *New England Journal of Medicine, Lancet,* or the *Journal of the American Medical Association.*

Virtually all healthcare professional school curricula in the United States address EBM in some manner, but few give the same emphasis to EBM that they do to subjects such as anatomy or physiology. Yet, EBM will likely play a greater role in the lives of most practitioners than the content of many of the courses emphasized during training. There is little incentive for healthcare professional school curricula to include an equitable segment addressing EBM because few professional boards emphasize evidence-based healthcare at this time. This is not the case in a number of other industrialized countries. We believe this must change and will change over the coming decade. Why? Because(evidence-based medical data enable clinicians to deliver higher quality care than care based upon anecdotal data.)

It has been estimated that from 1948 through 1994, the total sum of health-care knowledge increased 1,342 times.[6] This preceded the vast increase in com-municative ability given to us by personal computers and the Internet. Judging from the number of articles appearing in the healthcare literature to the present time, it has been suggested that the total sum of medical information now dou-bles in approximately 3.5 years.[6] Beginning in professional schools and extend-ing throughout our entire careers in healthcare, we must continue to learn new data and update our criteria for care. New clinical results change the standards of care on an ongoing basis. The "fact of the day" learned today in the classroom or hospital ward may very well not be dictum—or even correct—10 years hence. For example, 10 years ago, increased secretion of hydrochloric acid in the stom-ach was thought to be the essential cause of peptic ulcer disease. Now it is known that the bacterium *Helicobacter pylori* is responsible for initiating gastric damage in the majority of cases.[7] Twenty years ago, the diastolic measurement was believed to be the most important component of blood pressure for predicting subsequent cardiovascular and cerebrovascular adverse events. Today, there is general agreement that *systolic hypertension* is just as important as *diastolic hypertension*.[8]

> The total sum of medical information doubles in approximately 3.5 years

We strongly believe that learning about EBM greatly improves the efficacy with which healthcare professionals gather and process new and meaningful information during their careers. Once the terminology is learned, practitioners will be able to differentiate the level of evidence for interventions to facilitate delivery of the highest quality of care. They will be able to quickly discern whether a negative study is underpowered, the important difference between *rel-ative risk reduction* and *absolute risk reduction*, and the meaning of *numbers needed to treat*. Rather than blindly accepting an article at its face value, profes-sionals will scan the oft-dreaded "Methods" section to see whether it merits inclusion in their disease-fighting armamentarium. Instead of wasting time por-ing over information that may be poorly gathered or presented, they will quickly move on to information that is more worthy of their attention. We can see that beginning to occur now, and welcome the increased emphasis on evidence-based changes; they bode well for our patients.

Value-based medicine, however, takes EBM to yet a higher level. It is even more fruitful for patients, healthcare professionals, and the entire healthcare system in the United States. Why? A major reason is because VBM incorporates all patient-perceived quality-of-life variables associated with an intervention, thus allowing a more accurate measure of the overall worth of that intervention to a patient than obtained with solely a primary evidence-based outcome.

Consequently, a better understanding of the patient-perceived value conferred by an intervention allows practitioners to tailor care and deliver higher quality by giving patients what they value most.

A healthcare *intervention* is a treatment (medical, surgical, pharmaceutical, and so on) designed to provide benefit to a patient.

VALUE-BASED MEDICINE

Evidence-based medicine is the practice of medicine based upon the most accurate and reproducible medical facts, while *value-based medicine* is the practice of medicine based upon the patient-perceived value conferred by an intervention. Value-based medicine takes the best evidence-based data and converts these data into value form.

Value-based medicine also permits the luxury of comparing the value conferred by the intervention with the resources expended on that intervention.[9–12] The instrument that allows this conversion of evidence-based data to value-based form is *utility analysis,* and the instrument that further integrates the cost associated with the intervention is *cost-utility analysis.* Cost-utility analysis affords a *Consumer's Report* on nearly all medical interventions in healthcare by providing a cost-effective ratio for each intervention that will allow the creation of a comprehensive VBM database.

Value-based medicine integrates the best EBM data with the *patient-perceived quality-of-life* improvement conferred by a healthcare intervention. It also allows integration of the value given by an intervention with the resources expended for that intervention.

While EBM was the catchphrase of the last decade of the 20th century, we are convinced that VBM will supplant it in importance in the early 21st century. Value-based medicine[9–11] takes disparate evidence-based data—whether in terms of percent improvement in cardiac ejection fraction after coronary artery bypass grafting or Snellen visual acuity improvement after cataract surgery—and converts the data into patient-perceived *value* using a common outcome measure. This value conferred by treatments can then be compared on a common scale for almost every intervention in healthcare.

Many clinicians currently speak of evidence-based outcomes in terms of numbers. For example,

- coronary artery bypass improves the cardiac ejection fraction from 45% to 55% or
- cataract surgery improves a person's vision from 20/80 to 20/25.

The questions of additional importance, however, are:

1. what is the patient-perceived value of each of these interventions, and
2. how can two such dissimilar interventions be compared in value?

It is obvious that the numbers as described here cannot be directly compared. But they can be converted to a value-based form that allows them to be directly compared.

How Is Value Measured?

The *value* conferred by any healthcare intervention is measured by quantifying the improvement (or maintenance) it confers in:

- quality of life and/or
- length of life.

An objective measure of value, standardized across the diverse fields in healthcare, is highly desirable because it readily provides:

- the most accurate assessment of the patient-perceived worth of an intervention,
- the means to compare all healthcare interventions on the same scale, and
- a measure that can be combined with the cost of an intervention to arrive at a cost-utility ratio.

Utility analysis is the principal instrument that allows us to measure the quality of life associated with a health state (or disease) across all specialties in medicine. It objectively assesses the quality of life associated with a health state, as well as the improvement in quality of life conferred when a healthcare intervention is administered for that health state. By convention, a utility value of 1.0 = perfect health and a value of 0.0 = death.

Cost-utility analysis is the means by which the value conferred is integrated with the costs associated with intervention. This allows us to create the information system that provides the foundation for the practice of VBM. Value-based medicine can be viewed as a pyramid, with EBM serving as the base, the conversion of evidence-based interventional data to patient-perceived, value-based data serving as the intermediate tier, and cost-utility analysis combining the patient-perceived value with the associated costs occupying the top tier (Figure 1.1). Both the overall value gained from an intervention and the cost-utility

FIGURE 1.1

The Value-Based Medicine Pyramid. Evidence-based medicine comprises the foundation. The evidence-based data are converted to value form and then costs are integrated with value using cost-utility analysis to arrive at the top tier, value-based medicine. The value conferred by an intervention and the cost-utility ratio associated with that intervention are the two most important outcomes in value-based medicine.

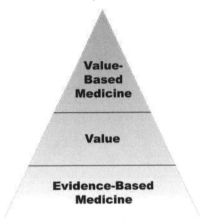

Figure courtesy Kathryn Brown.

ratio associated with that intervention are the two major outcomes of VBM we address throughout the book.

COST-UTILITY (COST-EFFECTIVENESS) ANALYSIS

Cost-utility analysis specifically refers to an economic analysis with an outcome measuring the resources (dollars) expended for the value (improvement in length of life and/or quality of life) conferred by an intervention.[13] The outcome measure is the dollars expended for a quality-adjusted life-year gained ($/QALY).*

> Cost-utility analysis refers to an economic analysis with the outcome of $/QALY, or dollars expended per quality-adjusted life-year gained.

Cost-effectiveness analysis refers to an economic analysis measuring a specific outcome such as the resources (dollars) expended per year of life gained, year of good vision granted, year of ambulation gained, and so on.

*By definition, the number of QALYs gained from an intervention equals the utility value gained from the intervention × the duration of the benefit in years. Thus, a gain in utility of 0.5 for 4 years equals 2.0 QALYs gained.

> Cost-effectiveness analysis refers to an economic analysis with an outcome of $/life-year (dollars expended per year of life gained), $/vision-year (dollars expended per year of good vision), and so on.

The Panel on Cost-Effectiveness in Health and Medicine, a panel appointed by the United States Public Health Service,[14] combined cost-utility analysis with other variants of cost-effectiveness analysis, and suggested that they all be referred to as *cost-effectiveness analysis*, a term with which most people have some familiarity. We believe this consolidation considerably confuses the literature for researchers and healthcare professionals, and that cost-utility analysis and cost-effectiveness analysis should be viewed as separate entities for the sake of clarity.

As we progress through this book, we primarily address cost-utility analysis. Despite the differentiation between *cost-utility analysis* and *cost-effectiveness analysis*, we still utilize the term *more cost-effective* when comparing the cost-utility of two interventions. While theoretically more correct, we believe that use of the term *more cost-utilitarian* would also confuse the literature and stakeholders in healthcare.

There are few industries in the world in which purchasers are unable to measure the value of what they purchase; historically healthcare has been the major one. Cost-utility analysis, the most sophisticated form of healthcare economic analysis, allows an objective measure of the value of healthcare services so that all persons with an interest in healthcare will be better able to appreciate the value of the services received for the dollars spent.

> There are few industries in which purchasers are unable to measure the value of what they purchase; historically healthcare has been the major one.

Some people perceive a system based upon cost-effectiveness and quality standards as rationing of care. It must be noted that VBM is not rationing. It is an *information system* that identifies treatments of substantial value and those that are of negligible value, of no value, or actually harmful. If an intervention is expensive, but works well, it is cost-effective. If an intervention has no benefit, it is not cost-effective at any price. In actuality, VBM is the *antirationing tool* in that it gives us ability to intelligently shift our resources to provide healthcare interventions that confer value to *all* of our citizens, including the 40+ million who currently lack healthcare insurance.[15,16]

Value-based medicine highlights interventions that provide considerable value and those that are of minimal benefit, of no benefit, or harmful. In this regard, it goes further than EBM in evaluating treatment benefit. In subsequent chapters we explain that VBM readily discerns which interventions can be harmful or of no value when EBM fails to differentiate an overall adverse or neutral outcome. Conversely, VBM can highlight therapeutic benefits not apparent with evidence-based data alone. How? Because VBM integrates *all* of the increments or decrements in quality of life associated with an intervention. These quality-of-life aspects are ignored more often than not in evidence-based clinical trials that typically measure outcomes such as survival, mortality, the incidence of stroke or myocardial infarction, the degree of pain, and other similar outcomes.

> Value-based medicine integrates all improvements or decrements in quality of life associated with an intervention. Value-based medicine allows a more accurate measure of the overall worth of an intervention to a patient than EBM alone.

Value-based medicine will not prevent patients in the United States from receiving medical interventions that work. Just the opposite: VBM will allow many more people to receive these interventions because it can be used to shift costs away from interventions that are shown to be ineffective or harmful. This ineffectiveness of therapies is a concept foreign to many policymakers and those not on the front lines of medical care. Nonetheless, there is not a healthcare professional in practice who does not realize that select therapies have no or negligible proven benefit and are possibly harmful.

With a VBM information system we will:

- improve the quality of healthcare and
- spend healthcare dollars more efficiently. ;

There are already more than enough resources devoted to healthcare services in the United States to allow the delivery of healthcare interventions that work to every citizen.[17] We just have to allocate them correctly.

WHY SHOULD WE CARE ABOUT VALUE-BASED MEDICINE?

Value-based medicine has several distinct advantages over EBM. Unlike EBM, VBM provides:

1. the most accurate assessment of the *patient-perceived* worth of an intervention,
2. a means to compare the value of all healthcare interventions using the same outcome measure, and
3. a measure of the total value conferred by an intervention that can be combined with the cost of an intervention to arrive at a cost-utility ratio.

What does this boil down to? Again, VBM offers the highest quality of care at the same time it saves dollars by maximizing the efficiency of the use of healthcare resources. By providing a more accurate measure of the value conferred by an intervention, VBM allows clinicians to practice the highest quality of healthcare. Why? Because it permits clinicians to selectively utilize interventions that deliver the greatest value from the viewpoints of patients who have lived in a health state.

Value-based medicine allows:
1. the highest quality care,
2. the maximization of healthcare dollars, and
3. the incorporation of *patient-based perceptions* of quality of life.

History

Famed American philosopher George Santayana is credited with the avowal that, "Those who cannot remember the past are condemned to repeat it." In this regard, physicians and other healthcare providers have a long history of opposing change (and forgetting the past). Many healthcare providers opposed the introduction of Medicare in the 1960s despite the need for a program to cover healthcare expenses of senior citizens. Consequently, the government moved ahead and provider input was minimal. And although healthcare costs in the United States spiraled at double-digit rates in the 1980s, most in healthcare did little to help stem the rise. Consequently, government policymakers promoted the concept of managed care because society demanded quality healthcare at a reasonable price.

> Although healthcare costs in the United States spiraled at double-digit rates in the 1980s, most in healthcare did little to help stem the rise.

Many providers opposed managed care, often with good reasons, but unfortunately did not offer alternatives to help provide quality care at a cost all could afford. Now, with healthcare inflation again rising at double-digit levels,[18] the healthcare community still has no collective plan for providing high quality care at an affordable cost. In this vacuum, others will surely come up with a solution—good or not—and prove Santayana right again.

What About the Educational Institutions?

The attitude of most healthcare professional schools toward healthcare costs is particularly striking. The great majority of schools have remained aloof in regard to healthcare economic issues, despite the great impact these issues will have upon their graduates and upon the most important people in the healthcare system—the patients.

We recently reviewed the curricula of the top ten medical schools[19] and found only one offered any formal introduction—a two-week course in the second year—to healthcare economics. The others had no formal teaching, and most did not even offer an elective available to medical students on the subject of healthcare economics or cost-effectiveness. Yet, addressing costs is critical, particularly when more than 40 million lack healthcare insurance;[15–17] those with insurance have difficulty affording pharmaceuticals, co-pays, and other charges;[20] and healthcare insurance inflation is well into the double digits.[18]

The Future

The understanding of cost-utility analysis requires knowledge of the efficacy of healthcare interventions, quality-of-life measures, and some basic economic principles. Once healthcare providers understand the economic principles, they are well equipped to evaluate the cost-utility of interventions because of their intimate knowledge of patient care and its complexities. It has been estimated that a system of VBM could potentially save more than $123 billion from the $1.77 trillion healthcare bill in the United States in 2004, while improving quality of care at the same time.[10,11,17]

It is our intent in this book to present an integrated vision of EBM and how it can be converted to VBM in a practical manner that is user-friendly to clinicians, including physicians, nurses, pharmacists, students, and other providers. There are other excellent texts that delve more into economic theory than we will address in this book,[13,21] but their complexity tends to intimidate practicing clinicians who, much like ourselves, deliver care "in the trenches."

We are convinced that providers must become fluent in the language of value, costs, and medical evidence. If clinicians do not lead in the development and promotion of these concepts, VBM will have a difficult, uphill course before being successfully incorporated into healthcare. Unless clinicians play an active role in the further development of VBM, we believe they will become little more than well-trained technicians in the healthcare system, while those more peripheral to actual patient care will be the policy decision makers. If this is the case, the United States public will surely suffer, because it is clinicians, with an intimate understanding of disease and health, who have the greatest potential to make positive contributions to VBM. Above all, the major goal of VBM is to promote what is best for patients.

> The major goal of VBM is to promote what is best for the most important people in healthcare—the patients.

CORE CONCEPTS

- Evidence-based medicine is the practice of medicine based upon the best scientific data available.
- Value-based medicine is the practice of medicine based upon the patient-perceived value conferred by an intervention.
- The value conferred by an intervention is measured in terms of improvement in length of life and quality of life.
- Value-based medicine allows clinicians to deliver higher quality patient care than EBM alone.
- The value conferred by a healthcare intervention can be integrated with the associated costs of that intervention using cost-utility analysis.

- Cost-utility analysis could save more than $120 billion from the United States annual healthcare expenditure at the same time it improves quality of care.
- The savings accrued from the adoption of VBM standards are sufficient to provide healthcare insurance to the current 40+ million uninsured in the United States.

REFERENCES

1. Chapman RH, Stone PW, Sandberg EA, Bell C, Neumann PJ. A comprehensive league table of cost-utility ratios and a sub-table of "panel-worthy" studies. *Med Decis Making.* 2000;20:451–467.

2. Evidence-Based Medicine Working Group. Evidence-based medicine: a new approach to teaching the practice of medicine. *JAMA.* 1992;268:2420–2425.

3. Neumann PJ, Stone PW, Chapman RH, Sandberg EA, Bell CM. The quality of reporting in published cost-utility analyses, 1976-1997. *Ann Intern Med.* 2000;132:964–972.

4. Sackett DL, Straus SE, Richardson WS, Rosenberg W, Haynes RB. *Evidence-Based Medicine: How to Practice and Teach EBM.* New York: Churchill Livingstone; 2000.

5. Stone PW, Teutsch S, Chapman RH, Bell C, Goldie SJ, Neumann PJ. Cost-utility analyses of clinical preventive services: published ratios, 1976-1997. *Am J Prev Med.* 2000;19:15–23.

6. Freitas R. Doubling of medical knowledge. Available at: http://discussforesight.org/critmail/sci_nano/5165/html. Accessed July 3, 2003.

7. Chan FK, Leung WK. Peptic-ulcer disease. *Lancet.* 2002;360:933–941.

8. Chobanian AV, ed. *The Seventh National Report on the Prevention, Detection Evaluation and Treatment of High Blood Pressure.* Bethesda, Md: National Heart Lung and Blood Institute, National Institutes of Health; May 2003. NIH Publication 03-5233.

9. Brown MM, Brown GC. Outcome of corneal transplantation: value-based health care. *Br J Ophthalmol.* 2002;86:2–3.

10. Brown MM, Brown GC, Sharma S, Landy J. Health care economic analyses and value-based medicine. *Surv Ophthalmol.* 2003;48:204–223.

11. Brown MM, Brown GC, Sharma S. Value-based medicine. *Evidence-Based Eye Care.* 2002;3(1):8–9.

12. Weinstein MC, Stason WB. Foundations of cost-effectiveness analysis for health and medical practices. *N Engl J Med.* 1977;296:716–721.

13. Drummond ME, O'Brien B, Stoddart GL, Torrance GW. *Methods for the Economic Evaluation of Health Care Programmes.* 2nd ed. New York, NY: Oxford University Press; 1999.

14. Torrance GW, Siegel JE, Luce BR. Framing and designing the cost-effectiveness analysis. In: Gold MR, Siegel JE, Russell LB, Weinstein MC, eds. *Cost-Effectiveness in Health and Medicine.* New York, NY: Oxford University Press; 1996:54–81.

15. Appleby J. Health-care premiums on rise again. *USA Today.* May 17, 1999:1.

16. Rundle RL. The outlook: can managed care manage costs? *Wall Street Journal.* August 9, 1999:1.

17. Brown GC, Brown MM, Sharma S. Health care in the 21st century: evidence-based medicine, patient preference-based quality and cost-effectiveness. *Qual Manage Health Care.* 2000;19:23–31.

18. Freudenheim M. CalPERS to vote on new health care rates. *New York Times.* June 16, 2003:C2.

19. *U.S. News and World Report Best Graduate Schools 2003.* Available at: www.usnews.com/usnews/edu/grad/ rankings/med/medindex.htm. Accessed March 29, 2003.

20. Carey J, Barrett A. Drug prices: what's fair? How we can encourage research and still keep prices within reach…for Cipro and beyond? *Business Week.* December 10, 2001:60–70.

21. Gold MR, Patrick DL, Torrance GW, et al. Identifying and valuing outcomes. In: Gold MR, Siegel JE, Russell LB, Weinstein MC, eds. *Cost-Effectiveness in Health and Medicine.* New York, NY: Oxford University Press; 1996:82–134.

Barriers to Entry

Despite the increasing popularity of cost-utility analysis in the healthcare literature,[1] it has not yet had a major impact on healthcare policy to date in the United States. This impact has failed to occur despite the fact that Klarman et al[2] described the quality-adjusted life-year (QALY) in 1968. Weinstein and Stasson[3] popularized cost-effectiveness analysis (today's cost-utility analysis) in 1977 and Sinclair et al[4] introduced the term *cost-utility analysis* in 1981.

In this chapter we discuss the issues that have impeded the incorporation of cost-utility analysis and value-based medicine (VBM) into mainstream healthcare practice. As well, we address how these issues can be resolved so that VBM can be integrated into healthcare practice.

PREVIOUS IMPEDIMENTS

Are there any current overriding drawbacks to performing cost-utility analysis?

1. Lack of standardization.
2. Lack of standardization.
3. Lack of standardization.

These three drawbacks may appear unnecessarily repetitive. But until standardization is undertaken, cost-utility analysis and VBM will not assume prominent roles in our healthcare system.

On a broad scale, a healthcare economic evaluation is not an exact science, and the methods used are typically not identical among analysts. An economic evaluation is, by definition, a multidisciplinary study design requiring input from the fields of clinical medicine, clinical epidemiology, economics and business, public policy, and mathematics. Subsequently, different analysts bring different expertise to their individual study designs, while possibly lacking knowledge in other areas. Also, methodological issues of controversy such as the decision perspective, the instruments used for measuring quality of life, the cost basis, and the rate used to account for the time preference of money have led to the employment of inconsistent study designs. Standardization of cost-utility analysis input variables will allow cost-utility analysis to be much more broadly applied in health policy.

CURRENT STANDARDS FOR THE
VARIABLES USED IN COST-UTILITY ANALYSIS

The guidelines currently used most often are those developed by the Panel for Cost-Effectiveness in Health and Medicine in 1996-1997.[5–8] The Panel for Cost-Effectiveness in Health and Medicine is a group organized by the United States Public Health Service to set standards of methodological practices a healthcare economic analyst should follow. The Panel for Cost-Effectiveness in Health and Medicine set forth some excellent recommendations, including the use of preferences in cost-utility analysis, the performance of reference case (the average person with the average variables associated with a disease) analysis, discounting costs and outcomes (QALYs, or quality-adjusted life-years gained) at a 3% annual rate, and the utilization of sensitivity analyses.

Despite the production of a comprehensive and learned academic treatise on cost-effectiveness (cost-utility) analysis,[9] the recommendations of the Panel for Cost-Effectiveness in Health and Medicine have had a negligible effect upon public policy and resource allocation in the United States as of this writing.

Why? We list what we believe are likely reasons in the section that follows and give possible solutions for each that we will detail throughout the book. We believe the work of others can almost always be improved with time. Just as we hope to improve upon the work presented by the Panel for Cost-Effectiveness in Health and Medicine, we believe that others will improve upon our work.

Reasons Why Current Recommendations Are Ineffective

The reasons we deem that cost-utility analysis and VBM have yet not assumed a major role in the United States healthcare system are listed as follows.

Reason 1   The recommendations of the Panel for Cost-Effectiveness in Health and Medicine are complex and written more from the point of view of economic researchers than clinicians who deliver care on a daily basis.

Solution   Healthcare providers have substantial expertise in the area of interventions and patient care, but they lack experience with economic and business principles (discounting, present value analysis, decision analysis, sensitivity analysis, incremental costs, and so on), as well as the variants of healthcare economic analysis, especially cost-utility analysis. In this book we introduce providers and other researchers to cost-utility analysis—the theory, terminology, and methodology in what we hope is a user-friendly fashion—and present feasible, specific guidelines for performing cost-utility analyses—even without an MBA or degree in economics.

Reason 2   Although the Panel for Cost-Effectiveness in Health and Medicine recommended the use of a preference-based instrument in cost-utility analysis, it did not recommend a specific type of preference-based instrument (standard gamble utility analysis, time tradeoff utility analysis, willingness-to-pay utility analysis, rating scales, and so on) to measure quality of life for use in cost-utility analysis.

Solution The development of a preference-based, quality-of-life measurement database is imperative for the establishment of VBM standards. The lack of a uniform quality-of-life database comprised of patient preferences has been a huge deterrent to the performance of comparable cost-utility analyses. Healthcare economic researchers often refer to utility values as *patient prefer-ences* because a patient is required to decide which health state he or she prefers:

- life in his or her specific health state, or
- the alternative of good health received in return for giving up or risking something of value (time of life, money, life itself, and so on).

The various types of utility value analysis fit this description, and thus are all considered to be preference-based. Rating scales that require a person to select a point estimate on a scale from 0 to 100 that corresponds to his or her health-related quality of life are also considered by some to be preference-based.

We believe that time tradeoff utility analysis is an excellent preference-based instrument to use for the acquisition of patient-based utility values, although the study of rating scale methodologies is also reasonable to pursue. Whatever validated instrument is used, almost any is preferable to the current chaos in the arena of quality-of-life measures utilized in cost-utility analysis.

> A patient preference-based, utility value database obtained using a single quality-of-life instrument is imperative for the creation of VBM standards.

Time tradeoff utility analysis is discussed in depth in Chapter 9. If another methodology is shown in the future to be definitively preferable and universally acceptable relative to time tradeoff utility analysis, then we will use it. But con-tinuing along the current path of using a myriad of incomparable quality-of-life measures only propagates healthcare economic analyses that are incomparable, of negligible help in creating value-based quality standards, and not useful for public policy decisions.

Reason 3 The Panel for Cost-Effectiveness in Health and Medicine did not rec-ommend that utility values *from patients* be employed for cost-utility analyses used in resource allocation decisions.

Solution Instead, the Panel for Cost-Effectiveness in Health and Medicine rec-ommended the use of *community preferences* (utility values obtained from the general community) when performing a reference case analysis due to the belief that patients with a health state have a tendency to positively overestimate their health-related quality of life due to their ability to adapt to illness.[5] Others have observed just the opposite—that utility values obtained from a community-based population are higher than those of patients[10,11]—suggesting that the general community does not appreciate the degree to which a health state can diminish a patient's quality of life.

Whether higher or lower, the fact exists that utility values obtained from surrogate respondents (physicians, researchers, the general community, and so on) asked to evaluate the quality of life associated with a health state often differ dramatically from utility values obtained from patients with that health state.[10–14] We believe, as do others,[15–17] that *patient-based preferences* (utility values) associated with a given health state should be the "criterion" or "gold standard" for use in cost-utility analysis, since patients are best able to judge firsthand the quality of life associated with their health state.

> *P*atient-based preferences should be the gold standard for use in cost-utility analysis.

Reason 4   The Panel for Cost-Effectiveness in Health and Medicine recommended the *societal* cost-utility analysis perspective be used in cost-utility analyses utilized to decide healthcare resource allocations rather than the *third-party insurer* perspective.

Solution   Most healthcare services in this country are paid for by healthcare insurers or managed care organizations that have little interest in societal costs such as the loss of productivity and the cost of caregiver time and disability benefits. Therefore, we recommend the use of a *third-party insurer perspective* for cost-utility analysis. This perspective includes all direct medical costs, including hospital costs, physician costs, and pharmaceutical costs, and measures outcome in terms of QALYs gained.

The *societal perspective* includes all costs, direct medical, direct non-healthcare (caregiver costs, babysitting costs, and so on), and indirect (loss of wages, disability payments, and so on), and also measures the outcome in terms of QALYs gained. While the societal perspective may ultimately be the best, the wide-ranging costs it introduces, as well as the lack of agreement on which costs to include, greatly increase the difficulty in developing a usable VBM database. Once a VBM database is created, it can then be further refined to include important societal costs. The key is to develop that initial database. Too many hurdles of uncertainty will not allow it to happen.

Reason 5   There are varying recommendations on how to treat comorbidities.

Solution   *Comorbidities* are diseases that accompany a primary disease or disease of interest. Certain healthcare quality-of-life measurement methodologies rate interventions as more valuable in an otherwise healthy patient than in a patient with comorbidities. Thus, a total hip arthroplasty in a patient with a renal transplant and the Guillian-Barre syndrome is valued less than a total hip arthroplasty in a person with no other health problems. This can be viewed as a form of discrimination against those who are disabled, in this case the individual with a renal transplant and Guillian-Barre syndrome. We are certain that legislative and judicial bodies in the United States would not allow this form of discrimination to enter into public policy, especially since it runs counter to the Americans with Disabilities Act of 1990,[18] which forbids federal agencies (Centers for Medicare and Medicaid Services) from participating with entities that discriminate on the basis of disability. Therefore, we recommend the performance of cost-utility analysis without using comorbidities in a fashion that causes them to decrease the value of an intervention. (This issue is discussed at greater length in Chapter 9.)

> The use of comorbidities in a fashion that assigns more value gain from an intervention for a relatively healthy patient than one for a generally unhealthy patient violates the Americans with Disabilities Act of 1990.

Not only does not taking comorbidities into account keep within the law, but also it substantially decreases the enormous number of cost-utility analyses that must be performed to have a usable VBM information system. Utilizing comorbidities, the example of cost-utility analysis for total hip arthroplasty theoretically would have to be calculated for a minimum of thousands of variants (for example, for patient populations with diabetes mellitus and osteoarthritis of the hip, those with hypertension and osteoarthritis of the hip, those with diabetes, hypertension, and osteoarthritis of the hip, and so on).[19] A cost-utility analysis for osteoarthritis of the hip incorporating thousands of comorbidity variants would be a daunting task, to say the least.

Reason 6   Individual case analyses favor the young over the elderly.

Solution   Cost-utility analysis inherently favors interventions in younger individuals when different ages are factored in because the duration of benefit is often longer for a younger person than for an older person. While some believe this is the best way to distribute scarce resources in theory, we do not believe it is acceptable in a country with the resources of the United States. In addition, policymakers would be most reluctant to institute age-based standards since lobbying groups would oppose age-based analyses with considerable political effectiveness.

The Panel for Cost-Effectiveness in Health and Medicine recommended that healthcare economic analyses generally be performed using a *reference case* (average case) for an interventional model. The age utilized for a cost-utility analysis is therefore the age of the average person who undergoes a particular intervention. We agree.

Reason 7   There are insufficient evidence-based clinical trials to assess many interventions.

Solution   This is true for some interventions. But many interventions have excellent evidence-based data available to allow the performance of superior cost-utility analyses. We should use the best data first, knowing that a cost-utility analysis need not be performed on every intervention immediately to have an extremely useful VBM database. As more evidence-based clinical trial data become available, the respective cost-utility analyses can be performed. If a clinical trial also incorporates quality-of-life measurement instruments that can be used in cost-utility analysis, so much the better.

Reason 8 Some incorrectly believe that VBM is rationing and is therefore unethical.

Solution There is a perception, especially among those with the most superficial understanding of cost-utility analysis and United States healthcare economics, that VBM will lead to rationing of healthcare. From the ethicist's point of view, this could be viewed as potentially pitting individual rights (protecting the welfare of the individual) against utilitarian rights (maximizing resources for the most benefit for the most people).[20] Nevertheless, the utilitarian would argue that cost-utility analysis actually decreases rationing by allowing the savings resulting from the deletion of ineffective treatments to be shifted to insure the 40+ million people lacking health insurance in this country. The latter argument is compelling, to say the least.

We believe that policymakers should be educated to the fact that there is already more than enough money in the United States healthcare system to pay for *all of the healthcare interventions that work effectively for everyone in the country.*[10,21] Value-based medicine is *not* a system of healthcare rationing. Instead, it should be viewed as the system of "antirationing" that will ameliorate the unintended rationing that currently exists in the United States with 40+ million uninsured. Value-based medicine is an *information system* that allows the creation of quality standards so that all stakeholders in healthcare will maximize the quality of care received for the resources spent. But those interventions that have no value or that cause harm should be carefully scrutinized and made better or deleted.

> Value-based medicine is not a system of healthcare rationing. It is the "antirationing" instrument.

A crucial factor that policymakers and critics fail to understand is that not all medical, surgical, or pharmaceutical interventions are of benefit to patients: there are a number of healthcare interventions with negligible or no value, or that are actually harmful. Value-based medicine identifies those that are of superior value, negligible value, or no value, or that are harmful more accurately than evidence-based medicine (EBM) because it factors in all aspects of quality of life that evidence-based, clinical trial, primary outcomes often ignore.

Reason 9 People incorrectly equate the Oregon Plan with VBM. Naysayers to healthcare economic analysis often incorrectly quote the "Oregon Plan," referring to the healthcare priority list used for Oregon's Medicaid population in the

> Value-based medicine, as compared to EBM, more accurately measures which interventions offer superior value, negligible value, or no value, or are actually harmful.

early 1990s. Seven hundred seven diagnoses were listed, with funding starting at number 1 and progressing until no additional funds remained.[22] Payment for treatment would not have been made for approximately the last 140 diseases on the list.

Solution We agree that the Oregon Plan was unacceptable and would ration care. (It would have theoretically led to the unnecessary death of one of us.) But the 1993 Oregon Plan ranked diseases on the basis of 5-year survival and provider judgment, rather than utilizing any type of patient-perceived values or VBM principles. A comparison between the Oregon Plan and VBM is therefore most *inappropriate*. Again, the assessment of value conferred by an interventions and cost-utility analysis provides the information system database for VBM, a *Consumer's Report* that will allow the best care for the most people, whether in the United States or another country.

> Value-based medicine is *not* a system of healthcare rationing. It dramatically differs from the unsatisfactory and unpopular "Oregon Plan."

Reason 10 Cost-utility analysis may run counter to some stakeholders' financial interests in the healthcare system. For example, a medical intervention or surgical intervention currently practiced might be shown to have negligible value or no value, or be harmful once its longevity benefits, quality-of-life benefits, and adverse effects are taken into account using decision analysis.

Solution The influence of stakeholder groups in healthcare cannot be overemphasized. If VBM is to be successful, buy-in from groups such as the American Association of Retired Persons (AARP), the American Medical Association (AMA), the American Nursing Association (ANA), and other professional and public advocacy groups will be necessary. Can this be done? Unequivocally yes. Why? Because the paradigm of VBM ultimately benefits patients greatly.

> The reason VBM should be incorporated into public policy: *value-based medicine greatly benefits patients.*

The overriding reason to promote or discourage an intervention is whether it is beneficial for or detrimental to the patient. Value-based medicine identifies interventions that are beneficial, or that are neutral or harmful, when they are not identified with evidence-based data by integrating the important quality-of-life parameters that many evidence-based studies ignore. While special interests could considerably slow the adoption of VBM, the facts that it:

- incorporates patient preferences,
- permits higher quality care, and
- maximizes the efficiency of expenditures

are features that will create a momentum to usher in VBM.

Possible additional reasons for the lack of impact of cost-utility analysis have been outlined by Brown and Fitzner.[23]

Reason 11 Healthcare insurance contracts do not include cost-effectiveness as a coverage criterion.

Solution Spiraling healthcare costs will facilitate the public acceptance of cost-utility analysis as a reasonable alternative to doubling the number of United States citizens unable to afford healthcare services.

Reason 12 There is no explicit cutoff between cost-effectiveness and lack of cost-effectiveness.

Solution Standards will be established once cost-utility analyses have been performed on a sufficient number of diseases to develop distribution curves. Whether lack of cost-effectiveness is established at two standard deviations above the mean or some other point estimate will be a societal decision.

Of critical importance is the fact that VBM will identify numerous interventions that deliver no value or have a net harmful effect and actually subtract value from a patient's remaining life. In these instances, the cutoff between cost-effectiveness and lack of cost-effectiveness is irrelevant since such interventions will not be cost-effective at any cost.

Reason 13 The values in cost-utility analyses change from year to year.

Solution Cost-utility analyses will be updated as interventions improve, new interventions are introduced, and costs change. Among all of the other drawbacks, this one can be readily addressed.

While we all desire perfection, we will never achieve a faultless healthcare system that pleases 100% of the population. But we can create a value-based healthcare system that will increasingly benefit patients and other stakeholders in healthcare. Once the public understands VBM and its rewards, the impetus to institute it will be considerable.

HOW DO WE MAKE VALUE-BASED MEDICINE HAPPEN?

Recent data suggest the healthcare system in the United States is heading toward severe fiscal distress.[24] Numerous remedies will be suggested, hopefully before this occurs.

We believe that VBM will provide the information system that allows the highest quality care to be delivered to the most people for the resources expended. Each of the drawbacks outlined can be readily addressed to make the system desirable, viable, and politically acceptable. For this to occur, however, the first step is to standardize the variables (patient preferences, costs, perspective, and so on) that go into cost-utility analysis.

In addition, the message must also be sent to the public and policymakers that VBM is advantageous because it will improve the quality of healthcare services for patients. Unfortunately, most papers in medicine are never read by other providers, much less the public. The information is lost or never taken from the laboratory or clinical trial setting to a point at which it helps actual patients. Value-based medicine cannot be allowed to go this route, and thus crossover writings into the lay literature will be necessary. To date, the concept of VBM has been extraordinarily well received by patient groups, healthcare professionals, and top healthcare policymakers.

When will we have a perfect methodology of cost-utility analysis? There is a surgical dictum that states "the enemy of good is perfect." We believe the same principle applies to healthcare economic analyses. So far, we have established no database of cost-utility analyses in the United States despite the fact that we have had quality-adjusted life-years for over 35 years[2] and a major public health push for healthcare economic analyses in the 1990s.[5] If we wait for the perfect methodology that meets everyone's standards for perfection, it will never come. Thus, we must start somewhere, and that is the reason for this book. Our recommendations will undoubtedly be improved over time, but unless we start with a standardized system at some point, we will continue to flounder with serious healthcare economic problems.

A Value-Based Medicine System Must Be Compatible With Current Reimbursement Methodology

We fully believe that we must create a system of VBM that is as compatible as possible with the present healthcare system. It is a system that should be compatible with the International Classification of Diseases (ICD) used for diagnoses,[19] the Current Procedural Terminology (CPT®) codes used for payment,[25] and the clinical trials that have already been performed. The cost of repeating trials to obtain utilities or other quality-of-life values is prohibitive, but repeating the trials is unnecessary since their data can be incorporated using a properly configured utility value database. In essence, we believe it is substantially easier to change the direction of the sails than change the course of the wind.

PEARL

It is far easier to change the direction of the sails than to change the course of the wind.

While the methods may not be perfect, they are far better than the arbitrary standards in place in the healthcare system at the current time. To let another quarter century pass before VBM is in widespread use would be unfortunate and

MEANING

We should incorporate a system of value-based parameters into our existing clinical trials and healthcare system.

unacceptable to those who require a strong and effective quality system of healthcare.

CORE CONCEPTS

- The lack of cost-utility input variable standards is a major deterrent to the widespread incorporation of VBM.
- Other deterrents to VBM include:
  - the complexity of the subject,
  - the lack of a standardized, patient preference-based, quality-of-life database,
  - the lack of standardized treatment for comorbidities,
  - the fact that VBM may run counter to the interests of select stakeholders in healthcare, and
  - the incorrect assumption that VBM will lead to healthcare rationing.
- Each of the deterrents can be overcome as described herein.
- There are healthcare interventions that provide negligible value or no value, or that are actually harmful.
- Value-based medicine is the "antirationing" instrument because it will allow the shift of resources from interventions that have negligible value or no value, or that are harmful to the provision of healthcare using interventions that work for all patients.
- Value-based medicine will be embraced by stakeholders in healthcare because it:
  - allows patient input in the form of preferences for health states and interventions to be included in treatment regimens,
  - improves the quality of patient care, and
  - maximizes the efficiency of the use of healthcare resources.

REFERENCES

1. Chapman RH, Stone PW, Sandberg EA, Bell C, Neumann PJ. A comprehensive league table of cost-utility ratios and a sub-table of "panel-worthy" studies. *Med Decis Making*. 2000;20:451–467.

2. Klarman H, Francis J, Rosenthal G. Cost-effectiveness applied to the treatment of chronic renal disease. *Med Care*. 1968;6:48–55.

3. Weinstein MC, Stasson WB. Foundations of cost-effective analysis for health and medical practice. *N Engl J Med*. 1977;296:716–721.

4. Sinclair J, Torrance GW, Boyle M, Horwood M, Saigal S, Sackett D. Evaluation of neonatal intensive care programs. *N Engl J Med*. 1981;305:489–494.

5. Gold MR, Patrick DL, Torrance GW, et al. Identifying and valuing outcomes. In: Gold MR, Siegel JE, Russell LB, Weinstein MC, eds. *Cost-Effectiveness in Health and Medicine*. New York, NY: Oxford University Press; 1996:82–123.

6. Siegel JE, Torrance GW, Russell LB, Luce BR, Weinstein MC, Gold MR. Guidelines for pharmacoeconomic studies: recommendations from the Panel on Cost-Effectiveness in Health and Medicine. *Pharmaeconomics*. 1997;11:159–168.

7. Siegel JE, Weinstein MC, Russell LB, Gold MR. Recommendations for reporting cost-effectiveness analyses: Panel on Cost-Effectiveness in Health and Medicine. *JAMA*. 1996;276:1339–1341.

8. Russell LB, Gold MR, Siegel JE, Daniels N, Weinstein MC. The role of cost-effectiveness analysis in health and medicine: Panel on Cost-Effectiveness in Health and Medicine. *JAMA*. 1996;276:1172–1177.

9. Gold MR, Siegel JE, Russell LB, Weinstein MC, eds. *Cost-Effectiveness in Health and Medicine*. New York, NY: Oxford University Press; 1996.

10. Brown GC, Brown MM, Sharma S. Difference between ophthalmologist and patient perceptions of quality-of-life associated with age-related macular degeneration. *Can J Ophthalmol*. 2000;35:27–32.

11. Fryback DG, Dasbach EJ, Klein R, et al. The Beaver Dam outcomes study: initial catalog of health-state quality factors. *Med Decis Making*. 1993;13:89–102.

12. Landy J, Stein JD, Brown GC, Brown MM, Sharma S. Patient, community and clinician perceptions of the quality of life associated with diabetes mellitus. *Med Sci Monitor*. 2002;8:543–548.

13. Stein J, Brown GC, Brown MM, Sharma S, Hollands H, Stein HD. The quality of life of patients with hypertension. *J Clin Hypertens*. 2002; 4:181–188.

14. Stein JD, Brown MM, Brown GC, Sharma S, Hollands H. Quality of life with macular degeneration: perceptions of patients, clinicians and community members. *Br J Ophthalmol*. 2003;87:8–12.

15. Angell M. Patients' preferences in randomized clinical trials. *N Engl J Med*. 1984;310:1385–1387.

16. Kassirer JP. Incorporating patient's preferences into medical decisions. *N Engl J Med*. 1994;330:1895–1896.

17. Kassirer JP. Adding insult to injury: usurping patients' prerogatives. *N Engl J Med*. 1983;308:898–901.

18. Gomez-Mejia LR, Balkin DB, Cardy RL. *Managing Human Resources*. Englewood Cliffs, NJ: Prentice Hall; 1995:134–136.

19. Hart AC, Hopkins CA. *International Classification of Diseases, 9th Revision, Clinical Modification*. Salt Lake City, Utah: Ingenix; 2003.

20. Desjardins JR, McCall JJ. *Contemporary Issues in Business Ethics*. 3rd ed. New York, NY: Wadsworth Publishing Company; 1996:23–41.

21. Brown MM, Brown GC, Sharma S, Landy J. Health care economic analyses and value-based medicine. *Surv Ophthalmol.* 2003;48:204–223.

22. Klevit HD, Bates AC, Castanares T, Kirk EP, Sipes-Metzler PR, Wopat R. Privatization of health care services: a progress report by the Oregon Health Services Commission. *Arch Intern Med.* 1991;151:912–916.

23. Brown E, Fitzner K. Cost-effectiveness and coverage policy. *Physician Exec.* 1999;25:75–77.

24. Freudenheim M. CalPERS to vote on new health care rates. *New York Times.* June 16, 2003:C2.

25. Davis JB. *Medical Fees in the United States 2004.* Los Angeles, Calif: Practice Management Information Corporation; 2003.

3

Healthcare Economics

Healthcare economics is a subject generally not addressed during the four-year curriculum of most medical schools or the subsequent years spent in residency programs. Nonetheless, once in practice, the majority of physicians and other providers find that healthcare economics plays a critical role in their professional lives and in the lives of their patients. In this chapter we present an overview of the aspects of healthcare economics pertinent to all providers, to other stakeholders, and to the subject of value-based medicine (VBM).

THE ESSENTIALS OF HEALTHCARE ECONOMICS IN THE UNITED STATES: A SYNOPSIS

Macroeconomics refers to the behavior of the economy as a whole. It deals with entities such as income, employment, productivity, and healthcare expenditures on a national level.[1] As the prefix *macro-* implies, macroeconomics is economics applied on a very large scale. The relation of macroeconomics to healthcare composes the majority of this chapter.

Microeconomics deals with the behavior of individual households and the laws of supply and demand.[1] In regard to supply and demand, we should know about *elasticity*. Elasticity signifies that *demand* changes concomitantly with *price*. For example, as the price of cars increases, the demand decreases, and the supply consequently decreases. As the price of cars decreases, the demand increases, and the supply consequently increases to meet the demand. A good illustration of elasticity is demonstrated by the sales of videocassette recorders (VCRs). As the price has decreased over the past decade, the demand has increased, as has the supply to the point that most households own a VCR.

Healthcare is generally considered to be *inelastic*, in that demand and supply respond slightly, or not at all, to changes in price.[1] Thus, although the price of insulin syringes increases, demand remains stable and the supply unchanged—rather than decreasing—as many diabetic patients cannot survive without insulin injections. They continue to purchase their syringes and will find some way to do so.

> Healthcare services are generally *inelastic,* meaning that as prices rise, the demand fails to decrease and the supply fails to decrease.

An important question arises given the previous information. How can healthcare inflation be brought down to a reasonable level while maintaining quality of care when the demand for healthcare services is inelastic and the normal market forces of supply and demand do not readily apply? We believe that VBM is the answer because it allows the maximization of the healthcare value received for the dollars expended.

WHY SHOULD PROVIDERS BE AWARE OF HEALTHCARE ECONOMICS?

There are some numbers that healthcare providers should know concerning the macroeconomics of the United States' healthcare system. There are not many, but a few basics are critically important.

In a recent poll of house officers and medical students, we found that only 10% had a vague concept of the annual United States expenditure on healthcare. When the question was asked in multiple-choice (five possible answers) fashion, 30% correctly answered, but 20% of responses were correct by chance alone. The obvious corollary that follows is: *why should physicians and other healthcare providers have any say in the allocation of healthcare dollars when their understanding of healthcare economics is so rudimentary?* Indeed, the thought is difficult to refute when data such as our physicians-in-training survey are presented.

> Only 10% of medical students and residents are aware of the annual United States national healthcare expenditure.

ANNUAL HEALTHCARE EXPENDITURE IN THE UNITED STATES

Actuaries from the Centers for Medicare and Medicaid Services (CMS), the parent organization of both Medicare and Medicaid formerly known as the Health Care Financing Administration (HCFA), have extensively studied annual healthcare expenditures in the United States.[2,3] In 1970, the total expenditure on healthcare in the United States was $73.1 billion (Figures 3.1 and 3.2), or approximately 7.0% of the gross domestic product (GDP). Adjustment of the 1970 expenditure for general inflation yields an expenditure of $356 billion in year 2004 dollars. The Centers for Medicare and Medicaid Services has estimated, however, that $1.773 trillion (15.3% of GDP) will be spent on healthcare services in 2004. Thus, the total healthcare expenditure grew at a rate five times that expected with general inflation from 1970 to 2004.

Put into another frame of reference, the estimated $1.773 trillion annual healthcare expenditure in 2004 is 4.7 times that of the fiscal year 2004 expenditure

($379.9 billion) of the United States Department of Defense.[4] The annual healthcare expenditure in the United States is estimated to rise to $2.639 trillion, or 16.8% of GDP, by 2010.[2]

> The estimated healthcare expenditure in the United States in 2004 is 4.7 times the expenditure for defense.

FIGURE 3.1

Annual United States Healthcare Expenditure

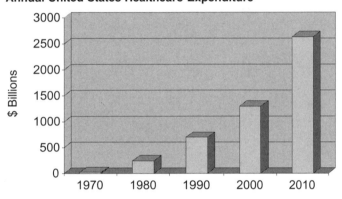

Source: The Office of the Actuary at the Centers for Medicare and Medicaid Services.[2]

FIGURE 3.2

United States Healthcare Expenditures as a Percent of the Gross Domestic Product

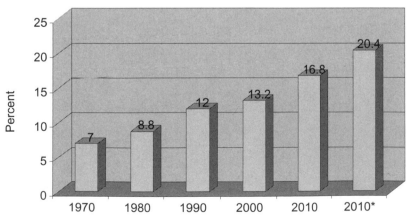

Source: The Office of the Actuary at the Centers for Medicare and Medicaid Services.[2]
* Estimate from the Center for Value-Based Medicine.[5]

> Approximately $1.773 trillion (15.4% of GDP) will be spent on healthcare in the United States in 2004. That figure is conservatively expected by the CMS to rise to $2.64 trillion (16.8% of GDP) by 2010.

THE RATE OF HEALTHCARE INFLATION

According to actuaries at Medicare,[3] healthcare expenditures over the 30-year period from 1970 through 1999 rose at an annual rate of approximately 10%, while general inflation rose at half that rate at an annual rate of 5%. A regression analysis from the Center for Value-Based Medicine suggests, however, that unless major healthcare policy changes are instituted, the 10% annual rate of healthcare inflation will continue in the foreseeable future with a 95% certainty.[5] If this trend does in fact continue, the total United States healthcare expenditure by 2010 will rise to $3.4 trillion, or 20.4% of GDP, rather than the Medicare estimate of $2.6 trillion,[2] or 16.8% of GDP.

PEARL

One might ask how economists can calculate the GDP for 2010. They can't. They know no better than we do what internal and external factors will affect the United States. It is an assumption game of guesses based on historical data.

The CMS actuaries have estimated that the yearly rate of healthcare inflation from 2000 through 2010 will range from 6.6% to 9.6%, with an average yearly healthcare inflation rate of 7.3% (versus 10% per year from 1970 through 1999). Nevertheless, healthcare insurance premiums for the California Public Employees' Retirement System (CalPERS) rose 25.1% in 2003 and will rise 18% for 2004.[6] Industry-wide figures for health insurance costs are estimated by Wall Street analysts to be 14% for 2003 and 12% for 2004, but the CalPERS data are widely viewed as an early indicator of national inflation rates in healthcare.[6] With a large number of aging baby boomers, the overall healthcare expenditure numbers have the potential to be forbidding. The time-bomb of baby boomers needing healthcare services is even more reason to incorporate the efficiency of the use of resources that VBM will offer.

PER CAPITA HEALTHCARE EXPENDITURES

The yearly per capita expenditure, or the amount spent on each person for healthcare services in the United States per year, has risen from $341 in 1970 to an estimated $6,126 nominal (face value or non–inflation adjusted) dollars in 2004 and is expected to rise to $8,704 nominal dollars by the year 2010.[2] (See Table 3.1.) Adjusting for the rate of general inflation (according to the Consumer Price Index) from 1970 through 2004, the real dollar expenditure in 1970 dollars equates to $1,662 in 2004. Thus, negating the influence of general inflation, the data show a 3.7 times ($6,126/$1,662) increase in healthcare expenditure per person above inflation over the past three decades. Put another way, the inflation-adjusted healthcare expenditure for the average person in the United States in 2004 is 3.7 times the amount expended for healthcare services for the average person in 1970. While the 2004 per capita healthcare costs are 3.7 times those of 1970,[2] the total 2004 healthcare costs are five times those of 1970 because of the concomitant increase in the United States population.[2,3]

PEARL

Real dollars are adjusted for inflation. Nominal dollars are not adjusted for inflation.

> After adjustment for inflation, the 2004 healthcare expenditure for the average person in the United States is approximately 3.7 times what it was in 1970.

Whether the 3.7 times inflation-adjusted increase in per capita healthcare expenditure from 1970 to 2004, or the annual doubling of overall healthcare inflation above general inflation over the same period, it is evident that healthcare expenditures have substantially outdistanced general inflation. There appears to be little evidence that the disconnect between healthcare inflation and general inflation will abate in the near future.

With the exception of the first four years of life, particularly the first year, healthcare expenditures per capita increase accordingly with age. Data from Older Americans 2000[7] show that in 1996 the average healthcare expenditure for a person aged 65 to 69 years was $5,864, compared with $9,414 among persons aged 75 to 79 and $16,465 among persons aged 85 or older. Approximately 1% of the Medicare population incurred over 13% of Medicare resources, while 5% incurred 37% of the resources.

Nursing home expenditures are particularly striking, with elderly patients living in institutions incurring approximately six times the healthcare expenditure per capita (mean = $38,906 in 1996) compared to those living in the community (mean = $6,360 in 1996).

TABLE 3.1

Per Capita Healthcare Expenditures in the United States

Year	Actual Expenditure	1970 Expenditure*
1970	$341	$341
1980	$1,067	$518
1990	$2,737	$769
2000	$4,637	$1,047
2004[†]	$6,126	$1,655
2005[†]	$6,519	NA
2010[†]	$8,704	NA

NA indicates not applicable (the rate of general inflation is not yet known).

* Inflation adjusted to 1970 real dollars.

[†] Estimate

THE DISTRIBUTION OF
HEALTHCARE EXPENDITURES

The distribution of healthcare expenditures in the United States since 1970 has
also changed and is anticipated to continue to change substantially (Figures 3.3
and 3.4).[2] In 1970, physician payments accounted for 19% of healthcare expenditures, while hospital payments accounted for 38% and prescription drugs for
8%. By 2000, physician payments had increased to 22%, hospital payments had
decreased to 32%, and drug costs had increased to 9%. It is estimated that by
2010, physician payments will decrease slightly to 21% and hospital payments
will continue to decrease substantially from a percentage perspective to 28%.
Prescription drug expenditures, however, are anticipated to increase to more
than 14% of the healthcare dollar by 2010.

In 2003, the three top healthcare item expenditures were hospital costs, physician services costs, and prescription drug costs. Hospital costs were $502 billion
(30.4% of the healthcare dollar), physician services cost $361 billion (21.8% of
the healthcare dollar), and prescription drugs cost $182 billion (11% of the
healthcare dollar) (Figure 3.4). Administration costs composed $112.2 billion, or
6.7%, of the healthcare dollar in 2003, while research costs composed only $29
billion, or 1.6% of the dollar. Nursing home care composed $107.1 billion, or
6.5% of the healthcare dollar.

> **P**rescription drug expenditures are anticipated to increase to 14% of
> the healthcare dollar by 2010.

FIGURE   3.3

**Percent Distribution of Healthcare Dollars in the United States in 1970, 2000,
and 2010**

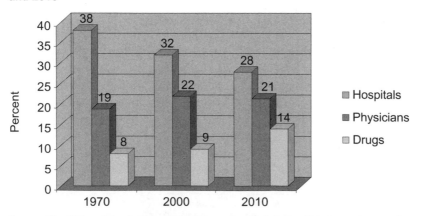

Source: The Office of the Actuary at the Centers for Medicare and Medicaid Services.[2]

FIGURE 3.4

Distribution of Healthcare Expenditures in the United States in 2003

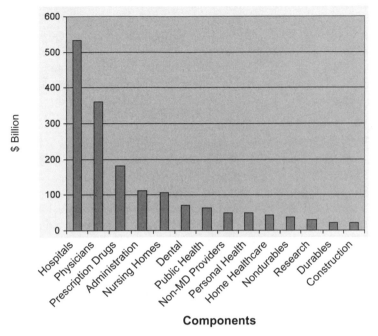

Components

WHO PAYS THE BILLS?

The 2003 United States healthcare expenditure was estimated to be $1.654 trillion.[2] This amount was equivalent to 78% of the total United States government expenditure of $2.1 trillion for fiscal 2003. Nonetheless, the federal government did not pay 78% of the United States healthcare bill. The federal government paid $511 billion from its total $2.1 trillion year 2003 budget, of which $270 went to the Medicare program. Accordingly, the 2003 expenditure for Medicare consumed 12.8% of the year 2003 federal budget. Other federal healthcare expenditures include those of the Medicaid program, administration, nursing homes, public health programs, the Veterans Administration health system, research, and construction.

States pay $230 billion for healthcare services, much of which goes to the Medicaid program. The Medicaid program, which is funded by state and federal subsidies to help economically disadvantaged citizens afford healthcare services, cost $266 billion in 2003,[8,9] an amount similar to the $270 billion spent on the Medicare program.

The $270 billion spent on the 2003 Medicare program is similar to the 2003 expenditure of $266 billion on the Medicaid program.

Approximately 45% ($741 billion) of all healthcare costs is funded through the public sector and 55% ($913 billion) is funded by the private sector (Figure 3.5).

There are two large publicly funded healthcare programs in the United States: Medicare and Medicaid. Medicare covers predominantly senior citizens and Medicaid covers predominantly lower-income individuals, but there is some crossover among who is covered in both of the programs. Some financially disadvantaged seniors are covered by Medicaid and some nonseniors, such as those with end-stage renal disease, are covered by the Medicare program.

Medicare

Originated concomitantly with Medicaid in 1965 as a result of the Social Security Act, Medicare was initially administered by the Social Security Administration. In 1977, Congress established the Health Care Financing Administration (HCFA) as a subsidiary of the Department of Health, Education, and Welfare (HEW) to administer both the Medicare and Medicaid programs. In 1980, HEW split into the Department of Education and the Department of Health and Human Services (HHS), with HCFA as a subsidiary of HHS. The Health Care Financing Administration changed its name to the Centers for Medicare and Medicaid Services (CMS) in 2001 and is still a subsidiary of HHS.[10]

The Medicare program covers approximately 40 million of the 292 million people in the United States in 2004. Included in the program are people aged 65 or older, disabled people under age 65, and people with end-stage renal disease (ESRD), defined as permanent kidney failure requiring dialysis, or kidney

FIGURE   3.5

Estimated United States Healthcare Costs in 2003

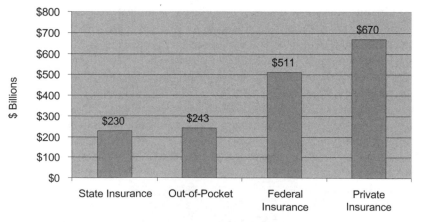

transplant. Medicare is essentially funded by the federal government. The distribution of all Medicare expenditures is shown in Table 3.2, while the distribution of Medicare dollars for provider healthcare services is shown in Table 3.3.[2]

The Medicare system of payment is the most standardized healthcare payment system in the United States. While all healthcare insurers in the United States have different reimbursement systems, the great majority are based upon the Medicare system, a factor that makes the Medicare payment system the best to use for healthcare economic analyses. Medicare alters payments for most interventions to account for geographic differences in costs. Thus, the average Medicare payment across the country is most suitable for use in economic analyses.[11]

Because Medicare will not incorporate a drug benefit to a significant degree prior to 2006, there is no standardized Medicare drug fee schedule at present. Thus, we currently use the Average Wholesale Price (AWP) from the *Red Book* for drug costs.[12] Nevertheless, this will likely change as the Medicare pharmaceutical program takes effect.

> The Medicare payment schedule is the most standardized system of healthcare payment in the United States It is therefore the best choice for use in healthcare economic analysis.

Prior to 2004, Medicare did not cover the costs for outpatient medications. It does, however, pay for some drugs (chemotherapeutic) injected in physicians' offices. The Medicare Prescription Drug Improvement and Modernization Act, which adds a prescription drug benefit to the Medicare program starting in 2006, is estimated to cost a minimum of $400 billion expended over a ten-year period.[13]

TABLE 3.2

Distribution of Medicare Expenditures in 2001

Healthcare Service	% of Medicare Expenditure
Hospital Inpatient, Acute	39
Managed Care	18
Physicians and Other Providers	17
Hospital Outpatient and Other Facilities*	8
Laboratory and Durable Medical Equipment	7
Skilled Nursing Care	5
Home Health	4
Hospice Care	1

Source: The Centers for Medicare and Medicaid Services.[9]

* Rehabilitation facilities and end-stage renal disease (ESRD) facilities.

TABLE   3.3

2004 Total Medicare-Allowed Charges for Various Provider Healthcare Services

Specialty	Medicare Allowed Charges ($ Millions)	Percent of All Provider Payments
Physicians		
Allergy/Immunology	$153	0.25
Anesthesiology	$1,327	2.20
Cardiac Surgery	$321	0.53
Cardiology	$5,759	9.54
Clinics	$1,167	1.93
Colon and Rectal Surgery	$101	0.17
Critical Care	$108	0.18
Dermatology	$1,708	2.83
Emergency Medicine	$1,444	2.39
Endocrinology	$246	0.41
Family Practice	$4,005	6.63
Gastroenterology	$1,513	2.51
General Practice	$954	1.58
General Surgery	$2,110	3.49
Geriatrics	$97	0.16
Hand Surgery	$46	0.08
Hematology/Oncology	$1,086	1.80
Infectious Disease	$336	0.56
Internal Medicine	$7,917	13.11
Interventional Radiology	$155	0.26
Nephrology	$1,187	1.97
Neurology	$1,072	1.78
Neurosurgery	$433	0.72
Obstetrics/Gynecology	$550	0.91
Ophthalmology	$4,291	7.11
Orthopedic Surgery	$2,645	4.38
Otolaryngology	$735	1.22
Pathology	$799	1.32
Pediatrics	$58	0.10
Physical Medicine	$594	0.98
Plastic Surgery	$274	0.45
Psychiatry	$1,073	1.78
Pulmonary Disease	$1,305	2.16
Radiation Oncology	$1,002	1.66
Radiology	$4,230	7.01
Rheumatology	$352	0.58

TABLE 3.3 continued

2004 Total Medicare-Allowed Charges for Various Provider Healthcare Services

Specialty	Medicare Allowed Charges ($ Millions)	Percent of All Provider Payments
Thoracic Surgery	$446	0.74
Urology	$1,540	2.55
Vascular Surgery	$429	0.71
Practitioners		
Audiologist	$25	0.04
Chiropractor	$589	0.98
Clinical Psychologist	$449	0.74
Clinical Social Worker	$277	0.46
Nurse Anesthetist	$452	0.75
Nurse Practitioner	$434	0.72
Optometry	$611	1.01
Oral/Maxillofacial Surgery	$33	0.05
Physical/Occupational Therapy	$835	1.38
Physician Assistant	$322	0.53
Podiatry	$1,307	2.16
Suppliers		
Diagnostic Testing Facility	$728	1.21
Independent Laboratory	$508	0.84
Portable X-ray Supplier	$82	0.14
Other		
All Other	$54	0.09
All Physician Fee Schedule	$60,385	100.00

Source: The Centers for Medicare and Medicaid Services.[10]

Medicaid

The Medicaid program, originated in 1965 with the Medicare program and now administered by the CMS in conjunction with each state, covers approximately 42.6 million economically disadvantaged patients.[8] There are five broad coverage groups among the economically disadvantaged:

1. children,
2. pregnant women,
3. adults in families with dependent children,
4. individuals with disabilities, and
5. individuals aged 65 or older.

Approximately 61% of Medicaid costs is covered by the federal government, while 39% of costs is covered by the state governments. Nonetheless, the percentage of costs covered by the federal government ranges from 50% to 83%, depending upon the affluence of the state.[14] States spend approximately 10% of their total budgets on Medicaid services.[14]

The overall Medicaid expenditure in 2003 was $266 billion.[8] A large proportion of Medicaid funding goes to nursing home care, an important program with wide public appeal to those in need of such services, as well as their families. Overall, Medicaid funded 46% of all nursing home costs in 1998, while Medicare funded 12% of nursing home costs, 33% of payments were out-of-pocket, and 9% came from miscellaneous sources.[15] All Medicaid funds were distributed as shown in Table 3.4. Compared to the Medicare program, hospital costs account for a considerably larger proportion of Medicaid dollars than do provider costs.

United States in Comparison With Other Countries

A comparison among healthcare expenditures in the United States and those of other countries is shown in Table 3.5. Per capita expenditures in 1997 United States dollars ranged from $4090 in the United States to $1347 in the United Kingdom, with a mean for industrialized countries of $1747.[16] As a percentage of GDP, the numbers in 1997 ranged from 13.6% for the United States to 6.7% for the United Kingdom. The mean percentage of GDP for industrialized countries was 7.6%.

Another methodology of comparing the healthcare costs of different countries is to use purchasing power parity (PPP), a ratio of healthcare prices in various countries for the same goods or services. It is composed of input measures into the medical care process that include pharmaceuticals, laboratory tests,

TABLE 3.4

Distribution of Medicaid Expenditures In 1998

Healthcare Service	% of Medicaid Expenditure
Hospital Inpatient, Accute	30.9
Disproportionate Share Hospitals (DSH)*	20.7
Prescription Drugs	16.1
Physicians and Other Providers	9.1
Hospital Outpatient	9.0
Clinics	6.0
Miscellaneous	5.0
Mental Health	3.2

Source: United States Department of Health and Human Services.[15]

* Hospitals that take care of a large proportion or poorer patients.

TABLE 3.5

International Healthcare Expenditures Per Capita in 1997[16]

Country	Expenditures (US Dollars)	% of GDP
United States	$4,090	13.6
Germany	$2,339	10.4
Canada	$2,096	9.3
France	$2,051	9.6
Australia	$1,805	8.3
Japan	$1,741	7.3
New Zealand	$1,352	7.6
United Kingdom	$1,347	6.7

office visits, appliances such as eyeglasses, supplies such as bandages, medical and surgical interventions, and the wages of healthcare occupations. A comparison of the PPP of various countries is shown in Figure 3.6.

A comparison of the healthcare expenditures of senior citizens in various countries also illustrates how the United States compares to other countries (Figure 3.7). The annual expenditure in the United States has been shown to be 3.35 times that in the United Kingdom for the average person aged 65 and older.

IS HEALTHCARE SPENDING BAD?

We do not mean to imply that spending an increasing proportion of GDP on healthcare services is necessarily bad for the economy. There is no hard and fast rule stating that spending a large amount for healthcare services is detrimental

FIGURE 3.6

Purchasing Power Parity of Multiple Countries in 1999. A healthcare service that costs $100 in the United States costs US $75 in Japan or US $39 in Greece.

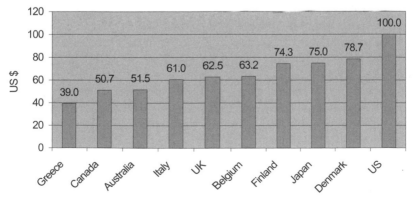

Source: Organization for Economic Cooperation and Development.[17]

FIGURE   3.7

Per Capita Health Expenditures for Adults Aged 65 Years and Older in 1997

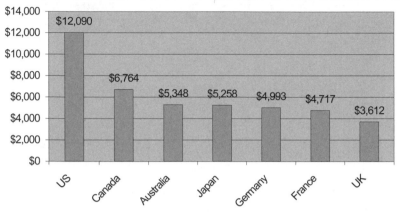

Source: The Commonwealth Fund.[18]

to the country. Despite the fact that healthcare services account for an increasing proportion of GDP, healthcare services contribute to an overall superior economy by directly contributing to GDP (the GDP is the sum of all goods and services produced in the United States during one year), improving worker productivity, and decreasing the economic burden of disease (lost wages, decreased disability costs, decreased caregiver costs, and so forth). These financial benefits occur in addition to the extraordinary benefits of improving quality of life and length of life. There is little doubt that pundits would applaud an increasing number of cars or other durable goods sold per capita. There is no compelling reason that healthcare services should be considered differently. Increasing healthcare service should fall under the praiseworthy category with one proviso—the dollars must be spent in the most efficient manner possible.

While efficient spending for healthcare services is good, spending healthcare dollars ineffectively is bad. We strongly believe that healthcare dollars should be spent for the highest return possible in terms of improving quality of life and length of life. Value-based medicine is the information system that allows for the highest return on investment for healthcare dollars spent.

Spending more money on healthcare services is good for the economy. Spending the money *inefficiently* is not.

The fact that improving quality of life and length of life also increases the productivity of United States workers should not be underestimated. This is a critical economic factor, as improving worker productivity enables our economy to expand and overall lifestyles to improve. In essence, improved productivity contributes to GDP (and thus the overall economy) while allowing more goods and services to be available without accompanying inflation. And which factors contribute more to increasing productivity than good health? Probably few.

Let us be very clear, however, about one other aspect: The 30-year annual rate of inflation of 10% for healthcare services far outdistances the average annual, general inflation rate of 5% as measured over the past 30 years.[5] Combined with the rate of rise of certain costs of the healthcare system, notably for pharmaceuticals and technological advances, the point at which many more people will be unable to maintain access to healthcare if the present system is left unchanged is looming. The writing on the wall is clear: reasonable control of costs due to greater efficiencies, while improving quality of care, is the desirable outcome for healthcare reform. Value-based medicine will facilitate these goals. It cannot come soon enough.

> Reasonable control of costs due to greater efficiencies, while improving quality of care, is the desirable outcome for healthcare reform. Value-based medicine will facilitate these goals.

WORLD HEALTH ORGANIZATION'S WORLD HEALTH REPORT 2000

In 2000, the World Health Organization published the World Health Report, a health system performance assessment of the 191 member states of the organization.[19] The United States ranked first in terms of the *level of responsiveness,* which was assessed using the parameters of:

- dignity,
- autonomy,
- confidentiality,
- prompt attention,
- quality of basic amenities of the health system,
- access to social support systems during care, and
- choice of provider.

The responsiveness level essentially pertains to what people *expect of the health system in terms of more peripheral health issues.*

Concerning overall actual *health attainment,* the United States ranked 15, between Germany (14) and Iceland (16). This was based upon a composite scale with the weighting of five components:

- 25% level of health,
- 25% distribution of health,
- 12.5% level of responsiveness,
- 12.5% distribution of responsiveness, and
- 25% fairness of financial contribution.

Level of health refers to attainment of overall health outcomes measured in disability-adjusted life expectancy, a relatively complex methodology developed by the World Bank to assess the burden of disease within a country.[20]

Regarding *health distribution,* or our ability to respond equally well to all citizens in obtaining these health outcomes, the United States fell to 32 out of the 191 member states. On the topic of *fairness of financial contribution,* measured by a country's ability to have the least amount of difference among groups or individuals in the hardship that health costs produce relative to a patient's ability to pay, the United States was assessed to be 54. Some have suggested, however, that the payment system aspects of the study were biased against the United States before the study was even undertaken. Perhaps that is the case, but the next aspect, *performance,* still mandates considerable attention.

Performance of a health system assesses how efficiently health systems translate expenditures into healthcare. The category, which correlates the actual level of health achieved for the dollars expended, places the United States in its worst ranking of the study: 72. Overall, the WHO evaluated the level of health that should be achieved by the level of expenditure in the most efficient health system, and the United States fared quite poorly. In essence, the report suggests that the United States spends an inordinate amount of money inefficiently for the healthcare its citizens receive. Bottom line: we are flushing buckets of money down the toilet.

> In the World Health Organization Report 2000, the United States ranked 72 among 191 member countries in the *efficiency of use* of healthcare resources.

We believe the United States can do much better in utilizing resources dedicated to healthcare. Serious consideration must be made to evaluate all medical interventions on the basis of their value and cost. Weeding out interventions of negligible value or no value, or those that are harmful, will shift resources to provide better, if not the best, treatments for all. This should be—at a minimum—our goal.

Should We Totally Revamp Healthcare Practice in the United States?

No. There are very compelling reasons to maintain many features of our healthcare system as we improve efficiency of resource use and improve quality of care for everyone. In addition to the privileges of access to care and choice of providers, survival with diseases such as cancer is the best in the world due to healthcare research, the availability of advanced treatments, and general practices already in place (Figure 3.8). We must be certain that such positive features remain in place.

How Big a Problem Is the Inefficient Use of Healthcare Resources?

Huge. The issue of ineffective use of healthcare dollars actually extends beyond healthcare because of the enormity of the healthcare service industry; it is by far

FIGURE 3.8

Five-Year Survival Percentages for All Cancers From 1987–1991

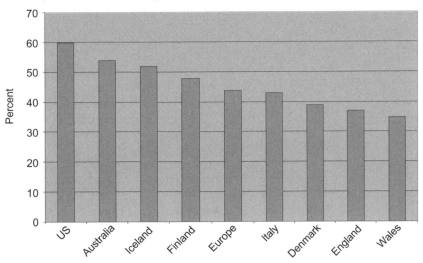

Source: Organization for Economic Cooperation and Development.[21]

the largest industry in the United States. But even the United States, with its vast resources, cannot expect to remain in a leadership position among the most influential nations on the globe when countless billions of dollars are misspent with no or little return. It is imperative for the overall well-being of the country that the United States achieve the maximum return on investment for its health-care dollars.

> It is imperative for the overall well-being of the country that the United States achieve the maximum return on investment for its healthcare dollars.

THE NEED FOR QUALITY STANDARDS

While many medical specialty organizations have practice guidelines[22] and other general healthcare organizations have made attempts at such,[23–25] there is no organized body that oversees quality standards for all of healthcare. Probably the closest one is the National Committee for Quality Assurance (NCQA),[26] a private nonprofit organization that establishes quality standards for managed care organizations.

The NCQA has worked to establish and refine the Health Plan Employer Data and Information Set (HEDIS),[26] but HEDIS encompasses only a small fraction of healthcare interventions and fails to adequately address the value conferred by interventions or the costs involved. Among the entities studied to date by HEDIS are aspects of heart disease, asthma, diabetes, cancer, smoking cessation, immunizations, and menopause counseling.

Managed Care Organizations

There are two basic managed care organization variants, the preferred provider organization (PPO) and the health maintenance organization (HMO). Each variant has a limited number of hospitals and providers within its panel, and patients pay a set yearly fee that essentially covers all of the health services they require. While the exact definition of each form of managed care organization varies from state to state, the HMO usually has a gatekeeper system in which a patient is first required to see a primary care doctor (family practice physician, internist, pediatrician, or obstetrician-gynecologist) before seeing a specialist. Capitation is frequently utilized, meaning that a provider takes care of a patient for a set yearly fee, whether the patient requires care one time per year or ten times per year. The system also often provides monetary discentives for primary physicians to refer patients to specialists for care. In a PPO system, a patient is allowed direct access to any physician in its panel.

As a principal in the establishment of a managed care organization, author Gary Brown quickly realized that the development of quality standards is among the greatest needs in healthcare in the United States.[27–31] At the present time, managed care organizations and other healthcare entities responsible for the brokering of healthcare services have only rudimentary knowledge of the services they are purchasing for their clients. These organizations establish cost limitations for specific interventions, as well as barriers to obtain care, yet they have little ability to evaluate and to compare the patient-perceived value conferred by these interventions. For example, how does one compare the value of anti-inflammatory medication for osteoarthritis of the knee with that of a transurethral resection of the prostate for severe benign prostatic hypertrophy? Or the treatment regimen for American Heart Association Functional Capacity Classification Class III congestive heart failure[32] with total knee arthroplasty for Class III American College of Rheumatology disease?[33] An information system that compares these interventions on an equal playing field simply does not exist at the present time. While the tools to create such a system are in progress,[28,29] the system itself is far from finished.

Managed care organizations currently look at the utilization of healthcare resources and attempt to reduce costs where their medical directors or committees believe that care may not be adversely affected. As there are few quality standards at the present, directors must use a variety of sources upon which to base their assessments, including their personal experiences, results of their evaluations of clinical studies, customary utilization figures, and perceived usual medical practices. Clearly, with no standards that quantify the value of healthcare interventions, the comparison of intervention decisions is haphazard within a medical specialty and nonexistent across specialties.

> With a lack of quality standards that quantify value, the comparison of healthcare intervention decisions is haphazard within a medical specialty and nonexistent across specialties.

With healthcare costs rising secondary to the advent of new technologies, an increasing elderly population, the inability of managed care organizations to further leverage providers, rising pharmacologic costs, and greater numbers of providers,[34] we firmly believe healthcare dollars must be utilized in the most efficient manner possible. Current healthcare standards and limited healthcare evaluation tools do not allow this. Value-based medicine does.

Managed care organizations are proficient in establishing the utilization of specific interventions, but they have little ability to evaluate and compare their patient-perceived value. They currently manage costs rather than care.

Managed care organizations have attempted to manage costs, rather than care, because they lack the tools to effectively manage care. In managing costs, they have leveraged providers to the point that many are unwilling or cannot afford to participate if further cuts occur. Thus, the easier cost cuts have already been made. In addition, there are no compelling reasons to believe that managed care organizations improve the overall quality of care of a patient population at this time. With VBM, the tools become available to improve quality of care at the same time unnecessary costs are reduced.

There is one answer to maximize the effective utilization of healthcare dollars to reflect the value placed on healthcare by society and its citizens—the development of value-based quality of care standards.

Clearly, care must be taken to apply the principles and assumptions of decision-making models consistently with the best EBM studies and patient perceptions of value measured in a constant, reproducible manner. Intuition and the pure availability of interventions as the determinants of healthcare are no longer acceptable methods when healthcare inflation outdistances other major components of our budget in the presence of 40+ million medically uninsured individuals.[35] The best care for all citizens will result when we apply the "four Cs" of improvement to *critically*, *conscientiously*, *consistently*, and *constantly* formulate and update quality standards upon which payers can appropriately design their priorities and go about the business of paying for the best quality healthcare.

A Special Note to Our Healthcare Colleagues

Providers balked at Medicare when the government first initiated the system, but it was developed because there was a need. Providers also shunned the implementation of managed care, but it also came because society recognized a need. Today, with rising healthcare costs and more than 40+ million uninsured, there is a need as well to make quality care available for everyone. We must not hesitate to embrace the concept of value-based quality standards, particularly because they allow healthcare quality to improve while they maximize the efficient use of our dollars. Healthcare providers must not relinquish the opportunity to be among the architects of a value-based system.

HOW MUCH CAN BE SAVED?

The savings allowed by VBM are difficult to estimate. Nevertheless, it has been suggested that approximately 7% of healthcare costs are inappropriate.[28] Assuming that VBM identifies this 7% of inappropriate interventions, approximately $123.9 billion could be saved from our total healthcare expenditure of $1.773 trillion in 2003.

> It is estimated that VBM could save $123.9 billion from the 2004 United States healthcare expenditure.

To put the potential savings into perspective, the estimated expenditure on the Medicare drug benefit included within the Medicare Prescription Drug Improvement and Modernization Act is $400 billion over a 10-year period, or approximately $40 billion per year.[13] Cost estimates of providing health insurance to the 40+ million uninsured in the United States range from $43 to $87.2 billion (in year 2004 dollars).[36] The cost of insuring the uninsured is less per capita ($1,075 to $2,180) than the average per capita healthcare cost in the country. (The 2004 national average is $6,126.) This is because senior citizens, who are already covered by Medicare, account for a larger proportion of healthcare expenditures than a younger population with commercial insurance (private, or non-Medicare and non-Medicaid insurance).

Combining the median cost of yearly health insurance costs for the 40+ million uninsured ($65.1 billion) with the yearly cost of the drug benefit included in the Medicare Prescription Drug Improvement and Modernization Act ($40 billion) yields a total annual sum of $105.1 billion. This is considerably less than the potential $123.9 billion savings incurred by the institution of VBM standards.

> The cost of providing healthcare insurance to the 40+ million uninsured in the United States in 2004 is estimated to range from $43 to $87.2 billion.

> The potential annual saving of $123.9 billion from VBM quality standards is more than enough to pay for health insurance for the 40+ million insured and the cost of the Medicare Prescription Drug Improvement and Modernization Act.

CORE CONCEPTS

- Healthcare is generally considered to be inelastic in that demand responds slightly, or not at all, to changes in price.
- The total United States annual healthcare expenditure for 2004 is estimated to be $1.773 trillion or 15.3% of gross domestic product (GDP).

- Only 10% of medical students and residents have any concept of the total United States annual healthcare expenditure.
- The estimated $1.773 trillion annual healthcare expenditure in 2004 is 4.7 times that of the fiscal year 2004 expenditure ($379.9 billion) of the United States Department of Defense.
- For the last three decades of the 20th century, healthcare inflation rose at approximately 10% per year while general inflation rose at approximately 5% per year.
- After adjustment for general inflation, the 2004 healthcare expenditure for the average person in the United States is approximately 3.7 times what it was in 1970.
- The 2003 Medicare expenditure was $270 billion, or 12.8% of the federal budget.
- The 2003 Medicaid expenditure was $266 billion.
- Forty-five percent of healthcare expenditures is paid by the public sector, while 55% is paid by the private sector.
- The World Health Report 2000 noted that the United States was first among 191 member countries in regard to choice of providers and access to providers but ranked 72 in the efficacy of the use of healthcare resources.
- It is imperative for the overall well-being of the country that the United States achieves the maximum return on investment for its healthcare dollars.

REFERENCES

1. Case KE, Fair RC. *Principles of Economics*. 4th ed. Upper Saddle River, NJ: Prentice Hall; 1996:1–165.
2. Office of the Actuary at the Centers for Medicare and Medicaid Services. National health care expenditures projections: 2001–2011. Available at: www.hcfa.gov. Accessed January 2, 2004.
3. National health care expenditures aggregate and per capita amounts, percent distribution, and average annual percent growth, by source of funds: selected calendar years 1960–1999. Available at: www.hcfa.gov. Accessed December 11, 2001.
4. Department of Defense. National defense budget estimate for FY 2004. Available at: www.defenselink.mil/news/Feb2003/b02032003_bt044-03.html. Accessed March 20, 2004.
5. Brown MM, Brown GC, Sharma S, Hollands H, Smith A. Physician manpower and health care expenditures in the United States: a thirty year perspective. *J Healthcare Finance*. 2001;27:55–64.
6. Freudenheim M. CalPERS to vote on new health care rates. *New York Times*. June 16, 2003:C2.
7. Federal Interagency Forum on Aging-Related Statistics. Older Americans 2000: Key Indicators of Well-Being. Indicator 25: Health Care Expenditures. Available at: www.agingstats.gov/chartbook2000/tables-healthcare.html. Accessed March 20, 2004.

8. Cauchon D. Medicaid rolls grow despite predicted cuts. *USA Today.* March 1, 2004:A1.

9. Centers for Medicare and Medicaid Services. Statistics and data. Available at: www.cms.hhs.gov. Accessed March 6, 2004.

10. Centers for Medicare and Medicaid Services. Medicare information resource. Available at: www.cms.hhs.gov. Accessed March 22, 2004.

11. Centers for Medicare and Medicaid Services. Program information on Medicare, Medicaid, SCHIP and other programs of the Centers for Medicare and Medicaid Services. Available at: www.cms.hhs.gov. Accessed March 6, 2004.

12. Flemming T, ed. *2004 Drug Topics Red Book.* Montvale, NJ: Medical Economics; 2004.

13. Goldstein A, Eilperin J. Medicare drug estimate rises: prescription benefit's price tag rises 33%. *Washington Post.* January 30, 2004:A01.

14. Cauchon D. For states, Medicaid too lucrative to cut: federal subsidy of up to 80% discourages cost-trimming, encourages inflated costs. *USA Today.* March 1, 2004:A3.

15. DeParle NA. *A Profile of Medicaid: Chart Book 2000.* Washington, DC: US Dept of Health and Human Services; 2000:1–87.

16. Anderson GF. Multinational comparisons of health care: expenditures, coverages, and outcomes. The Center for Hospital Finance and Management, Johns Hopkins University; 1998. Available at: www.cmwf.org/programs/international/ihp_1998_multicompsurvey_29. Accessed March 18, 2001.

17. Triplett JE. Integrating the cost-of-disease studies into purchasing power parities. In: Martin JP, ed. *A Disease-based Comparison of Health Systems.* Paris, France: Organization for Economic Cooperation and Development; 2003.

18. Anderson D, Hussey P. *Health and Population Aging: A Multinational Comparison.* The Commonwealth Fund; October 1999.

19. World Health Organization Report 2000. Available at: www.who.org. Accessed December 10, 2001.

20. The World Bank. *World Development Report 1993: Investing in Health.* New York, NY: Oxford University Press; 1993.

21. Stevenson C, Madden R, Gibson D, Goss J. Information needs and the implications for monitoring health systems: the Australian experience. In: Martin JP, ed. *A Disease-based Comparison of Health Systems.* Paris, France: Organization for Economic Cooperation and Development; 2003:317–337.

22. American Academy of Pediatrics Committee on Quality Improvement, Subcommittee on Attention-Deficit/Hyperactivity Disorder. Diagnosis and evaluation of the child with attention-deficit/hyperactivity disorder (AC0002). *Pediatrics.* 2000;105:1158–1170.

23. Update Software, Ltd. *The Cochrane Library.* Issue 4. Oxford, England: Update Software, Ltd; 2003.

24. Sackett DL, Straus SE, Richardson WS, Rosenberg W, Haynes RB. *Evidence-Based Medicine: How to Practice and Teach EBM.* 2nd ed. Philadelphia, Pa: Churchill Livingstone; 2000:1–12.

25. Evidence-Based Medicine Working Group. A new approach to teaching the practice of medicine. *JAMA.* 1992;268:2420–2425.

26. National Committee for Quality Assurance. Available at: www.ncqa.org. Accessed March 20, 2003.

27. Brown MM. The greatest need in medicine: quality standards. *Evidence-Based Eye Care.* 2000;1:69–71.

28. Colman K. Education: key for eye M.D.s in face of fraud crackdown. *EyeNet* 1999;3:19-20.

29. Brown GC, Brown MM, Sharma S. Quality and cost-effectiveness in health care: a unique approach. *J Ophthalmic Nurs & Technol.* 2000; Jan–Feb:26–30.

30. Brown GC, Sharma S, Brown MM, Garrett S. Evidence-based medicine and cost-effectiveness. *J Healthcare Fin.* 1999;26:14–23.

31. Brown MM, Brown GC, Sharma S, Garrett S. Evidence-based medicine, utilities, and quality of life. *Curr Opin Ophthalmol.* 1999;10:221–226.

32. American Heart Association. American Heart Association Functional Capacity Classification. Available at: www.americanheart.org. Accessed September 4, 2003.

33. Hochberg MC, Chang RW, Dwosh I, Lindsey S, Pincus T, Wolfe F. The American College of Rheumatology revised criteria for the classification of global functional status in rheumatoid arthritis. *Arthritis Rheum.* 1992;35:498–502.

34. Brown GC, Brown MM. The perils of health care: when is it too much? *Evidence-Based Eye Care.* 2000;1:133–135.

35. Cowley G, Turque B, Hager M, King P. Critical condition. *Newsweek.* November 8, 1999:59–61.

36. Hadley J, Holahan J. Insuring the uninsured: How much would it cost? The cost of additional medical care used by newly insured Americans would be lower than most people think, this analysis confirms. *Health Affairs* [serial online]. June 2003. Available at: www.kff.org/uninsured/index.cfm. Accessed March 17, 2004.

2

Evidence-Based Medicine

The Foundation of the Value-Based Medicine Pyramid

Chapter 4   Total Quality Management and Evidence-Based Medicine

4

Total Quality Management and Evidence-Based Medicine

Total quality management can be defined as managing an organization so that it excels on all relevant dimensions of products and services that are important to the customer. It is a philosophy behind Japan's remarkable recovery following World War II and has become a source of competitive advantage for many United States companies, including Motorola, DuPont, and General Electric. In fact, Jack Welch, the former chairman of General Electric, believed that its Six Sigma program, an embodiment of total quality management, had the potential to save the company nearly $10 billion over the next decade.

How can healthcare managers adopt the principles of total quality management to ensure the programs they offer are of excellent quality? One way is to selectively choose the best evidence-based medicine (EBM) practices to convert to value-based form (Figure 4.1). This process has the potential to dramatically improve how medicine is practiced.

THE EVIDENCE-BASED MEDICINE PARADIGM

Traditionally, the practice of medicine has been based on principles that are deeply rooted in pathophysiology, deductive reasoning, and clinical experience.[1] We are, however, entering a new era in medicine, where patients, clinicians, and governments demand that medical practice no longer be based on hypothetical thinking but be scientifically validated. Accordingly, a new movement in healthcare questions the way clinicians practice medicine. This initiative, termed *evidence-based medicine,* represents the philosophy that medical practice should be based on the best scientific evidence.

Evidence-based medicine is the practice of medicine based upon the highest level of scientific evidence.

According to the EBM doctrine, each practice, be it a surgical or a medical intervention, should be based on research that applies the principles of the scientific method.[1] Tactically, EBM involves incorporation of the latest medical

FIGURE 4.1

The Value-Based Medicine Pyramid. Evidence-based data are first converted to value-based format in the middle tier. The addition of cost-utility analysis in the upper tier completes the triangle and results in value-based medicine.

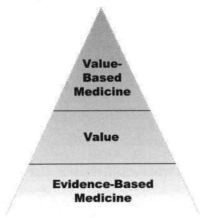

Figure courtesy Kathryn Brown.

research into clinical practice. It leverages a rapidly expanding global database and state of the art communication systems to allow instantaneous access to information to make healthcare decisions. It is a process that is being adopted by medical educators across the world and requires all users to develop their own critical filters to determine which medical practices are of the highest quality.

THE TRADITIONAL HEALTHCARE MODEL NEEDS A MAKEOVER

Some may wonder why we should abandon the traditional healthcare system based on deductive reasoning and supported by "expert opinion." The answer is that clinical practices are fraught with numerous biases and cannot in any way be considered surrogates for clinical trials. Would the Food and Drug Administration (FDA) allow a drug to be available to the United States public without unbiased, rigorous scientific evidence to support its efficacy? Of course not.

Recommendations based upon evidence derived solely from expert opinion are flawed for the following five reasons:

1. Compliance is not adequately controlled in clinical practice.
2. Patients who are lost to follow-up are not factored into analyses in clinical practice.
3. Unusual results frequently regress toward the mean.
4. Randomization does not occur in clinical practice.

5. Patients and clinicians are not masked in clinical practice.

Each of these facets merits additional explanation.

1. **Compliance is not adequately controlled in clinical practice.** Favorable treatment responses are more likely to be noted and recalled by clinicians when patients comply with physician recommendations and keep follow-up appointments.[2] However, compliance in itself has been proven to be a powerful effector of outcome. In no fewer than five clinical trials,[3-7] compliant placebo groups had a significantly improved outcome when compared to treatment groups. Thus, as compliance with our interventions is known to have a positive effect with respect to outcomes, our clinical experiences represent uncontrolled trials where this effect serves as a bias.

2. **Patients who are lost to follow-up are not factored into analyses in clinical practice.** A second problem with clinical practice is that a clinician typically has no way to monitor the clinical response of those patients who are lost to follow-up (that is, those who do not return for follow-up after initial treatment has been recommended). Since it is known that compliant patients fare better than those who are noncompliant, this bias can make treatments appear more efficacious than they really are.

3. **Unusual results frequently regress toward the mean.** Unusual patterns of symptoms, signs, or laboratory values tend to regress toward the mean with the passage of time.[8] Due to this trend of regression toward the mean, one would expect an extreme factor to improve somewhat on its own. Thus, any therapy that is initiated in the interim can appear efficacious regardless of its real effect.[8] A treatment effect may indeed exist, but in extreme values a combination of factors may be responsible for this effect. Clinical trials compare groups of patients who receive treatments to those who do not; thus, the possibility of regression toward the mean is eliminated.

4. **Randomization does not occur in clinical practice.** Randomization is a technique that is used in clinical trials to ensure that the "third alternative" is eliminated.[9] Without randomization, there are three possible explanations for a given therapeutic effect: (a) chance alone, (b) the intervention being tested, and (c) the means by which the groups were constituted.[9] Randomization aims to eliminate alternative c from the list of possibilities to explain an observed effect. In clinical practice, randomization of interventions does not occur; thus, differences in the patient population may account for differences observed in treatment responses.

5. **Patients and clinicians are not masked in clinical practice.** *Blinding* or *masking* is a principle used in research to eliminate potential bias.[9] By necessity clinical practice is never blind, as both the clinician and the patient know when treatment is received. In fact, this knowledge is necessary for informed consent to take place. As a result, both the placebo effect and the desire of the clinician and the patient for a successful outcome tend to overestimate treatment efficacy.[2]

For these reasons, expert opinion alone should be considered an imperfect system for making health policy decisions. Because it attempts to correct the deficiencies of expert opinion alone, the movement advocating EBM is rapidly gaining momentum.

INTERVENTIONAL STUDIES

If we create critical filters to develop quality standards, what should these filters look like? Two critical hallmarks can be used to measure the quality of a given intervention: the *level of evidence* upon which it was based, and the *clinical importance* of the intervention itself. The clinical importance can be ascertained by measuring the *total value* conferred by an intervention, a parameter we will discuss at length in Chapter 11. In the following section we discuss levels of evidence.

Levels of Evidence

Sackett[2] proposed a set of guidelines for grading the level of evidence presented to support authors' recommendations for interventional studies. These guidelines were adopted by the participants in the Canadian Consensus Conference on Coronary Thrombolysis and are now being used across the globe to determine the quality of evidence for clinical studies that involve interventions.

In this scheme, evidence levels range from Level I, which is the most scientifically reproducible, to Level V, which is the weakest form of evidence for grading the clinical effectiveness of a given intervention. The guidelines are summarized in Table 4.1.

Evaluation of the level of evidence upon which an intervention is based is critical, for a cost-utility analysis and value-based medicine database is only as strong as its weakest link.

TABLE 4.1

Summary of Hierarchical Levels of Evidence for Interventional Studies[2,10]

Level of Evidence	Interventional Study
Level I	Randomized clinical trial with low type 1 error (≤ 0.05) and low type 2 error ($\leq 20\%$) or meta-analysis
Level II	Randomized clinical trial with high type 1 error (>0.05) and/or high type 2 error (>0.20)
Level III	Uncontrolled, nonrandomized clinical trial (treatment group compared to no treatment group without randomization)
Level IV	Intervention on a series of patients with no comparison group
Level V	Interventional case report

Level V evidence. Case reports are classified as Level V evidence. In an interventional case report, one patient who is managed with a new treatment or who experiences a variant in treatment effect is described. As an example of an intervention based on Level V evidence, Giner and associates[11] reported a case of thrombocytopenia associated with levodopa treatment. Does this mean that patients treated with levodopa are at high risk of developing thrombocytopenia? Not by any means. The limitation of a single case report is that the reader is unsure if the next patient subjected to the same intervention will obtain the same result.

Level IV evidence. Level IV evidence comes in the form of a case series without a control group. In an interventional study, authors report on how patients respond to an intervention without comparing them to another group. An example of Level IV evidence is the study by Clark and associates[12] in which seven consecutive patients with cleft palate underwent repair using decellularized dermal grafting. Two patients experienced dehiscence of the oral mucosa, but the authors concluded the procedure was safe and effective. The question is, safe and effective compared to what? The decision to offer an intervention to a patient should not be based on Level IV evidence alone. These studies do, however, play an important role as they often result in hypothesis generation and are necessary precursors to an analytical study. A consecutive case series is more illuminating and valued than a series that does not include consecutive patients treated with an intervention.

A *consecutive* case series is more illuminating than a nonconsecutive case series.

Level III evidence. Level III evidence is derived from nonrandomized, uncontrolled clinical trials. In these studies, patients who receive an intervention are compared to those who do not receive the intervention. Often, consecutive patients receiving a novel therapy are compared to historical controls in the literature. Unfortunately, randomization techniques are not employed in these trials. Given these facts, the third alternative may play a role here, since a significant therapeutic effect may occur secondary to demographic or other differences that exist between the two groups. Often, those selected for treatment also have a more favorable prognosis than those not receiving therapy.

Wang and colleagues[13] recently described the protection of the intervention of running against disability and early mortality in the elderly population. In their nonrandomized clinical trial, a cohort of elderly runners was compared with a control group of community control subjects who were not long-distance runners. Controls had a death rate three times higher than runners, but there were significant differences between the two groups in gender, age, smoking, and alcohol consumption. With randomization, it is much more likely the two groups would have been similar with respect to potential confounders. Very likely these inequities between the groups biased the results. Without major inequities, we can be more confident in the results.

Level II evidence.   Reviewing a clinical trial is very similar to serving as a juror in a criminal trial. Both involve weighing evidence and making educated guesses about reality. In both situations errors can be made. In the criminal justice system, errors are made when jurors either convict an innocent person or erroneously set a criminal free. Similarly, in a clinical trial, a mistake can be made if a methodologist either:

- determines that a treatment works when in reality it does not (akin to wrongfully convicting an innocent person), or
- erroneously fails to detect a difference when one exists (akin to setting a criminal free).

The former error is referred to as a Type 1 error and the latter as a Type 2 error.

The *null hypothesis* is a hypothesis that states there no is difference between two populations in regard to a specific parameter.[14] The absence of a difference between a drug and a placebo confirms the null hypothesis. If we demonstrate a real difference, we discard the null hypothesis and adopt the *alternative hypothesis.*

A Type 1 error occurs if the null hypothesis is rejected when it is true. It can also be viewed as a *false-positive* result. The probability of making a Type 1 error is statistically noted as an *alpha* error; by convention, it is also the level at which statistical significance occurs in a study. Traditionally, high quality trials are usually designed around an alpha of less than or equal to 0.05, which means the chance of having a false-positive treatment effect is less than or equal to 1/20. In essence, the probability of finding a statistically significant difference due to chance alone is less than or equal to 5% ($P \leq 0.05$).

A Type 2 error occurs when the null hypothesis is accepted and it is false and should be rejected. It can also be viewed as a *false-negative* result. A Type 2 error is known as a *beta* error.

Assuming that we are evaluating a new drug, the Type 1 error is the chance of accepting the drug to be effective when it actually is ineffective (false-positive outcome). The Type 2 error is the chance of rejecting the drug as ineffective when it actually is effective (false-negative outcome).

Type 1 error = chance of accepting a false-positive outcome

Type 2 error = chance of accepting a false-negative outcome

The *power* of a study is defined as 1.0 – beta. For example, a study with a beta of 0.20 would have an 80% (1.0 – 0.20) power, or 80% chance, of detecting a significant difference between treatment and control groups for a given sample size. If the beta is 0.10, the power of detecting a significant difference between treatment and control groups for a given sample size is 90%.

Level II evidence comes from a randomized clinical trial but, unlike Level I evidence, has either a high alpha (Type I error of >5%) or beta (Type II error of >20%). In Level II studies, a trend toward patient improvement may be noted with treatment, but the overall results are not statistically significant, and the *P*-value is greater than 0.05, or the confidence interval includes 1. In a negative Level II study (a study where there is no difference between treatment and control groups), a sample size that is too small to detect a clinically significant difference may have been used. One should always search for or attempt to calculate the Type 2 error or power (power = 1.0 – beta) of a negative study, as a study may have missed a treatment difference due to a small sample size.

> ## Level II evidence: randomized clinical trial with
> ## Type 1 error (alpha) > 0.05 and /or Type 2 error (beta) > 0.20

In a pilot study, Bressler and colleagues[15] noted that a group of patients with exudative (wet) macular degeneration and poorly demarcated new blood vessels under the retina who were treated with laser therapy fared no better than a control group. Assuming that 40% of patients with no treatment will develop severe visual loss, an alpha of 0.05, and a beta of 0.2, 83 patients would have been necessary in each treatment arm to detect a 50% reduction in severe visual loss. With only 29 patients in the treatment arm (and 26 in the control arm), this Level II study was underpowered, and a treatment effect may have been missed by having too few patients evaluated for the treatment effect.

Level I evidence.   Level I evidence represents the highest caliber of research and is characterized by randomized clinical trials with low Type 1 (< 0.05) and Type 2 (≤ 0.20) errors. An example of Level I evidence is the treatment of adolescent obesity trial, in which Berkowitz and colleagues[16] demonstrated that the addition of sibutramine to behavioral therapy in obese adolescents results in an outcome of more weight loss than behavioral therapy alone ($P = 0.001$). This randomized clinical trial is categorized as Level I evidence due to randomization and the fact that the chance of erroneously demonstrating a treatment effect is only 0.001.

> ## Level I evidence: randomized clinical trial with
> ## Type 1 error (alpha) ≤ 0.05 and Type 2 error (beta) ≤ 0.20

Positive treatment effects need not always be demonstrated for a study to be classified as Level 1 evidence. In a negative study, one in which no treatment effect is noted, a low beta (high power) ensures that a large enough sample was used to detect a clinically relevant difference if one had been present. In the previously mentioned study by Berkowitz and colleagues[16] on treatment of obese adolescents, the authors calculated a 93% power that a body mass index (BMI) reduction as small as 4% between the two treatment groups would be detected. Thus, the beta in this instance was 0.07, assuring us that if the study was negative, the chance of missing the 4% difference in BMI is small (7% or less). Again, when reading a study with a negative result, one must search for (or calculate) the Type 2 error or power (1.0–Type 2 error). Traditionally, high quality studies have a beta error of less than or equal to 0.2 (or a power greater than 80%).

> In a negative study, it is important to know the *power* to ascertain the possibility that a positive treatment effect might have been missed.

Meta-analysis

The advent of meta-analysis has had an important role in synthesizing Level II evidence into Level I evidence. Meta-analysis is a research technique that combines randomized clinical trials in an attempt to increase the overall power to answer a research question. Although it is a powerful research tool, two potential problems may arise when performing a meta-analysis: publication bias and heterogeneity.

Publication bias refers to the fact that journals tend to publish studies that have a positive result (that is, treatment is better than placebo). If one were to use only published articles, he or she might miss including negative results (that is, treatment is no better than placebo) and artificially skew the results toward demonstrating a treatment effect. One way to minimize publication bias is to use unpublished research abstracts presented at international meetings in the meta-analysis.

Heterogeneity refers to the fact that different randomized clinical trials may differ with respect to inclusion criteria or design features. Some may argue that different trials should not be combined and that, by doing so, one is comparing apples to oranges. Despite these potential drawbacks and given fiscal limitations situation, meta-analysis is emerging as a cost-effective alternative to expensive, multicenter, randomized clinical trials.

An example of a meta-analysis derived from the cardiology literature is one demonstrating the benefit of streptokinase for the treatment of acute heart attack. In this study the results of eight randomized clinical trials were combined to demonstrate that patients receiving this treatment have a 20% reduction in mortality over the two-week period following their event when compared to patients receiving no therapy.[17]

> Meta-analysis is emerging as a cost-effective alternative to expensive, multicenter, randomized clinical trials.

Other Critical Aspects of a Study

In addition to the level of evidence, there are other relevant aspects to consider when reviewing a clinical trial. These include:

1. the dropout rate,
2. an intent to treat approach,
3. masking,
4. the study population, and
5. the source of funding.

Dropout rate. Sackett and associates[18] adhere to the *five and 20* rule regarding dropout rate. If less than 5% of patients drop out of a trial, there is likely little bias, whereas if greater than 20% dropout, the validity of the study is threatened because severe bias is possible. For example, if a study demonstrates a positive outcome in 10% of subjects and there is a 5% dropout rate, the highest possible incidence of a positive outcome if all subjects who dropped out also had a positive outcome would be 15%, a 50% increase over 10%. With a 20% dropout rate and a 10% incidence of a positive outcome, the potential incidence of a positive outcome if all subjects who dropped out also had a positive outcome could be 30%, a 200% increase over 10%.

Intent to treat. To preserve the value of randomization, an *intent to treat (intention to treat)* analysis should be performed. In an intent to treat analysis, all patients who are initially randomized are analyzed within the group to which they were randomized, regardless of whether they receive their assigned intervention.[18] For example, let us assume that in a study to assess whether hip prosthesis A or hip prosthesis B results in better ambulation, a patient is randomized to the hip prosthesis B group. Let us also assume that the patient experiences a myocardial infarction on the operating table just prior to the start of surgery, and that the infarction precludes the hip surgery and any further chance of hip surgery. Although the patient did not and will not undergo the surgery, randomization did take place and the patient data should be included in the final study analysis. In this instance, pertinent patient data from follow-up visits can be utilized. If the patient is unable to return for any future visits, the pertinent data at the time of randomization can be carried forward.[19]

Masking. Additionally, the *ideal* randomized clinical trial is *double blind* or *double masked* so that neither patients nor treating physicians know who receives the study treatment and who receives the control treatment. While double masking is reasonable with pharmaceutical trials, it may not be possible with surgical interventions. A trial is *single blind* or *single masked* if either the treating physicians or the study subjects do not know who is receiving the real intervention. In settings in which the intervention is known by the treating physicians, there is theoretically greater confidence in the data if the results are analyzed by a different group of researchers uninvolved in providing direct care.[10,18]

Study population. The population from which the study sample is enrolled in a study must be carefully defined, since populations that differ in baseline demographics are generally not strictly comparable. Demographic factors that often define a population include age, gender, ethnicity, and level of income.

A study that includes a representative cross section of a community population of interest is often referred to as a *population-based study*. The population can be stratified according to geographical, cultural, age, or other parameters.

Source of funding. The source of funding of a clinical trial remains controversial. Those trials funded by for-profit entities have a greater chance of demonstrating a positive result than those funded by nonprofit entities.[20,21] Negative findings have been noted in 35% of non–industry-funded studies but in only 13% of industry-funded studies.[21] It is difficult to ascertain whether negative studies are not published at the discretion of the authors, whether journals have a bias for publishing more positive studies, or whether industry studies are designed to have a greater chance of obtaining a positive result. Likely, all three reasons play a role.

OBSERVATIONAL STUDIES

Data from studies other than interventional studies are commonly used for healthcare economic analyses.[22,23] Among these are observational studies, which observe the natural course of a health state or disease.

Included in the observational study category are the case-control study, the cross-sectional study, and the cohort study. A *case-control study* is typically retrospective. Individuals with a disease or aspect(s) of a disease *(cases)* are studied and compared to individuals without a disease *(controls)*. Research often examines an effect or effects in regard to cause. For example, the retrospective lipid profiles obtained in a group of subjects with coronary artery disease (cases) could be compared to lipid profiles obtained in a group of age-matched subjects without coronary artery disease (controls).

In a *cross-sectional study*, also referred to as a *prevalence study*, individuals with a condition of interest are studied at a single point in time. As an example, utility values could be obtained from a group of consecutive patients undergoing hemodialysis.

In a *cohort study*, individuals with a condition or parameter of interest (study group) are observed longitudinally, typically prospectively, and compared to those without that condition or parameter (control group) in regard to the effect on disease outcome. Patients in both the study and control groups come from the same cohort. A *cohort* is simply a group of individuals who share a common condition or parameter. An example of a cohort study is one in which age-matched patients who smoke (study group) are compared to nonsmokers and the incidence of subsequent cancer(s) is studied in each.

With *observational studies* we observe the course of a disease or a health state. Observational studies include:

1. **Case-control:** retrospective
2. **Cross-sectional:** point in time
3. **Cohort:** prospective

USE OF LEVELS OF EVIDENCE

To ensure that healthcare is of the highest quality, policy standards should be considered that reward healthcare practitioners who practice medicine based on scientific evidence. Does this mean clinical practice should only be based on randomized clinical trials? No. However, all treatments that are offered in a system should be evaluated on a line-by-line basis. In the setting where no randomized clinical trials currently exist, policymakers can take one of two routes:

1. suggest implementation of a treatment based on a scientific study that contains a lower level of available evidence, or
2. support the concept that no treatment be offered by physicians until evidence from a randomized clinical trial has been created.

Once the level of evidence of a study has been determined, one must turn to evaluating the relevance of the study. More specifically, to what extent will a specific intervention reduce mortality and morbidity from a disease, or what is the value of the intervention? An interventional study may contain Level I evidence, but if the patient value it confers is negligible, its worth to society may also be negligible. The value of interventions will be discussed extensively in subsequent chapters.

WHAT IS THE RISK IN RISK REDUCTION?

Other evidence-based parameters useful in evaluating clinical data for analysis with VBM include *relative risk reduction* and the *absolute risk reduction.*[18] The difference between the two is often unappreciated by providers when interpreting a clinical trial, but the difference is of critical importance to patients.

Relative Risk Reduction

Traditionally, treatment efficacy has been measured in relative terms. A common measure of efficacy is therefore *relative risk reduction.*[24] The relative risk reduction (RRR) conferred by an intervention is defined as the Control Event Rate (CER) – Treatment Event Rate (TER)/Control Event Rate (CER).

> ### Relative Risk Reduction
> $$RRR = (CER - TER)/CER$$
> in which CER is the control event rate and TER
> is the treatment event rate.

The relative risk reduction conveys the quantity of disease or adverse outcome reduction in relative terms. In essence, the relative risk reduction measures the percentage decrease of an adverse outcome among a subgroup of treated *patients who would have definitely had an adverse outcome without treatment.*

For example, among 100 patients with cancer who are randomized to observation without treatment X, the one-year death rate is 5%. In a cohort randomized to treatment X, the death rate is 3%. The relative risk reduction associated with treatment X is therefore (5% − 3%)/5%, or 40%.

Absolute Risk Reduction

The *absolute risk reduction* (ARR) conferred by an intervention is the percentage decrease of an adverse outcome among *all patients who are treated*. It is defined as the Control Event Rate (CER) − Treatment Event Rate (TER).

Among the 100 patients with cancer, the absolute risk reduction is therefore 3% (5% − 2%), dramatically different from the relative risk reduction.

Absolute Risk Reduction

ARR = (CER − TER)

in which CER is the control event rate and TER is the treatment event rate.

Relative measures of efficacy, however, do not adequately convey real or absolute reductions in risk, as relative reductions are derived through ratios. For instance, we may be told that a new treatment for heart attack reduces one's risk of death by 50%, as does a new treatment for cancer. But one's risk of death, if untreated, may be dramatically different in these two situations; one's risk of death without treatment may only be 2% in the setting of cancer but be 40% in the situation of the heart attack. A 50% relative risk reduction for a patient with cancer would mean dropping the absolute risk from 2% to 1%, whereas in the situation of a heart attack, a 50% relative risk reduction would mean dropping the absolute risk from 40% to 20%. Although both treatments would yield a 50% reduction in relative risk, the absolute risk reductions of 1% for cancer and 20% for heart attack are drastically different.

The difference between relative and absolute risk reduction is critical, and one that all clinicians should appreciate because of its practical importance to patients. To better understand the limitation of relative measures of therapeutic efficacy, let us consider another example in which we evaluate a hypothetical medication developed to decrease development of new blood vessels on the iris, a potentially blinding complication of patients with blocked retinal veins or severe carotid artery obstruction. The medication prevents the development of new blood vessels in 50% (RRR = 50%) of patients who develop this complication, regardless of whether the patient has a blocked vein or severe carotid artery obstruction. The magnitude of the treatment effect can be reported as a relative risk of 0.5 or a relative risk reduction of 50%. However, since the risk of new blood vessel formation is quite different in these two groups (16% in the venous occlusion group and 66% in the carotid artery obstruction group),[25,26] the absolute reduction of new blood vessel formation conferred by treatment is quite different in the two groups. Specifically, if medication were administered to 100 patients who had blocked veins, one would anticipate that an additional eight patients (ARR = 8%), or half of the 16 that were expected to develop this complication, would be spared from it. If, however, this treatment were given to 100 patients with severe carotid artery obstruction, one would anticipate that an additional 33 patients (ARR = 33%), or half of the 66 that were expected to develop the complication, would be spared from it.

An even more striking difference between relative risk reduction and absolute risk reduction is seen with data from the Clopidogrel Versus Aspirin in Patients at Risk of Ischemic Events (CAPRIE) Trial.[27] The CAPRIE trial compared the annual risk of ischemic event outcomes (ischemic stroke, myocardial infarction, or vascular death) in high-risk groups treated using either aspirin (annual risk = 5.83%) or clopidogrel (annual risk = 5.32%), both inhibitors of platelet aggregation. In this instance, we are considering the control rate as that obtained with aspirin and the Treatment Event Rate as that obtained with clopidogrel. Thus, the annual relative risk reduction is (Control Event Rate – Treatment Event Rate)/Control Event Rate, or 8.7% ([5.83 – 5.32]/5.83) in favor of clopidogrel. The absolute risk reduction, however, is Control Event Rate/Treatment Event Rate, or 0.51% (5.83 – 5.32).

Typically, it is the absolute risk reduction that is most appropriate and useful for cost-utility analysis. Since the difference between absolute and relative risk reduction can be dramatic, it is critical that the type of risk reduction utilized from the evidence-based data be specified.

> Comparing absolute risk reduction and relative risk reduction is analogous to comparing night and day. The form used in a cost-utility analysis must be specified. Usually *absolute risk* reduction is more enlightening and a more valuable statistic.

Number Needed to Treat

An alternate method to help determine the clinical relevance of therapeutic trials utilizes the absolute risk reduction and is referred to as *number needed to treat*.[28,29] This index refers to how many patients with a given disease need to be treated to prevent one person from developing an adverse outcome. The number needed to treat (NNT) is defined as 1/ARR, or the inverse of the absolute risk reduction.

> **Number Need to Treat**
> NNT = 1/ARR
> in which ARR is the absolute risk reduction (in %).

Accordingly, if a hypothetical clinical trial demonstrates that ten patients need to be treated to prevent one stroke, the number needed to treat (NNT) is ten (10/1). This index not only considers treatment effects in absolute terms, but it also allows the clinical importance of various therapeutic trials with similar outcomes to be compared to one another. Employing CAPRIE trial data on clopidogrel, with an absolute risk reduction of 0.51% of clopidogrel over aspirin, it can be seen that the NNT is 200 (1.0/0.0051). Therefore, 200 people would have to be treated for one year with clopidogrel, as compared with aspirin, to prevent one adverse ischemic event.

Another clinically relevant example is demonstrated with the North American Symptomatic Carotid Endarterectomy Trial (NASCET) data.[30] The NASCET was a multicenter, randomized clinical trial designed to answer numerous questions, including whether carotid endarterectomy is beneficial in symptomatic patients (those with a previous nondisabling stroke, transient ischemic attack and/or amaurosis fugax) with a high-grade (70% to 99%) ipsilateral carotid stenosis. In this study, patients with symptomatic, high-grade carotid stenosis received either surgical endarterectomy or medical treatment with antiplatelet therapy (aspirin). The incidence of stroke at two years after randomization was 26% in the aspirin-treated patients and 9% in the surgical patients. Thus, surgery results in a *relative risk reduction* ([Control Event Rate – Treatment Event Rate]/Control Event) of 65% ([26% – 9%]/26%) for stroke with endarterectomy compared to antiplatelet therapy.

The absolute risk reduction (Control Event Rate – Treatment Event Rate) at two years conferred by surgery versus aspirin therapy is 17% (26% to 9%). Accordingly, endartectomy prevents 17% of patients from developing a stroke compared to aspirin over a two-year period. Based upon the NASCET results, if 100 patients with a symptomatic 70% to 99% carotid stenosis underwent carotid endarterectomy, 17 patients should be expected to be spared a stroke within a two-year period (as compared to antiplatelet treatment). By taking the inverse of the absolute risk reduction derived from this study, one can calculate the number of patients with symptomatic, high-grade carotid stenosis who need to be treated with endarterectomy to have one treatment success. Since the absolute risk reduction equals 17%, or 0.17, the NNT equals 1/ARR, or 1/0.17, or 5.9. This means that five or six patients with a symptomatic, high-grade carotid stenosis must be treated with endarterectomy to prevent one patient from having a stroke within two years after the onset of symptoms.

Numbers needed to treat have also been calculated for various other therapies frequently administered for the treatment of systemic vascular disease.[31] Specifically, 41 patients with nonvalvular atrial fibrillation need to be treated with blood thinners to prevent one stroke, 24 patients with peripheral vascular disease need to be treated to prevent one critical cardiac event, and 128 patients with diastolic blood pressures between 90 and 109 mm Hg need to be treated to prevent one major vascular event. The greater the absolute risk reduction conferred by an intervention, the lower the number needed to treat.

Confidence Interval

The confidence interval is another important parameter in EBM. The confidence interval is defined as the interval range within which the *mean* for a sample of normally distributed data will fall a given percentage of time if a study was to be repeated on the same population. A 95% confidence interval signifies there is a 95% chance the mean of a sample will lie within this interval if the study was repeated on the same population, whereas a 99% confidence interval signifies there is a 99% chance the mean will be within the interval. As an example, if a cohort has a mean diastolic blood pressure of 80 mm Hg after administration of an antihypertensive drug, with a 95% confidence interval from 70 mm Hg to 90 mm Hg, there is a 95% chance that if the study were to be repeated, the resultant mean diastolic blood pressure would be between 70 mm Hg and 90 mm Hg.

Confidence intervals are as the name implies. They give us confidence in the reproducibility of data.

WHY IS EVIDENCE-BASED MEDICINE ONLY THE FIRST STEP?

Total quality management has been transforming the United States business landscape over the past decades. Evidence-based medicine is a philosophy that can be used to improve the quality of the healthcare delivered in this country. Tactically, it can be considered an application of total quality management as applied to healthcare. Its specific tactics include the interpretation of the levels of evidence contained within scientific articles and determining the importance of a treatment effect in absolute terms.

While EBM improves the quality of medical care, it still does not allow us to quantify or compare the value of interventions. For example, what is the value of total hip arthroplasty to a patient who is barely able to walk due to osteoarthritis of the hip? And what is the value to a patient of cardiac bypass graft surgery that improves a cardiac ejection fraction from 45% to 50%? Furthermore, how do each of these interventions compare to the other? EBM does not answer these important questions, but it does provide the underlying information necessary to do so. Using the best evidence-based information, we can take the data to a higher level, VBM, that will allow a direct comparison of the value conferred by each of these interventions.

CORE CONCEPTS

- Evidence-based medicine is the practice of medicine based upon the highest level of scientific evidence.
- There are five levels of interventional evidence.
  — Level 1: randomized clinical trial with low Type 1 and Type 2 errors
  — Level 2: randomized clinical trial with higher Type 1 and Type 2 errors
  — Level 3: nonrandomized clinical trial
  — Level 4: case series
  — Level 5: case study
- A meta-analysis combines two or more clinical trials that may be underpowered. As such, it can convert Level II interventional evidence to Level I evidence.

- The power (chance of detecting a specified difference of interest) should be stated if the results of a clinical trial are negative.
- If less than 5% of subjects drop out of a clinical trial, there is little chance for bias, whereas if more than 20% of subjects drop out of a study, there is considerable chance for bias.
- There are three types of observational studies that model the natural course of a disease or parameter of interest.
  — Case-control: retrospective analysis of a group with a disease compared to a group without that disease
  — Cross-sectional: individuals with a condition of interest are studied at a point in present time
  — Cohort study: subjects from the same cohort with a condition are followed prospectively and compared to those from the same cohort without that condition.
- Absolute risk reduction = control event rate (%) – treatment event rate (%).
- Relative risk reduction = (control event rate – treatment event rate)/control event rate.
- Numbers needed to treat = 1/ARR. The number needed to treat is the number of patients that must be treated to prevent one adverse outcome.
- The 95% confidence interval is the range (bounded by a lower limit and an upper limit) within which the mean value of a normally distributed condition will fall 95 out of 100 times if the study is repeated.

REFERENCES

1. Rafuse J. Evidence-based medicine means MDs must develop new skills, attitudes, CMA conference told. *Can Med Assoc J.* 1994;150:1479–1481.
2. Sackett D. Rules of evidence and clinical recommendations. *Can J Cardiol.* 1993;9:487–489.
3. Asher WL, Harper HW. Effect of human chorionic gonadotropin on weight loss, hunger and feeling. *Am J Clin Nutr.* 1973;26:211–218.
4. Coronary Drug Project Research Group. Influence of adherence treatment and response of cholesterol on mortality in the Coronary Drug Project. *N Engl J Med.* 1980;303:1038–1041.
5. Fuller R, Roth H, Long S. Compliance with disulfiram treatment of alcoholism. *J Chronic Dis.* 1983;36:161–170.
6. Hogarty GE, Goldberg SC. Drug and sociotherapy in the aftercare of schizophrenic patients. *Arch Gen Psychiatry.* 1973;28:54–64.
7. Pizzo PA, Robichaud KJ, Edwards BK, Schumaker C, Kramer BS, Johnson A. Oral antibiotic prophylaxis in patients with cancer: a double blinded randomized placebo-controlled trial. *J Pediatr.* 1983;102:125–133.

8. Sackett DL, Haynes RB, Guyatt GH, Tugwell P. *Clinical Epidemiology: A Basic Science for Clinical Medicine.* 2nd ed. Boston, Mass: Little, Brown & Co; 1991:39, 205–209.

9. Pocock SJ. *Clinical Trials: A Practical Approach.* Chichester, England: John Wiley and Sons; 1983:50.

10. Sharma S. Levels of evidence and interventional ophthalmology. *Can J Ophthalmol.* 1997;32:359–362.

11. Giner V, Rueda D, Salvador A, Hernandez JC, Esteban JE, Redon J. Thrombocytopenia associated with levodopa treatment. *Arch Intern Med.* 2003;163:735–736.

12. Clark JM, Saffold SH, Israel JM. Decellularized dermal grafting in cleft palate repair. *Arch Facial Plast Surg.* 2003;5:40–44.

13. Wang BWE, Ramey DR, Schlettler MS, Hubert HB, Fries JF. Postponed development of disability in elderly runners. *Arch Intern Med.* 2002;162:2285–2294.

14. Coggon D. *Statistics in Clinical Practice.* London, England: BMJ Books; 2003:60.

15. Bressler NM, Maguire MG, Murphy PL, et al. Macular scatter ("grid") laser treatment of poorly demarcated subfoveal choroidal neovascularization in age-related macular degeneration: results of a randomized clinical trial. *Arch Ophthalmol.* 1996;114:1456–1464.

16. Berkowitz RI, Wadden TA, Tershakovec AM, Cronquist JL. Behavior therapy and sirbutamine for the treatment of adolescent obesity: a randomized controlled trial. *JAMA.* 2003;289:1805–1812.

17. Stampler MJ, Goldhaber SZ, Yusuf S, Peto R, Hennekens CH. Effect of intravenous streptokinase on acute myocardial infarction: pooled results from randomized trials. *N Engl J Med.* 1982:307:1180–1182.

18. Sackett DL, Straus SE, Richardson WS, Rosenberg W, Haynes RB. *Evidence-Based Medicine: How to Practice and Teach EBM.* 2nd ed. Philadelphia, Pa: Churchill Livingstone; 2000:95–153.

19. Treatment of Age-Related Macular Degeneration with Photodynamic Therapy (TAP) Study Group. Photodynamic therapy of subfoveal choroidal neovascularization in age-related macular degeneration with verteporfin: two-year results of 2 randomized clinical trials. *Arch Ophthalmol.* 2001;119:198–207.

20. Kjaergard LL, Als-Nielsen B. Association between competing interests and authors' conclusions: epidemiological study of randomized clinical trials published in the BMJ. *BMJ.* 2002;325:249.

21. Yaphe J, Edman R, Knishkowy B, Herman J. The association between funding by commercial interests and study outcome in randomized controlled drug trials. *Fam Pract.* 2001;18:565–568.

22. Hennekens CH, Buring JE. *Epidemiology in Medicine.* Boston, Mass: Little Brown & Co; 1987.

23. Last JM. *A Dictionary of Epidemiology.* 3rd ed. New York, NY: Oxford University Press; 1995.

24. Schulzer M, Mancini GB. 'Unqualified success' and 'unmitigated failure': number-needed-to-treat related concepts for assessing treatment efficacy in the presence of treatment-induced adverse events. *Int J Epidemiol.* 1996;25:704–712.

25. Brown GC, Magargal LE. The ocular ischemic syndrome. *Int Ophthalmol.* 1988;11:239–251.

26. Central Vein Occlusion Study Group. Natural history and clinical management of central retinal vein occlusion. *Arch Ophthalmol.* 1997;115:486–491.

27. CAPRIE Steering Committee. A randomized, blinded, trial of clopidogrel versus aspirin in patients at risk of ischaemic events (CAPRIE). *Lancet.* 1996;328:1329–1339.

28. Cook RJ, Sackett DL. The number needed to treat: a clinically useful measure of treatment effect. *BMJ.* 1995;310:452–454.

29. Laupacis A, Sackett DL, Roberts RS. An assessment of clinically useful measures of the consequences of treatment. *N Engl J Med.* 1988;318:1728–1733.

30. North American Symptomatic Carotid Endarterectomy Trial Collaborators. Beneficial effect of carotid endarterectomy in symptomatic patients with high-grade carotid stenosis. *N Engl J Med.* 1991;325:445–453.

31. McQuay HJ, Moore RA. Using numerical results from systemic reviews in clinical practice. *Ann Intern Med.* 1997;126:712–720.

PART

3

Value in Medicine

The Intermediate Tier of the Value-Based Medicine Pyramid

5

How to Evaluate Health-Related Quality-of-Life Instruments

We perform, or should perform, only one relevant service in healthcare: we deliver *value*. How is value measured? By two means. When we deliver value, we improve (or maintain):

- length or life, and/or
- quality of life.[1-3]

Interventions that do neither should be discarded or improved so they do provide value. The improvement in length of life conferred by an intervention can often be garnered from the evidence-based literature, but the improvement in quality of life has been more difficult to measure.

We perform only one relevant service in healthcare: we deliver *value*.

The outcomes in evidence-based clinical trials are typically expressed in scientific terms such as millimeters of mercury to assess blood pressure, IgG antibody titer levels to assess the degree of influenza A immunization, or the percentage obstruction in a carotid artery in a person with a transient ischemic attack. While these numbers can reveal substantial information about health states and the outcomes of interventions, there are major drawbacks in regard to their applicability for stakeholder groups in healthcare. Specifically, these numbers often fail to address the following:

1. **An objective measure of improvement in quality of life.**

   For example, exactly how much does decreasing the diastolic blood pressure from 110 mm Hg to 80 mm Hg improve quality of life? Or how much does an influenza immunization improve quality of life for the average person?

2. **A comparison of the quality-of-life improvement conferred by interventions in disparate specialties.**

Using the previous example, which is more valuable to a patient? The improvement in blood pressure or the influenza immunization? And by how much?

3. **The ability to incorporate data into cost-utility analysis to assess the value conferred by an intervention for the resources expended.**

   If two interventions provide the same value, are they equally desirable? From the therapeutic point of view, yes. But if one intervention costs 50 times the cost of the other, how much should a society with limited resources invest in each?

Obviously, measuring the improvement in quality of life and length of life that interventions confer is critically important. But how do we measure quality of life?

THE IDEAL HEALTH-RELATED QUALITY-OF-LIFE INSTRUMENT

Theoretically, the ideal health-related quality-of-life instrument should be one that is:

1. all-encompassing in regard to the variables that compose quality of life,
2. sensitive to small changes in health,
3. reliable (reproducible),
4. applicable across all medical specialties,
5. able to be completed within a reasonable time period,
6. understandable by patients,
7. able to demonstrate construct validity (the ability to measure what it is intended to measure), and
8. able to be integrated with healthcare costs for the performance of healthcare economic analyses

No instrument is ideal, but we believe utility analysis—especially the time tradeoff methodology—amply fulfills these criteria. Scaling methodologies also appear to have substantial potential for use, although more research is necessary in this area. Both of these instruments will be discussed in detail. We also believe, however, that those with an interest in cost-utility analysis and value-based medicine should have an appreciation of how to evaluate some of the multiple quality-of-life instruments commonly used in healthcare. This chapter and the next three address different health-related quality-of-life instruments.

What Is a Health State?

Before we go further, it is helpful to define a *health state*. It is a confusing term frequently used by researchers but rarely used by clinicians in practice.

A *health state* is simply the state of a person's health at a particular point in time. It is theoretically more inclusive than disease in that it includes normal health and death as well as all combinations of multiple diseases with varying severity along the spectrum between normal health and death. *Disease* generally refers to one entity and its continuum of degrees of severity. If the patient has health problems in addition to a primary disease, these are referred to as *comorbidities.*

The term *health state* is often used synonymously with *disease.* When a person is affected by only one disease, the substitution of health state for disease, and vice versa, makes little difference. For example, a person with diabetes mellitus and no other health problems can be referred to as having the health state of diabetes or as having diabetic disease.

When we speak about a state of well-being in the clinical context, we usually refer to a particular disease and its severity, such as mild coronary artery disease, severe pulmonary hypertension, or total renal failure. Rarely does a clinician use the term *health state.* Additionally, the healthcare reimbursement system in the United States is specifically tied to the diagnosis of single specific diseases,[4] rather than a health state composed of multiple diseases. For these reasons, and others to be discussed, we generally study a specific disease (with a specified degree of severity) in healthcare economic analyses, whether we call the disease a health state or not.

What Is the Current State of the Health-Related Quality-of-Life Arena?

It can be readily described in two words: unequivocal chaos. There is no standardized quality-of-life database despite the recommendations of the Panel for Cost-Effectiveness in Health and Medicine.[5] Furthermore, newer quality-of-life measuring instruments are appearing so fast in many specialties that it is virtually impossible to keep abreast with them.

Tengs and Wallace[6] performed a superb and exhaustive study of 1,000 health-related quality-of-life estimates in 2000. What they demonstrated was numerous incomparable studies and the desperate need for a standardized, single-instrument, health-related quality-of-life database. (See Table 5.1.) It is of note that Tengs and Wallace found that the most commonly used quality-of-life measure was subjective judgment by the authors of a manuscript (25.4%). As we demonstrate, this a very poor measure of health-related quality of life compared to the perceptions of patients who actually experience a disease firsthand.

What About Disease Severity?

It is critical that the severity of a disease be specified when the quality of life associated with that disease is measured. To illustrate, researchers in the Beaver Dam Health Outcomes Study,[7] a population-based, cross-sectional study of people living in Beaver Dam, Wisconsin, obtained time tradeoff utility values from patients with specific diseases. The mean time tradeoff utility value associated with asthma in the Beaver Dam Study was 0.82. Data from the Center for Value-Based Medicine indicate that people with asthma and no limitation on quality of life have a mean time tradeoff utility value of 0.98, while those with a severe

TABLE   5.1

Results of 1,000 Quality-of-Life Studies in the Healthcare Literature

QOL Instrument	Authors	Experts	Community	Patients	Proxy	Total
TTO	2 (1%)	8 (4.1%)	5 (2.6%)	26 (13.4%)	2 (1%)	22%
SG	0 (0%)	9 (4.7%)	1 (0.5%)	11 (5.7%)	0 (0%)	11%
RS	3 (1.6%)	12 (4.7%)	1 (0.5%)	19 (9.8%)	2 (1%)	18%
Judgment	49 (25.4%)	12 (6.2%)	0 (0%)	0 (0%)	0 (0%)	32%
Other QOL Instruments	6 (3.1%)	6 (3.1%)	1 (0.5%)	18 (9.3%)	2 (1%)	17%
Total	**31%**	**23%**	**4%**	**39%**	**3%**	**100%**

Proxy indicates a respondent who lives with or cares for a patient; QOL, quality-of-life; RS, rating scale; SG, standard gamble utility analysis; TTO, time tradeoff utility analysis.
Adapted from Tengs and Wallace.[6]

limitation have a utility value 0.53. Needless to say, a cost-utility analysis of an inhaled corticosteroid used for the treatment for asthma would be dramatically different depending upon which values were used. For cardiac angina, the Beaver Dam Study found a mean time tradeoff utility value of 0.79, while we have noted mild, or American Heart Association Functional Class I, angina to be associated with a mean utility value of 0.92 and severe, or American Heart Association Functional Class IV, angina to be associated with a mean utility value of 0.53. Again, the difference in the results between healthcare economic analyses can be dramatic, depending upon which utility values are used.

> When the quality of life associated with a disease is measured, the severity of the disease should be specified.

A system of value-based medicine built upon almost any standardized, patient preference-based, quality-of-life database would be preferable to the current incomparable clutter. Unfortunately, incomparable quality-of-life databases consequently lead to equally incomparable cost-utility analyses. The key is creating a uniform quality-of-life database that addresses the spectrum of diseases across healthcare.

HOW DO WE EVALUATE QUALITY-OF-LIFE INSTRUMENTS?

A number of parameters can be used to evaluate the worthiness of health-related quality-of-life instruments. A brief discussion of these parameters follows.

Reliability

Reliability is simply the *reproducibility* of an examination measure. Froberg and Kane[8] refer to three types of reliability:

1. intrarater reliability,
2. interrater reliability, and
3. test-retest reliability.

Intrarater reliability refers to the reproducibility of the same rater rating a parameter more than once. *Interrater reliability* refers to the reproducibility of a measure by more than one rater asking the same question(s), and *test-retest reliability* assesses the reproducibility of a measure at different points in time.

The *intraclass correlation coefficient* (ρ), also known as the *reliability coefficient*, is frequently utilized to measure the reproducibility of variables, such as utility values, obtained at different times. Rosner[9] notes that $\rho < 0.4$ indicates poor reproducibility, $0.4 \leq \rho < 0.75$ indicates fair to good reproducibility, and $\rho \geq 0.75$ indicates excellent reproducibility.

> *Reliability* is the reproducibility of a quality-of-life evaluation measure.

Validity

Validity is the ability of an instrument to measure a given effect—in our case, the quality of life associated with a health state. Petitti[10] divides validity into two variants:

1. criterion validity and
2. construct validity.

Criterion validity. *Criterion validity* assesses how well a tool measures up to the gold standard. For example, in regard to the diagnosis of carotid artery obstruction, the gold standard, or criterion, in the North American Symptomatic Carotid Endarterectomy Trial was arteriography in which contrast dye was injected into the carotid arteries through a catheter passed up through the femoral artery.[11] Thus, other measurement instruments, such as ultrasonography and Doppler imaging, were compared to the criterion (arteriography). In the field of health-related quality of life there is, however, no universally accepted gold standard. Therefore measuring the criterion validity of a quality-of-life instrument is not possible.

> *Criterion validity* assesses how well a tool measures up to the gold standard.

> There is no *criterion* among health-related quality-of-life instruments.

Construct validity. Construct validity assesses how well a tool measures what it is intended to measure. In essence, how well does utility analysis or the Medical Outcomes Study Short Form-36 measure health-related quality of life? Unfortunately, there is no general agreement on exactly which parameters comprise quality of life and which are the most important. As much as we would like to precisely measure the construct validity of our health-related quality-of-life instruments, the task is extraordinarily difficult because of the lack of quality-of-life standards and the weighting of standards according to their degree of importance.

Construct validity assesses how well a tool measures what it is intended to measure.

A list of health-related quality-of-life variables we consider important is shown in Table 5.2. While extensive, it is by no means complete. Theoretically, any instrument that measures one or more of the parameters listed in Table 5.2 could be included under the broad umbrella of a health-related quality-of-life instrument.

TABLE 5.2

Variables Composing Health-Related Quality of Life*

Cognitive Function

- Short-term memory
- Long-term memory

Motor Function

- Vocational (work-related)
- Avocational (recreation-related)
- Dependency
    — Basic needs (washing, dressing, eating)
    — Toileting needs
    — Grooming needs
    — Medication needs
- Mobility
- Level of energy: decreased or hyperactivity

Psychological Function

- Anxiety
- Uncertainty and/or fear of the future
- Depression
- Self-image perception
- Self-satisfaction
- Hypomanic health state

TABLE 5.2 continued

Variables Composing Health-Related Quality of Life*

Psychological Function continued

- Manic health state
- Perception of psychological well-being

Sensory Function

- Visual
- Auditory
- Tactile
- Loss of smell
- Loss of taste

Social Function

- Relating socially to family and friends
- Relating socially to the opposite gender
- Relating socially to vocational colleagues
- Relating socially to institutional or home caregivers
- Relating socially to healthcare professionals

Caregiver Support

- Is it available?
- How does illness affect the caregiver?
- How does illness affect the family as caregivers?

Economic

- Ability to afford healthcare costs
- Ability to afford domiciliary costs
- Ability to afford caregiver costs
- Indirect costs: the opportunity cost of illness, or lost wages
- Ability to provide for dependents
- Ability to afford future healthcare and nonhealthcare costs

Lifestyle Changes Necessitated by Illness

Pain

Pain Variants

- Paresthesias
- Dysesthesias
- Burning
- Temperature Intolerance
- Itching

* The order of the variables does not necessarily imply their relative importance.

To assess construct validity, an instrument can be compared to other well-accepted measures of clinical status. According to Torrence,[12] the construct validity of a quality-of-life instrument can also be demonstrated by predicting events or behaviors. In essence, the scores from a quality-of-life measure should correlate appropriately with the clinical symptoms and signs along the continuum of a disease from milder to more severe stages. For arthritis, the American College of Rheumatology Classification of Global Function Status in Rheumatoid Arthritis[13] is a basic comparison standard, and for angina, the American Heart Association Functional Capacity Classification[14] is an elementary comparison instrument. For visual health states, the visual acuity is a reasonable measure, while for hearing disorders, the degree of decibel loss is a good measure. As the vision in the better-seeing eye or the hearing in the better-hearing ear diminishes, the quality-of-life instrument decreases concomitantly.[1-3]

If a quality-of-life instrument demonstrates good correlation with clinical disease evaluation parameters commonly in use, we can have confidence in the construct validity of the instrument. Specific construct validity examples are addressed in detail in Chapter 9.

> If a quality-of-life instrument demonstrates good correlation with clinical disease evaluation parameters commonly in use, we can have confidence in its construct validity.

CORE CONCEPTS

- We perform one relevant service in healthcare: we deliver value.
- The *value* delivered by an intervention is measured by the improvement it confers in:
  — length of life and/or
  — quality of life
- A *health state* is the state of a person's health. A health state can include one or more diseases and different degrees of severity of the diseases, as well as death and normal (perfect) health.
- A good health-related quality-of-life instrument should be:
  — all-encompassing in regard to the variables that compose quality of life,
  — sensitive to small changes in health,
  — reliable (reproducible),
  — applicable across all medical specialties,
  — able to be completed within a reasonable time period,
  — readily understandable by patients,
  — able to demonstrate construct validity (the ability to measure what it is intended to measure) and
  — able to be integrated with healthcare costs for the performance of healthcare economic analyses.

- Quality-of-life instruments are evaluated according to reliability (reproducibility) and validity.
- There are three variants of reliability:
  — *Intrarater* reliability refers to the reproducibility of the same rater repeatedly measuring a parameter.
  — *Interrater* reliability refers to reproducibility of different raters measuring the same parameter.
  — *Test-retest* reliability refers to the reproducibility of a parameter at different points in time.
- There are two variants of validity:
  — *Criterion* validity assesses how well a quality-of-life instrument measures up to the gold standard or *criterion*. There currently is no criterion for health-related quality-of-life instruments.
  — *Construct* validity assesses how well a quality-of-life instrument measures what it is intended to measure. The construct of an instrument is assessed by how well the instrument predicts future events and behaviors, and how it compares to other well-accepted measures of clinical status.

REFERENCES

1. Brown GC, Brown MM, Sharma S. Health care in the 21st century: evidence-based medicine, patient preference-based quality and cost-effectiveness. *Qual Manage Health Care.* 2000;19:23–31.

2. Brown MM, Brown GC. Outcome of corneal transplantation: value-based health care. *Br J Ophthalmol.* 2002;86:2–3.

3. Brown MM, Brown GC, Sharma S. Value-based medicine. *Evidence-Based Eye Care.* 2002;3:8–9.

4. Hart AC, Hopkins CA, eds. *International Classification of Diseases, 9th Revision, Clinical Modification.* Salt Lake City, Utah: Ingenix; 2003.

5. Gold MR, Patrick DL, Torrence GW, et al. Identifying and valuing outcomes. In: Gold MR, Siegel JE, Russell LB, Weinstein MC, eds. *Cost-Effectiveness in Health and Medicine.* New York, NY: Oxford University Press; 1996:82–134.

6. Tengs TO, Wallace MA. One thousand health-related quality-of-life estimates. *Med Care.* 2000;38:583–637.

7. Fryback DG, Dasbach EJ, Klein R, et al. The Beaver Dam Health Outcomes Study: initial catalog of health-state quality factors. *Med Decis Making.* 1993;13:89–102.

8. Froberg DG, Kane RL. Methodology for measuring health state preferences, II: scaling methods. *J Clin Epidemiol.* 1989;42:459–471.

9. Rosner B. *Fundamentals of Biostatistics.* 5th ed. Pacific Grove, Calif: Duxbury Thomson Learning; 2000:451–453, 562–565.

10. Petitti DB. *Meta-Analysis, Decision Analysis and Cost-Effectiveness Analysis.* 2nd ed. New York, NY: Oxford University Press; 2000:169–181.

11.   Moneta GL, Edwards JM, Chitwood RW, et al. Correlation of North American Symptomatic Carotid Endarterectomy Trial (NASCET) angiographic definition of 70% to 99% internal carotid artery stenosis with duplex scanning. *J Vasc Surg.* 1993;17:152–157.

12.   Torrence GW. Social preference for health states: an empirical evaluation of three measurement techniques. *Socioecon Plann Sci.* 1976;10:129–136.

13.   Hochberg MC, Chang RW, Dwosh I, Lindsey S, Pincus Y, Wolfe F. The American College of Rheumatology 1991 revised criteria for the classification of global functional status in rheumatoid arthritis. *Arthritis Rheum.* 1992;35:498–502.

14.   American Heart Association. Classification of functional capacity and objective assessment. Available at: www.americanheart.org. Accessed April 29, 2003.

6

Classification of Health-Related Quality-of-Life Instruments

As noted in Chapter 5, the improvement in length of life can be acquired from the evidence-based literature. The measurement of quality of life is considerably more difficult to ascertain. Thus, the critical question is, *how do we measure the quality of life associated with health states so we can assess the value conferred by healthcare interventions?*

A key point is that no one has definitively defined a *health-related quality-of-life instrument* and the specific features necessary for an instrument to be included within the definition of a health-related quality-of-life instrument. Consequently, we will err on the side of discussing instruments that are considered by some to be health-related quality-of-life instruments, while others may disagree. Included within this realm are some of the categorical scales used by subspecialty groups, such as the American Heart Association Functional Capacity Classification,[1] the American College of Rheumatology Classification of Global Functional Status,[2] and the Modified Rankin Scale[3] used in neurology. Because there is no criterion or gold standard for a health-related quality-of-life instrument, one could argue that any instrument with construct validity that measures one or more of the variables listed in Table 5.2 in Chapter 5 should be included within the broad category of health-related quality-of-life instruments.

TYPES OF INSTRUMENTS

Many instruments have been developed to measure the quality of life associated with a health state, and numerous additional instruments are developed every year. While there is unequivocal crossover in classification for many instruments, we believe that most health-related quality-of-life instruments can be divided into two basic variants:

■ function-based instruments and
■ preference-based instruments.

Function-Based Instruments

Function-based instruments primarily measure the functional level of a patient with a given disease or health state. Encompassed within the spectrum of function is the ability to function cognitively, vocationally (in work-related activities), avocationally (recreationally), physically, socially, psychologically, and with pain. An example of a limited function-based instrument is the Modified Rankin Scale,[3] which assesses the function of a patient after a stroke.

Function-based health-related quality-of-life instruments primarily measure the functional capability associated with a health state or disease.

Included within the realm of function-based activities is the ability to function cognitively, vocationally, avocationally, physically, socially, and psychologically.

Preference-Based Instruments

Preference-based instruments require that a subject make a decision regarding his or her preference (desirability or undesirability) for his or her health state. Included within in the broad category of patient preference–based instruments, or patient preferences, are both utility analysis and rating scales. With utility analysis, patients typically choose (prefer) to live with their current disease or choose (prefer) freedom from their disease in return for trading something of value (money, time of life) or risking something of value (life itself).

Preference-based instruments require that patients make a decision regarding their preference (desirability or undesirability) for their health state.

Generic Instruments

In addition to being function-based or preference-based, health-related quality-of-life instruments can be classified according to whether they are applicable across all specialties in medicine, and thus are considered *generic*, or whether they can only be applied to one disease or a limited number of diseases, in which case they are generally referred to as *specialty-specific*. Generic instruments are also referred to as *multispecialty instruments*. Table 6.1 lists some of the more commonly used health-related quality-of-life instruments.

Generic quality-of-life instruments measure the quality of life associated with health states across all specialties of medicine.

TABLE 6.1

Quality-of-Life Measurement Instruments

Function-Based Instruments

Generic (Multispecialty)

1. Medical Outcomes Study 36-Item Short-Form Health Survey (SF-36)
2. Medical Outcomes Study 12-Item Short-Form Health Survey (SF-12)
3. Sickness Impact Profile (SIP)
4. Quality-of-Well-Being (QWB) Scale
5. Karnofsky Performance Status Scale
6. Eastern Cooperative Oncology Group (ECOG) Performance Status Scale
7. Activities of Daily Living (ADL) Scale
8. Categorical scales

Specialty-Specific

1. American Heart Association Functional Capacity Classification
2. American College of Rheumatology Classification of Global Functional Status in Rheumatoid Arthritis
3. Modified Rankin Scale
4. Hamilton Rating Scale for Depression
5. National Eye Institute Visual Functioning Questionnaire (NEI-VFQ-25)

Preference-Based Instruments (All Are Generic)

1. Utility analysis
    — Willingness-to-pay method
    — Standard gamble method
    — Time tradeoff method
2. Rating scales
3. Multiattribute utility analysis instruments
    — Euro-QOL 5-D
    — Health Utilities Index

Specialty-specific quality-of-life instruments measure the quality of life associated with one disease or a limited number of diseases.

APPLICABILITY OF INSTRUMENTS

New health-related quality-of-life instruments, particularly those that are specialty-specific, appear in the literature on almost a weekly basis. While they may be helpful in assessing the efficacy of interventions within a specialty, specialty-specific instruments are not often helpful for guiding healthcare policy. Their lack of widespread applicability greatly limits their usefulness.

We believe it is critical for a health-related quality-of-life instrument to be applicable across all specialties. Why? Because policymakers and payers will not carve out one specialty or another for preferential financial treatment; the effort is too great. *Carveouts* are arbitrary, create divisiveness within the patient and provider communities, and require additional administration and information systems, both features that equate to increased expense.

It is likely that quality-of-life measures will be linked in some fashion to the reimbursement of healthcare interventions in the future. Having been intimately involved with managed care, we believe it is exceedingly unlikely that an instrument that is not widely applicable will be utilized in any manner for asset allocation. The obstacles we point out make the task too difficult.

While on the subject of applicability, we believe that clinical trials should incorporate health-related quality-of-life instruments that:

- are comparable across specialties and
- can be used in cost-utility analysis.

Utility analysis instruments and rating scales fit both of these criteria. Considering the amount of money spent on clinical trials, the additional cost of incorporating utility analysis measurements is negligible.

Why Are There So Many Different Quality-of-Life Instruments?

To date, researchers in diverse specialties have used dramatically different outcome measures. This is because the majority of instruments have been developed by investigators in different subspecialties of medicine. The American Heart Association Functional Capacity Classification,[1] which evaluates the decrease in pain and dyspnea associated with cardiac interventions, differs from the National Eye Institute Visual Functioning Questionnaire (NEI-VFQ-25),[4] which is used to measure improvement associated with ophthalmic interventions. Different aspects of quality of life are emphasized by each, although there is overlap. The American Heart Association Functional Capacity Classification assesses the overall ability of a person with angina and/or dyspnea to perform work-related and recreational activities, while the NEI-VFQ-25 assesses whether a person with impaired vision can perform work-related and recreational activities as well.

Upon closer inspection, seemingly disparate interventions such as coronary artery bypass graft and cataract extraction may actually have more in common than first appreciated. Both interventions allow a person to resume normal activity, including working, earning an income, socializing, and participating in recreational activity. They can also decrease dependency and help reverse depression and decrease fear of the future. Nonetheless, there is still enough difference (with pain, mobility, cognition, self-image, dependency, level of energy, and others) that many health-related quality-of-life instruments are not able to effectively compare the two interventions.

Does the Method of Administration of a Health-Related Quality-of-Life Instrument Matter?

Yes. The results can be considerably different when the same health-related quality-of-life instrument is *self-administered* vs *interviewer-administered*.[5–10] It is possible that interviewers may introduce bias, but self-administered instruments can do the same. Self-administered instruments have the advantage of being less labor intensive; nonetheless, we believe that interviewer-administered health-related quality-of-life instruments are superior to self-administered health-related quality-of-life instruments. Why? For several reasons:

1. With self-administered instruments, such as mail surveys, the response rate is typically far below the 20% dropout rate we would accept for a clinical trial. There can therefore be an especially large bias in self-administered exams. For example, patients who have a good outcome after total hip arthroplasty are more likely to fill out a lengthy questionnaire for research purposes than those who are dissatisfied with the outcome, thus giving a false perception that the intervention has a better outcome than it does.

2. With interviewer-administered examinations, it is possible to obtain a more consecutive sample.

3. Subjects can interpret the same question very differently. For example, if a patient is asked to evaluate a postoperative health state, does that mean with pain medication or without pain medication? And which medication? How much? With constant caregiver support or not? The patient-perceived variations can be infinite. Interviewers can remedy these uncertainties and describe the exact health state.

4. Subjects may not understand a self-administered question. Interviewers can explain them.

Despite the difference in results between self-administered tests and interviewer-administered tests, it has been shown that interviewer-administered tests over the telephone and face-to-face give similar values.[11]

Interviewer-administered tests given face-to-face or by telephone produce the same results.

Do We Have to Repeat Clinical Trials to Obtain Quality-of-Life Data?

Clinical trials are increasingly attempting to incorporate health-related quality-of-life instruments as part of the primary trial. But just as clinical trials have diverse outcomes, many utilize diverse health-related quality-of-life instruments. Unfortunately, a good number of the health-related quality-of-life instrument data employed cannot be used as utility values in cost-utility analysis.

Additionally, there is a vast amount of superior clinical trial data that has already been incorporated into the evidence-based literature at a cost of hundreds of billions of dollars.

It is not possible to repeat extremely expensive and time-consuming clinical trials for the sole purpose of obtaining health-related, quality-of-life data for use in cost-utility analysis. Instead, it is easier to convert the evidence-based outcome(s) of a clinical trial, or the associated quality-of-life measure, to a form in which it can be used in cost-utility analysis. Familiarity with the more common health-related quality-of-life instruments, including their strengths and weaknesses, allows the health economic researcher to better appreciate their relevance and whether they can be used in place of patient preferences in cost-utility analysis.

Some health-related quality-of-life instruments can be used directly in cost-utility analysis, while others cannot or have not been used. Table 6.2 lists the quality-of-life measures that have been used and not used for cost-utility analysis.

Do Some Instruments Fit Into More Than One Category?

Yes. For example, the Quality of Well-Being Scale[12,13] is primarily a function-based scale, but is comparable to a continuous rating scale in that the rating can occur anywhere on a continuum from 0.0 to 1.0. Thus it has been utilized as a substitute for the preferences used with cost-utility analysis. Theoretically this could also be done with the SF-36,[14] SF-12,[15] or the Sickness Impact Profile,[16] although we are unaware that these tests have been used in cost-utility analysis. Categorical scales place subjects into a limited number of groupings (categories), and thus are *insensitive*, meaning that they are unable to differentiate health states or diseases and severities of diseases unless there is a considerable difference separating them. A scale dividing diseases on the basis of mild affliction, moderate affliction, or severe affliction can be considered a rudimentary categorical scale. We elected to include categorical rating scales in the function-based category rather than in the preference-based category, as they deal primarily with basic function and cannot be used as substitutes for utilities in cost-utility analysis.

A number of the instruments we have listed as function-based, including the Karnofsky Performance Status Scale,[17] the Eastern Cooperative Oncology Group Performance Status Scale,[18] the American College of Rheumatology Classification of Global Functional Status in Rheumatoid Arthritis,[2] the American Heart Association Functional Capacity Classification,[1] and the Modified Rankin Scale,[19] can also be considered as categorical rating scales; this means study participants are divided into a limited number of categories rather than placed on any point along a continuum.

TABLE 6.2

Common Health-Related Quality-of-Life Instruments in Clinical Practice and Their Use in Cost-Utility Analysis

Instrument	Use	Preference Based	Use in CUA
Function-Based Instruments			
Generic			
— SF-36	Generic	No	No
— 2SF-12	Generic	No	No
— 3SIP	Generic	No	No
— QWB Scale	Generic	No	Yes
— ADL Scale	Generic	No	No
— Karnofsky Scale	Generic	No	No
— ECOG Performance Status Scale	Generic	No	No
— Categorical Scale (mild, moderate, severe)	Generic	No	No
Specialty-Specific			
— American Heart Association Functional Capacity Classification	Specialty (cardiology, pulmonary)	No	No
— American College of Rheumatology of Global Functional Status in Rheumatoid Arthritis	Specialty (rheumatology, orthopedics)	No	No
— Modified Rankin Scale	Specialty (neurology)	No	No
— Hamilton Rating Scale for Depression	Specialty (psychiatry)	No	No
— NEI-VFQ-25	Specialty (ophthalmology)	No	No
Preference-Based Instruments			
Utility Analysis			
— Standard gamble	Generic	Yes	Yes
— Willingness-to-pay	Generic	Yes	Yes
— Time tradeoff	Generic	Yes	Yes
Rating Scale			
Rating scales, continuous	Generic	Yes	Yes
Multiattribute Utility Analysis			
— Euro-QOL5-D	Generic	Yes	Yes
— HUI	Generic	Yes	Yes

ADL indicates Activities of Daily Living; CUA, cost-utility analysis; ECOG, Eastern Cooperative Oncology Group; HUI, Health Utilities Index; Karnofsky, Karnofsky Performance Status Scale; NEI-VFQ-25, 25-item National Eye Institute Visual Functioning Questionnaire; QWB, Quality of Well-Being; SF-12, Medical Outcomes Study 12-Item Short Form Health Survey; SF-36, Medical Outcomes Study 36-Item Short Form Health Survey; SIP, Sickness Impact Profile; specialty, specialty-specific.

Can Different Instruments Be Correlated?

In many instances, correlating utility values associated with a disease with another measure of disease severity, such as the Karnofsky Performance Status Scale,[17] allows clinical trial data to be configured to value-based form. For example, data from our center show that the average patient with irritable bowel syndrome who improves from Karnofsky 70 (cares for self, but unable to carry on normal activity or do active work) to Karnofsky 90 (able to carry on normal activity; minor signs or symptoms) with treatment goes from a utility value of 0.68 to a utility value of 1.00. It should be readily apparent that a database correlating utility values for a specific disease with a common categorical scale such as the Karnofsky Scale would be very valuable since data correlated in this fashion could likely be applied to numerous clinical trials.

Why Are Preference-Based Instruments Important?

To satisfy the quality-adjusted life-year (QALY) concept, the Panel for Cost-Effectiveness in Health and Medicine stated that quality weights must be preference-based.[20] We agree, since preference-based instruments all allow a ready measure of value and all:

- encompass all possible variables that contribute to quality of life,[21]
- are reproducible,[22]
- range on a continuum from 0.0 to 1.0 (or 0 to 100),
- have been shown to have good construct validity (as discussed in Chapter 9), and
- can be used in cost-utility analysis.

As mentioned, preference-based instruments include utility analysis models that typically require a subject to decide which health state they prefer:

1. their present health state or
2. return to a normal health state for which they take a risk or give up something of value in return.

The risk can include premature death and the loss can include time of life or monetary resources. Utility analysis instruments are considered to be preference-based and range on a continuum scale from 0.0 to 1.0.

Continuous rating scales also compare on a continuum from 0.0 to 1.0, or 0 to 100, but ask the patient to choose a point that corresponds to their quality of life on a scale, rather than to select one of two alternatives. As such, continuous rating scales ask a patient what point along the scale he or she prefers to associate with his or her health-related quality of life.[23,24] Continuous rating scale values are therefore considered to be preference-based and can be substituted for utility values in cost-utility analysis.

CORE CONCEPTS

■ Health-related quality-of-life instruments can be broadly categorized into two basic types.

— *Function-based instruments* include the measurement of function in various arenas of daily living, including vocational, avocational, physical, cognitive, psychological, social, and with pain.

— *Preference-based instruments* require a subject to make a decision between his or her current health state and the alternative of trading or risking something of value (time of life, money, or life itself) for a return to perfect health. Utility analysis measurement instruments are preference-based.

■ Quality-of-life values obtained with preference-based instruments should be used in cost-utility analysis.

■ All preference-based instrument values can be used in cost-utility analysis.

■ Most function-based instruments cannot be used in cost-utility analysis.

■ *Generic* quality-of-life instruments are applicable across all specialties in medicine. All utility analysis instruments are generic.

■ *Specialty-specific* quality-of-life instruments are applicable to one disease or a small number of diseases.

■ Quality-of life values obtained using an interviewer-administered technique appear to be preferable to those obtained with a self-administered technique.

■ Face-to-face, interviewer-administered, quality-of-life values are similar to those obtained by telephone interview.

REFERENCES

1. American Heart Association. Classification of functional capacity and objective assessment. Available at: www.americanheart.org. Accessed April 29, 2003.

2. Hochberg MC, Chang RW, Dwosh I, Lindsey S, Pincus Y, Wolfe F. The American College of Rheumatology 1991 revised criteria for the classification of global functional status in rheumatoid arthritis. *Arthritis Rheum.* 1992;35:498–502.

3. Bonita R, Beaglehole R. Modification of Rankin Scale: recovery of motor function after stroke. *Stroke.* 1988;19:1497–1500.

4. National Eye Institute Visual Functioning Questionnaire–25 (NEI-VFQ-25). Available at: www.nei.nih.gov. Accessed April 2, 2001.

5. Andresen EM, Bowley N, Rothenberg BM, Panzer R, Katz P. Test-retest performance of a mailed version of the Medical Outcomes Study 36-Item Short-Form Health Survey among older adults. *Med Care.* 1996;34:1165–1170.

6. Grootendorst PV, Fenny DH, Furlong W. Does it matter whom and how you ask? Inter-rater and intra-rater agreement in the Ontario Health Survey. *J Clin Epidemiol.* 1997;50:127–135.

7. Hobart JC, Williams LS, Moran K, Thompson AJ. Quality of life measurement after stroke: uses and abuses of the SF-36. *Stroke.* 2002;33:1176–1177.

8. Linder M, Chang TS, Scott IU, et al. Validity of the visual function index (VF-14) in patients with retinal disease. *Arch Ophthalmol.* 1999;117:1611–1616.

9. Meletiche DM, Doshi D, Lofland JH. Medical Outcomes Study Short Form 36: a possible source of utilities? *Clin Ther.* 1999;21:2016–2026.

10. Parker SG, Peet SM, Jagger C, et al. Measuring health status in older patients: the SF-36 in practice. *Age Ageing.* 1998;27:13–18.

11. Van Wijck EE, Bosch JL, Hunink MG. Time-tradeoff values and standard-gamble utilities assessed during telephone interviews versus face-to-face interviews. *Med Decis Making.* 1998;18:400–405.

12. Kaplan RM, Anderson JP. The general health policy model: an integrated approach. In: Spikler B, ed. *Quality of Life and Pharmacoeconomics in Clinical Trials.* 2nd ed. Philadelphia, Pa: Lippincott-Raven; 1996:309–322.

13. Kaplan RM, Ganiats TG, Sieber WJ, Anderson JP. The Quality of Well-Being Scale: critical similarities and differences with the SF-36. *Int J Qual Health Care.* 1998;10:509–520.

14. Ware JE, Sherbourne CD. The MOS 36-item short-form health survey (SF-36), I: conceptual framework and item selection. *Med Care.* 1992;30:473–483.

15. Gandek B, Ware JE, Aaronson NK, et al. Cross-validation of item selection and scoring for the SF-12 Health Survey in nine countries: results from the IQOLA Project. International Quality of Life Assessment. *J Clin Epidemiol.* 1998;51:1171–1178.

16. Bergner M, Bobbitt RA, Carter WB, Gilson BS. The Sickness Impact Profile: Development and final revision of a health status measure. *Med Care.* 1981;119:787–805.

17. Karnofsky DA, Abelmann WH, Craver LF, Burchenal JH. The use of nitrogen mustards in the palliative treatment of cancer. *Cancer.* 1948;1:634–656.

18. Oken MM, Creech RH, Toomey DC, et al. Toxicity and response criteria of the Eastern Cooperative Oncology Group. *Am J Clin Oncol.* 1982;5:649-655.

19. National Institute of Neurological Disorders and Stroke rt-PA Stroke Study Group. Tissue plasminogen activator for acute ischemic stroke. *N Engl J Med.* 1995;333:1581–1587.

20. Gold MR, Patrick DL, Torrance GW, et al. Identifying and valuing outcomes. In: Gold MR, Siegel JE, Russell LB, Weinstein MC, eds. *Cost-Effectiveness in Health and Medicine.* New York, NY: Oxford University Press; 1996:82–134.

21. Redelmeier DA, Detsky AS. A clinician's guide to utility measurement. *Med Decis Making.* 1995;22:271–280.

22. Read JL, Quinn DM, Berwick DM, Fineberg HV, Weinstein MC. Preferences for health outcomes: comparisons of assessment methods. *Med Decis Making.* 1984;4:215–329.

23. Jampel HD, Friedman DS, Quigley H, Miller R. Correlation of the binocular visual field with patient assessment of vision. *Invest Ophthalmol Vis Sci.* 2002;43:1059–1067.

24. Drummond MF. *Methods for the Economic Evaluation of Health Care Programmes.* Oxford, England: Oxford University Press; 2000:139–199.

7

Function-Based Quality-of-Life Instruments

Function-based instruments are what the name implies: health-related quality-of-life instruments that primarily assess function in normal daily activities. Although the concept of function equates with physical activity for some, it should be recognized that functional instruments can assess how a person functions:

1. cognitively,
2. vocationally (at work),
3. avocationally (recreationally),
4. physically,
5. psychologically,
6. socially, and
7. with pain.

Each function-based instrument may or may not include all of these variables; each also weights the variables differently. These activities are interrelated and overlap in that cognitive, social, and psychological proficiency, as well physical activity attributes, contribute to the ability to perform vocational or avocational activities.

A list of primarily function-based instruments is shown in Table 7.1, as is the category of each instrument (generic or specialty-specific) and whether it has been used for cost-utility analysis. The quality-of-life instruments listed are commonly used, although the list should be considered far from complete. From this point forward in the book we will refer to health-related quality-of-life instruments as simply quality-of-life instruments. The "health-related" part of the term will be considered to be implied.

Most of the instruments in this chapter cannot be utilized alone to provide utility values for use in cost-utility analysis. Nonetheless, results from the categorical instruments (designated by ** in Table 7.1) can often be correlated with the results of clinical trials and also correlated with utility values. These categorical instruments separate diseases into a finite number of categories based upon

TABLE 7.1

Function-Based Quality-of-Life Instruments

Instrument	Category	Preference-Based	Use in CUA
Generic			
1. SF-36	Generic	No	No
2. SF-12	Generic	No	No
3. SIP	Generic	No	No
4. QWB Scale*	Generic	+/-	Yes
5. ADL Scale	Generic	No	No
6. Karnofsky Scale**	Generic	No	No
7. ECOG Performance Status Scale**	Generic	No	No
8. Categorical Scales**	Generic	No	No
Specialty-Specific			
9. American Heart Association Functional Capacity Classification**	Specialty (cardiology, pulmonary)	No	No
10. American College of Rheumatology Classification of Global Functional Status in Rheumatoid Arthritis**	Specialty (rheumatology, orthopedics)	No	No
11. Modified Rankin Scale**	Specialty (neurology)	No	No
12. NEI-VFQ-25	Specialty (ophthalmology)	No	No
13. Hamilton Rating Scale for Depression	Specialty (psychiatry)	No	No

ADL indicates Activities of Daily Living; CUA, cost-utility analysis; ECOG, Eastern Cooperative Oncology Group; HUI, Health Utilities Index; Karnofsky, Karnofsky Performance Status Scale; NEI-VF-25, 25-item National Eye Institute Visual Functioning Questionnaire; QWB, Quality of Well-Being; SF-12, Medical Outcomes Study 12-Item Short Form Health Survey; SF-36, Medical Outcomes Study 36-Item Short-Form Health Survey; SIP, Sickness Impact Profile.

* Can be considered as either a function-based or a preference-based instrument.

** Categorical rating scale.

clinical criteria of severity, and can act as intermediaries between clinical trial data and utility values (Figure 7.1). While the penchant in a perfect world would be to measure primary utility values directly within the context of a clinical trial, this obviously cannot be done for trials that have already been performed. Since the vast majority of evidence-based data come from clinical trials that have

FIGURE 7.1

Categorical Quality-of-Life Instruments. Categorical quality-of-life instruments can act as intermediaries between evidence-based clinical trial data and utility values.

Clinical Trial Data	Utility Values
Categorical Instruments	

already been performed, there must be some mechanism(s) to correlate clinical trial data with utility values. This is one way.

Clinical trial data can often be correlated with function-based categories, which in turn can be correlated with utility values. By this method, the data from previously performed clinical trials can be converted to utility value (value-based) format.

GENERIC QUALITY-OF-LIFE INSTRUMENTS

Generic quality-of-life instruments are those that can be applied across most or all specialties in medicine. In contrast, specialty-specific quality-of-life instruments are those that primarily apply to a single specialty, a limited number of specialties, and a finite number of diseases. The instruments that immediately follow are generic and, therefore, widely applicable to most diseases.

The 36-Item Short-Form Health Survey

The 36-Item Short-Form Health Survey (SF-36) was initially developed by Ware and Sherbourne[1] in 1992 as a part of the Medical Outcomes Study, a multiyear, multisite study undertaken to explain variations in patient outcomes.[1] The SF-36 is probably the most commonly used of the generic quality-of-life instruments.[1-3] It has 36 questions and takes approximately ten minutes to complete according to Edelman et al,[4] but we have found that it can take a good deal longer to complete, especially in the elderly population. A sample questionnaire of the variant used by the RAND Corporation[3] is provided in Table 7.2 to give the reader an appreciation of a generic quality-of-life instrument of moderate length.

Among the health concepts the SF-36 addresses are (the numbers of questions in each subcategory are shown in parentheses):

1. physical functioning (10)
2. role functioning (7)
3. social functioning (1)
4. mental health (5)
5. health perceptions (2)
6. energy or fatigue (4)
7. pain (2)
8. general health perception (5)

TABLE 7.2

36-Item Short-Form Health Survey (SF-36)*

1. In general, would you say your health is:

Excellent	1
Very good	2
Good	3
Fair	4
Poor	5

2. Compared to one year ago, how would you rate your health in general now?

Much better now than one year ago	1
Somewhat better now than one year ago	2
About the same	3
Somewhat worse now than one year ago	4
Much worse now than one year ago	5

The following items are about activities you might do during a typical day. Does your health now limit you in these activities? If so, how much? (Circle one number on each line.)

	Yes, Limited a Lot	Yes, Limited a Little	No, Not Limited at All
3. Vigorous activities, such as running, lifting heavy objects, participating in strenuous sports	1	2	3
4. Moderate activities, such as moving a table, pushing a vacuum cleaner, bowling, or playing golf	1	2	3
5. Lifting or carrying groceries	1	2	3
6. Climbing several flights of stairs	1	2	3
7. Climbing one flight of stairs	1	2	3
8. Bending, kneeling, or stooping	1	2	3
9. Walking more than a mile	1	2	3
10. Walking several blocks	1	2	3
11. Walking one block	1	2	3
12. Bathing or dressing yourself	1	2	3

During the past four weeks, have you had any of the following problems with your work or other regular daily activities as a result of your physical health? (Circle one number on each line.)

	Yes	No
13. Cut down the amount of time you spent on work or other activities	1	2
14. Accomplished less than you would like	1	2

TABLE 7.2 continued

36-Item Short-Form Health Survey (SF-36)*

	Yes	No
15. Were limited in the kind of work or other activities	1	2
16. Had difficulty performing the work or other activities (for example, it took extra effort)	1	2

During the past 4 weeks, have you had any of the following problems with your work or other regular daily activities as a result of any emotional problems (such as feeling depressed or anxious)? (Circle one number on each line.)

	Yes	No
17. Cut down the amount of time you spent on work or other activities	1	2
18. Accomplished less than you would like	1	2
19. Didn't do work or other activities as carefully as usual	1	2

20. During the past 4 weeks, to what extent has your physical health or emotional problems interfered with your normal social activities with family, friends, neighbors, or groups? (Circle one number.)

Not at all	1
Slightly	2
Moderately	3
Quite a bit	4
Extremely	5

21. How much bodily pain have you had during the past 4 weeks? (Circle one number.)

None	1
Very mild	2
Mild	3
Moderate	4
Severe	5
Very severe	6

22. During the past 4 weeks, how much did pain interfere with your normal work (including both work outside the home and housework)? (Circle one number.)

Not at all	1
A little bit	2
Moderately	3
Quite a bit	4
Extremely	5

These questions are about how you feel and how things have been with you during the past 4 weeks. For each question, please give the one answer that comes closest to the way you have been feeling.

How much of the time during the past 4 weeks . . . (Circle one number on each line.)

continued

TABLE 7.2 continued

36-Item Short-Form Health Survey (SF-36)*

All of the Time	Most of the Time	A Good Bit of the Time	Some of the Time	A Little of the Time	None of the Time
23. Did you feel full of pep?					
1	2	3	4	5	6
24. Have you been a very nervous person?					
1	2	3	4	5	6
25. Have you felt so down in the dumps that nothing could cheer you up?					
1	2	3	4	5	6
26. Have you felt calm and peaceful?					
1	2	3	4	5	6
27. Did you have a lot of energy?					
1	2	3	4	5	6
28. Have you felt downhearted and blue?					
1	2	3	4	5	6
29. Did you feel worn out?					
1	2	3	4	5	6
30. Have you been a happy person?					
1	2	3	4	5	6
31. Did you feel tired?					
1	2	3	4	5	6

32. During the past 4 weeks, how much of the time has your physical health or emotional problems interfered with your social activities (like visiting with friends, relatives, and so on)? (Circle one number.)

All of the time	1
Most of the time	2
Some of the time	3
A little of the time	4
None of the time	5

How TRUE or FALSE is each of the following statements for you? (Circle one number on each line.)

Definitely True	Mostly True	Don't Know	Mostly False	Definitely False
33. I seem to get sick a little easier than other people.				
1	2	3	4	5
34. I am as healthy as anybody I know.				
1	2	3	4	5
35. I expect my health to get worse.				
1	2	3	4	5
36. My health is excellent.				
1	2	3	4	5

* The 36-Item Short-Form Health Survey was developed at the RAND Corporation as a part of the Medical Outcomes Study. Reprinted with permission from the RAND Corporation.[3]

The SF-36 was created to provide a practical quality-of-life evaluation sufficiently short to be used in a clinical setting.[3] Although shorter than the Sickness Impact Profile (SIP), it similarly emphasizes functional status, rather than patient preferences, associated with a particular health state. While ten questions are ostensibly involved with function directly,[5] closer examination reveals at least 22 of the 36 are readily applicable to physical function.

The SF-36 has been utilized in assessing numerous health states, with good validity and reproducibility (test-retest reliability), but some researchers believe it unsatisfactory for patients who have experienced a stroke,[6] as well as older hospitalized patients.[7,8] In people with multiple comorbidities, such as hypertension, hypothyroidism, breast cancer, rheumatoid arthritis, and so on, the SF-36 is not sensitive to differentiating the magnitude of the effect of each disease upon quality of life. In addition, the instrument does not address health-related economic status, caregiver status, or sensory deprivation. SF-36 values appear to cluster over a similar range on a scale for common ailments such as arthritis, hypertension, diabetes, stroke, and so on, whereas time tradeoff utility values are spread over a wider spectrum.[9]

Attempts have been made to derive utility values from the SF-36 since it can be put on a scale from 0 to 100, but they have been largely unsuccessful.[10] Although a formula based on linear regression analysis has been developed to convert SF-36 values to utility scores, the Pearson correlation has been shown to range from 0.39 to 0.70.[9] SF-36 scores have therefore not been generally used in cost-utility analysis as substitutes for utility values.

Does it matter how the SF-36 is administered? Yes! The SF-36 can yield substantially different results when self-administered as compared to administration by an interviewer.[2,6,8,10] This is the case with many quality-of-life instruments, as we have noted in patients undergoing utility analysis. The degree of difference can be sufficiently dramatic that—unless a close correlation is shown—data from the same instrument incorporating self-administered values and those elicited by an interviewer generally should not be lumped together for the performance of cost-utility analysis.

The 12-Item Short-Form Health Survey

A modification of the SF-36, the shorter 12-Item Short-Form Health Survey (SF-12) has 12 questions and been shown to be a practical alternative in the United States and multiple countries.[11] When compared to the SF-36, the SF-12 achieves an r^2 of 0.91, meaning that the SF-12 accounts for 91% of the variance encompassed by the SF-36.[12] Thus, despite its abbreviated form, it appears to closely capture the information elicited by the 36-question SF-36. The SF-12 appears to be as good for the measurement of arthritic diseases as the SF-36,[13] but has been specifically criticized in regard to reproducibility with stroke

PEARL

Beware of comparing quality-of-life instrument values obtained through interview with those that are self-administered.

patients.[14] As is the case with the SF-36, we are unaware that results from the SF-12 have been used in cost-utility analysis.

The Sickness Impact Profile

The Sickness Impact Profile (SIP) has 136 questions in 12 categories and takes approximately 30 minutes to complete.[15] The instrument has high test-retest reliability ($r = 0.92$).[16] It assesses physical health well as it evaluates ambulation, mobility, body care, and movement. Nevertheless, the correlation for psychological aspects has been noted to be only fair.[16] It has been used as a quality-of-life instrument for chronic obstructive pulmonary disease, asthma, arthritis, hip arthroplasty, angina, and glaucoma.[15–17]

The SIP behaviors can be scored on a scale of 0 to 100, but the instrument has not been generally used for cost-utility analysis. The SIP defines a functional state for a particular person, rather than a preference for a particular health state. The numerous questions and the substantial amount of time required for the test are major factors that prevent this test from being used on a large scale.

> With the exception of the Quality of Well-Being Scale, the results from function-based instruments are not generally used for cost-utility analysis.

The Quality-of-Well-Being Scale

The Quality-of-Well-Being (QWB) Scale is a generic health instrument that classifies patients according to four functional components:

1. mobility,
2. physical activity,
3. social activity, and
4. difficulties associated with symptom/problem complexes.

If a patient has multiple problems, the most undesirable situation is examined. We believe this is an excellent approach to the overall evaluation of a person's health state, since with utility analysis research we have noted that the vast majority of patients with multiple comorbidities rate their overall health-related quality of life at the same level as that associated with their most severe disease.

Scoring for the QWB Scale is based upon a rating scale measurement from a sample of the general public. This rating scale places each individual on a continuum from 0.0 (death) to 1.0 (perfect health). Thus, it could theoretically also be considered as a preference-based instrument. The QWB Scale has been used to calculate quality-adjusted life-years.[18,19] It has been criticized, however, for not offering a mental health component[19] and for being difficult to administer.[17,20] While it can be applied in cost-utility analysis, its use is not widespread.

Activities of Daily Living Scale

Originally utilized to evaluate patients with fractured hips, the Activities of Daily Living (ADL) Scale has been in use for several decades,[21] primarily as a test to assess function in an older population.[22] As described by Katz and coworkers in 1963, the scale was based on six criteria[21]:

1. bathing (sponge, bath, or shower),
2. dressing,
3. toilet use,
4. transferring (in and out of chair and/or bed),
5. urine and bowel continence, and
6. eating.

Each criterion was graded as:

1. performs independently,
2. performs with assistance, or
3. unable to perform.

An overall score was then calculated, ranging from A (independent) to G (dependent for all functions).

The ADL Scale has been modified by numerous authors to include other activities. Gill et al[23] added grooming to the previously listed six activities, but Lawton and Brody[22] used the following completely different criteria:

1. using the telephone,
2. getting to places beyond walking,
3. grocery shopping,
4. preparing meals,
5. doing housework or handyman work,
6. doing laundry,
7. taking medications, and
8. managing money.

Thus, there is great variation in the test. The ADL Scale is applicable across all specialties, but the scale lacks sensitivity, especially for less serious diseases. To our knowledge, the results have not been used as a substitute for utility values in cost-utility analysis. In addition, it ignores the important quality-of-life parameters of psychological interactions, social interactions, pain, caregiver support, and economic issues.

Karnofsky Performance Status Scale

The Karnofsky Performance Status Scale is a widely used categorical scale that assesses a patient's functional status and independence. It rates well-being on a scale from 10 to 100 as shown in Table 7.3.

TABLE 7.3

The Karnofsky Performance Status Scale

100	Normal, no complaints, no evidence of disease
90	Able to carry on normal activity; minor signs or symptoms
80	Normal activity with effort; some signs or symptoms of disease
70	Cares for self; unable to carry on normal activity or do active work
60	Requires occasional assistance but is able to care for most of his/her needs
50	Requires considerable assistance and frequent medical care
40	Disabled, requires special care and assistance
30	Severely disabled; hospitalization indicated. Death not imminent
20	Very sick; hospitalization indicated. Death not imminent
10	Moribund, fatal process progressing rapidly

Originated as an instrument for use with primarily bronchogenic carcinoma patients undergoing palliative nitrogen mustard therapy,[24] its spectrum of use has since broadened dramatically.[25] The interobserver correlation coefficient is excellent at 0.85 to 0.91 and the intraobserver correlation coefficient is also excellent, ranging from 0.95 to 0.99.[26,27]

The Karnofsky Performance Status Scale is a categorical scale.

Categorical scales separate diseases into a finite number of categories based upon clinical severity.

According to Rosner,[28] a correlation coefficient (r) of greater than 0.75 indicates excellent reproducibility, a coefficient between 0.40 and 0.75 indicates good reproducibility, and a coefficient less than 0.40 indicates poor reproducibility. When the evaluation of patients is performed by clinicians, the Karnofsky Performance Status Scale has excellent reliability and allows for an optimal selection of patients for inclusion in clinical trials.[26]

Correlation coefficients:
> 0.75   Excellent reproducibility
0.40–0.75   Good reproducibility
< 0.40   Poor reproducibility

Simplistic as a quality-of-life instrument, the Karnofsky Scale has not been used in healthcare economic analysis. While the Karnofsky Scale has not been directly used in cost-utility analysis, it has been used in numerous clinical trials and is applicable to almost any health state or disease at different levels of severity.

The fact that Karnofsky scores for patients with a specific disease can be correlated with utility values facilitates the conversion of clinical trial data to utility value form. For example, osteoarthritis patients with a Karnofsky score of 90 due to the arthritis (able to carry on normal activity; minor signs or symptoms) have a mean time tradeoff utility value of 0.99, while a Karnofsky value of 40 (disabled; requires special care and assistance) due to osteoarthritis correlates with a mean utility value of 0.46. With congestive heart failure (CHF), a Karnofsky value of 90 (able to carry on normal activity; minor signs or symptoms) from the CHF correlates with a mean utility value of 0.93 and a Karnofsky value of 40 (disabled; requires special care and assistance) due to the CHF correlates with a mean utility value of 0.45. As seen, utility values for the same Karnofsky scale level differ for different diseases, although the difference is often small.

Eastern Cooperative Oncology Group Performance Status Scale

Also derived originally for use with cancer patients, the Eastern Cooperative Oncology Group (ECOG) Performance Status Scale (Table 7.4) is a simplistic categorical scale similar to the Karnofsky Scale in that it has functional divisions.[29] However, the ECOG has six grades rather than ten, and the distinction between Grades 1 and 2 can be blurred. Tables to transform the Karnofsky Scale to the ECOG Scale, and vice versa, have been proposed but are difficult to implement.[29-31] The ECOG Scale has not been used directly in cost-utility analysis but, as with the Karnofsky Scale, can be correlated with utility values for a particular disease and its levels of severity, thus facilitating the conversion of clinical trial data into utility value form.

TABLE 7.4

The Eastern Cooperative Oncology Group Performance Status Scale

Grade 0	Fully active, no restriction
Grade 1	Restricted in strenuous physical activity but ambulatory and able to carry out light work
Grade 2	Ambulatory and capable of all self-care but unable to carry out any working activities. Up and about more than 50% of waking hours
Grade 3	Capable of only limited self-care, confined to bed or chair more than 50% of waking hours
Grade 4	Completely disabled. Cannot carry on any self-care. Totally confined to bed or chair
Grade 5	Dead

> The Eastern Cooperative Oncology Group Performance Status Scale
> is a categorical scale.

Categorical Scales

Categorical scales classify quality of life into a finite number of categories. The Karnofsky Performance Status Scale, the Eastern Cooperative Oncology Group Performance Status Scale, the American Heart Association Functional Capacity Classification, the American College of Rheumatology Classification of Global Functional Status in Rheumatoid Arthritis, and the Modified Rankin Scale are all function-based scales that are also categorical scales. Categorical scales, unless correlated with utility values associated with specific diseases, are not used in cost-utility analysis.

A scale that subjectively defines a disease or health state as mild, moderate, or severe is a rudimentary categorical scale as well. We have not found the results from this form of categorical scale to be consistent as there is a wide variance in subjectivity.

SPECIALTY-SPECIFIC QUALITY-OF-LIFE INSTRUMENTS

As the name implies, specialty-specific quality-of-life instruments were developed to assess the severity of a single disease or a limited number of diseases treated by specialty groups of professionals. They can also function as basic quality-of-life instruments. By no means does the list in this chapter include all specialty-specific instruments, but several are presented as illustrations. Some specialty-specific instruments (American Heart Association Functional Capacity Classification, American College of Rheumatology Classification of Global Functional Status in Rheumatoid Arthritis, and the Modified Rankin Scale) have applicability across multiple specialties, while others (National Eye Institute Visual Functioning Questionnaire) are single-specialty-specific. None of the specialty-specific instruments is an effective instrument to use across all specialties in healthcare.

> Specialty-specific quality-of-life instruments evaluate diseases usual-
> ly encountered by professionals in predominantly one specialty.
> They are not applicable across all specialties or diseases.

Cardiology

The American Heart Association (AHA) Functional Capacity Classification[32,33] was developed as a revision of the New York State Heart Association functional criteria in 1994. The classification stratifies cardiac patients into four functional classes depending upon symptoms associated with activity, as shown in Table 7.5. We have found it useful for the evaluation of pulmonary patients as well.

The AHA Functional Capacity Classification by itself does not determine the utility of any health state and cannot be used for cost-utility analysis until a utility value correlation has been undertaken in association with it. Like the Karnofsky Scale and the ECOG Scale, the AHA Functional Capacity Classification can be correlated with utility value measurements to allow data from clinical trials that utilize it to be employed for cost-utility analysis. As examples, we have found that patients with Class IV disease with angina have a mean associated time tradeoff utility value of 0.53, while those with Class IV congestive heart failure and predominantly dyspnea have a mean associated utility value of 0.57. When the average patient improves to Class II angina, the associated utility value improves to 0.86, while improvement to Class II congestive heart failure is associated with a utility value improvement to 0.85. As might be anticipated, the utility values associated with various diseases evaluated with one specialty-specific instrument are often similar at the same stage or class.

Rheumatology

Revised in 1991,[34,35] the American College of Rheumatology Classification of Global Functional Status in Rheumatoid Arthritis was developed to measure the function of patients with rheumatoid arthritis. (See Table 7.6.) It can also be used to assess function with osteoarthritis and other forms of arthritis, as well as the results of orthopedic interventions such as total hip and total knee arthroplasty.[36] It is not particularly helpful, however, for assessing the quality of life associated with cardiac disease or pulmonary disease, renal dialysis, sensory abnormalities, and numerous other disease entities.

As is the case with cardiac utility values, the utility values associated with each American College of Rheumatology Class can be correlated with individual

TABLE 7.5

American Heart Association Functional Capacity Classification

Class I	Patients with cardiac disease, but without resulting limitation of physical activity. Ordinary physical activity does not cause undue fatigue, palpitation, dyspnea, or anginal pain.
Class II	Patients with cardiac disease resulting in slight limitation of physical activity. Ordinary physical activity results in fatigue, palpitation, dyspnea, or anginal pain.
Class III	Patients with cardiac disease resulting in marked limitation of physical activity. Less than ordinary activity causes fatigue, palpitation, dyspnea, or anginal pain.
Class IV	Patients with cardiac disease resulting in inability to carry on any physical activity without discomfort. Symptoms of heart failure or the anginal syndrome may be present even at rest. If any physical activity is undertaken, discomfort increases.

TABLE 7.6

American College of Rheumatology Classification of Global Functional Status in Rheumatoid Arthritis

Class	Description
Class I	Completely able to perform usual activities of daily living (self-care, vocational, and avocational*)
Class II	Able to perform usual self-care and vocational activities but limited in avocational activities
Class III	Able to perform usual self-care activities but limited in vocational and avocational activities
Class IV	Limited in ability to perform usual self-care, vocational, and avocational activities

* Usual self-care activities include dressing, feeding, bathing, grooming, and toileting. Vocational (work, school, homemaking) and avocational (recreational and/or leisure) activities are patient-desired and age- and sex-specific.

diseases and their level of severity. We have found that with Class II arthritic disease, the time tradeoff utility value associated with osteoarthritis of the hip is 0.95, while the value for osteoarthritis of the knee is 0.93. For Class IV arthritic disease, the time tradeoff utility value for patients with osteoarthritis of the hip is 0.52, exactly the same as for osteoarthritis of the knee.

Neurology

The Modified Rankin Scale shown in Table 7.7 is among the most common scales utilized in the evaluation of functional disability associated with stroke.[37-39] Despite the development of other instruments, such as the National Institutes of Health (NIH) Stroke Scale,[40] the Modified Rankin Scale remains in wide use.[41] It has been noted to have good interrater agreement ($r = 0.91$).[39] While originated for stroke patients, it can be applied to more generalized neurologic diseases and neurosurgical diseases. As is the case with most of the other specialty-specific instruments, the Modified Rankin Scale[37] is categorical and focuses primarily on physical function.

The scale has seven categories ranging from 0 (no symptoms) to 6 (dead). Duncan and colleagues[42] have noted time tradeoff utility values ranging from 0.88 for a Rankin score of 1 to 0.34 for a Rankin score of 5 at six months after acute stroke. Tengs and coworkers,[43] however, noted a time tradeoff utility value of 0.20 for a Rankin score of 5 for stroke at 10 years after the initial event. The different values for a score of 5 in the two studies may be accounted for by the fact that severely affected stroke patients have more hope of recovery at 6 months after the event than at 10 years after the event.

TABLE 7.7

The Modified Rankin Scale for the Evaluation of Stroke Patients

Score	Description
0	No symptoms
1	No significant disability despite symptoms. Able to carry out all usual duties and activities
2	Slight disability. Unable to carry out all previous activities but able to look after own affairs without assistance
3	Moderate disability. Requiring some help but able to walk without assistance
4	Moderately severe disability. Unable to walk without assistance and unable to attend to own bodily needs without assistance
5	Severe disability. Bedridden, incontinent, and requiring constant nursing care and assistance
6	Dead

The NIH Stroke Scale is also an instrument that evaluates the symptoms and signs of a stroke to assess clinical function. It has high interrater reliability ($r = 0.95$)[44] and evaluates the following 11 parameters:

1. level of consciousness,
2. best gaze,
3. visual field loss,
4. facial palsy,
5. arm palsy,
6. leg palsy,
7. limb ataxia,
8. sensation,
9. best language,
10. dysarthria, and
11. extinction and inattention.

Anywhere from zero to three points are given in an area, with the higher total score indicating more severe dysfunction. The test score can be estimated retrospectively from medical records with a high degree of reliability and validity.[45] We are unaware that the NIH Stroke Scale has yet been correlated with utility values, but such a correlation could provide a more sensitive scale than the Modified Rankin Scale.[42]

Depression

Depression can be a primary disease of interest, but can also accompany other diseases. A disease may decrease quality of life, but when depression is present as well the quality of life often decreases further. An important corollary to remember is that, even though treatment of a primary disease may be ineffectual, treatment of the accompanying depression can confer considerable value to a patient. Probably the most commonly utilized scale for evaluating the change in depression is the Hamilton Rating Scale for Depression.[46–48]

Hamilton Rating Scale for Depression: Measuring Change in Depression.
The most widely used instrument to assess change in the severity of depression is the Hamilton Rating Scale for Depression,[46–49] which comes in variants ranging from 17 questions to 21 questions.[48] Among the variables it assesses are mood, guilt, suicide, insomnia, psychomotor retardation, agitation, anxiety, somatic symptoms, hypochondriasis, insight, depersonalization, paranoid symptoms, and obsessive-compulsive symptoms. Considering that the instrument evaluates a number of the quality-of-life variables included in Table 5.2, it is most reasonable to consider this tool a quality-of-life instrument.

The test, shown in Table 7.8, was designed to be administered to those already diagnosed with depression, and is frequently employed to evaluate the benefit of pharmaceuticals used to treat depression. It has been suggested that the modified Hamilton Rating Scale for Depression six-item instrument also gives an accurate score for the rating of antidepressant drugs.[46]

While the Hamilton Rating Scale measures changes in the severity of depression, other instruments are used to screen for the presence of depression.

The Center for Epidemiological Studies Depression Scale: Screening for Depression.   The Center for Epidemiological Studies Depression (CES-D) Scale is used primarily as a screening test for depression.[50–53] The instrument has a 100% sensitivity for detecting major depression compared to the "gold standard" of major depression as per the Structured Clinical Interview for the *Diagnostic and Statistical Manual of Mental Disorders, Fourth Edition.*[50] It can be administered in several minutes and comes in a 20-question format and in a ten-question format that is 97% as sensitive as the 20-question variant.[51] A weakness of the instrument is that the specificity has been shown to range from 70% to 93%, meaning that in 7% to 30% of cases, it reads positive when major depression is not present.

A shorter version of the CES-D Scale using five of the 20 questions with high sensitivity and good specificity has recently been developed to screen for depression.[52] This short version is reproduced here in Table 7.9. Assessed against the 20-question scale, the five-item CES-D Scale has a sensitivity of 99% and a specificity ranging from 81% to 89%. Thus, it is an excellent instrument to screen for the presence of depression.

A very simple screening test for depression is to ask a patient. Lee et al[54] reported that the question, "Do you feel sad or depressed?" detects clinical depression with a sensitivity of 78% and a specificity of 80%.

TABLE 7.8

The Hamilton Rating Scale for Depression (Clinician Administered)*

To rate the severity of depression in patients who are already diagnosed as depressed, administer this questionnaire. The higher the score, the more severe the depression. For each item, write the correct number on the line next to the item. (Only one response is allowed per item.)

_____ 1 DEPRESSED MOOD (feelings of sadness, hopelessness, helpless-ness, worthlessness)

  0 = Absent

  1 = These feeling states indicated only on questioning

  2 = These feeling states spontaneously reported

  3 = Communicates feeling states nonverbally (ie, through facial expression, posture, voice, and tendency to weep)

  4 = Patient reports virtually only these feeling states in his or her spon-taneous verbal and nonverbal communication

_____ 2 FEELINGS OF GUILT

  0 = Absent

  1 = Self-reproach, feels he or she has let people down

  2 = Ideas of guilt or rumination over past errors or sinful deeds

  3 = Present illness is a punishment; delusions of guilt

  4 = Hears accusatory or denunciatory voices and/or experiences threatening visual hallucinations

_____ 3 SUICIDE

  0 = Absent

  1 = Feels life is not worth living

  2 = Wishes he or she were dead or any thoughts of possible death to self

  3 = Suicidal ideas or gesture

  4 = Attempts at suicide (any serious attempt rates 4)

_____ 4 INSOMNIA EARLY

  0 = No difficulty falling asleep

  1 = Complains of occasional difficulty falling asleep (ie, more than 30 minutes)

  2 = Complains of nightly difficulty falling asleep

_____ 5 INSOMNIA MIDDLE

  0 = No difficulty

  1 = Patient complains of being restless and disturbed during the night

  2 = Waking during the night (any getting out of bed rates 2 except for purposes of voiding)

_____ 6 INSOMNIA LATE

  0 = No difficulty

  1 = Waking in early hours of the morning but goes back to sleep

  2 = Unable to fall asleep again if he or she gets out of bed

continued

TABLE   7.8 continued

The Hamilton Rating Scale for Depression (Clinician Administered)*

_____   7   WORK AND ACTIVITIES

0 = No difficulty

1 = Thoughts and feeling of incapacity, fatigue, or weakness related to activities, work, or hobbies

2 = Lost of interest in activity, hobbies, or work—either directly reported by patient, or indirect in listlessness, indecision, and vacillation (feels he or she has to push self to work or activities)

3 = Decrease in actual time spent in activities or decrease in productivity

4 = Stop working because of present illness

_____   8   RETARDATION: PSYCHOMOTOR (Slowness of thought and speech, impaired ability to concentrate, decreased motor activity)

0 = Normal speech and thought

1 = Slight retardation at interview

2 = Obvious retardation at interview

3 = Interview difficult

4 = Complete stupor

_____   9   AGITATION

0 = None

1 = Fidgetiness

2 = Playing with hands, hair, and so on

3 = Moving about, can't sit still

4 = Hand wringing, nail biting, hair-pulling, biting of lips

_____   10   ANXIETY (PSYCHOLOGICAL)

0 = No difficulty

1 = Subjective tension and irritability

2 = Worrying about minor matters

3 = Apprehensive attitude apparent in face or speech

4 = Fears expressed without questioning

_____   11   ANXIETY SOMATIC (Physiological concomitants of anxiety [ie, effects of autonomic overactivity, "butterflies," indigestion, stomach cramps, belching, diarrhea, palpitations, hyperventilation, paresthesia, sweating, flushing, tremor, headache, urinary frequency]. Avoid asking about possible medication side effects [ie, dry mouth, constipation])

0 = Absent

1 = Mild

2 = Moderate

3 = Severe

4 = Incapacitating

_____   12   SOMATIC SYMPTOMS (GASTROINTESTINAL)

0 = None

1 = Loss of appetite but eating without encouragement from others; food intake about normal

TABLE 7.8 continued

The Hamilton Rating Scale for Depression (Clinician Administered)*

		2 = Difficulty eating without urging from others; marked reduction of appetite and food intake
_____	13	SOMATIC SYMPTOMS GENERAL
		0 = None
		1 = Heaviness in limbs, back, or head; backaches, headache, muscle aches; loss of energy and fatigability
		2 = Any clear-cut symptom rates 2
_____	14	GENITAL SYMPTOMS (Symptoms such as loss of libido, impaired sexual performance, menstrual disturbances)
		0 = Absent
		1 = Mild
		2 = Severe
_____	15	HYPOCHONDRIASIS
		0 = Not present
		1 = Self-absorption (bodily)
		2 = Preoccupation with health
		3 = Frequent complaints, requests for help, and so on
		4 = Hypochondriacal delusions
_____	16	LOSS OF WEIGHT
		When rating by history:
		0 = No weight loss
		1 = Probably weight loss associated with present illness
		2 = Definite (according to patient) weight loss
		3 = Not assessed
_____	17	INSIGHT
		0 = Acknowledges being depressed and ill
		1 = Acknowledges illness but attributes cause to bad food, climate, overwork, virus, need for rest, and so on
		2 = Denies being ill at all
_____	18	DIURNAL VARIATION
		Note whether symptoms are worse in morning or evening; if no diurnal variation, mark none
		0 = No variation
		1 = Worse in AM
		2 = Worse in PM

When present, mark the severity of the variation; mark "None" if no variation

		0 = None
		1 = Mild
		2 = Severe
_____	19	DEPERSONALIZATION AND DEREALIZATION (such as feelings of unreality; nihilistic ideas)
		0 = Absent

continued

TABLE   7.8 continued

The Hamilton Rating Scale for Depression (Clinician Administered)*

		1 = Mild
		2 = Moderate
		3 = Severe
		4 = Incapacitating
_____	20	PARANOID SYMPTOMS
		0 = None
		1 = Suspicious
		2 = Ideas of reference
		3 = Delusion of reference and persecution
_____	21	OBSESSIONAL AND COMPULSIVE SYMPTOMS
		0 = Absent
		1 = Mild
		2 = Severe

Total Score _____

Adapted from Hedlund and Vieweg.[49] Reprinted courtesy of the Department of Veterans Affairs.

* The variant shown here is a 21-question modification utilized by the Department of Veterans Affairs.

> The five-item CES-D Scale is an excellent instrument to screen for depression.

We are unaware that either the Hamilton Rating Scale for Depression or the CES-D Scale has been converted to utility value form. We have observed depression, however, to affect utility values, with diabetes as a prime example. A mean time tradeoff utility value of 0.88 was found for diabetes in general, but was 0.83 in the same population for diabetics with depression.[55]

Relatively little attention has been given to cost-utility analysis for depression.[56,57] Bennett and colleagues[57] from McMaster University, however, obtained utility values on a group of 105 patients with remission of depression, but at least one episode of major unipolar depression within the past two years. The utility value for mild hypothetical depression was 0.58, while that for moderate depression was 0.32, and that for severe depression was 0.04. Of particular note is the fact that 56% of patients considered severe depression to be worse than death. Needless to say, depression produces an extraordinary diminution in quality of life.

Ophthalmology

Traditionally, visual acuity using either the Snellen or logMAR (log of the minimal angle or resolution) system has been used as the parameter most closely associated with quality of life.[58] It has been demonstrated that ocular utility

TABLE 7.9

Center for Epidemiological Studies Depression (CES-D) Scale*
For each of the following, please indicate how often you felt that way during the past week, using the following ratings. (A total score of 4 or more is a positive depression screen.)

Score for Statements 1–4 Only

Rarely or none of the time (less than one day)	0
Some or a little of the time (one to two days)	1
Moderately or much of the time (three to four days)	2
Most or almost all the time (five to seven days)	3

Item	Statement	Score
1	I felt that I could not shake off the blues even with help from my family or friends.	0 1 2 3
2	I felt depressed.	0 1 2 3
3	I felt fearful.	0 1 2 3
4	My sleep was restless.	0 1 2 3

Score for Statement 5 Only

Most of the time	0
Moderately or much of the time	1
Some of the time	2
Rarely	3

5	I felt hopeful about the future.	0 1 2 3

* This screening instrument is derived from the CES-D,[53] courtesy of the Robert Wood Johnson Foundation.

values—thus quality of life—most closely correlate with visual acuity in the better-seeing eye.[59–65] As the visual acuity in the better-seeing eye decreases, the associated ocular utility value decreases accordingly.[59] Importantly, it is the vision in the better-seeing eye, rather than the causes of visual loss (diabetic retinopathy, age-related macular degeneration, cataract, and so on), that most closely correlates with utility values.[59, 66]

The most widely used ophthalmic quality-of-life instrument other than vision is the VF-14, a questionnaire that measures primarily function.[67] It was modified by the National Eye Institute from a 14-item instrument to a 51-item instrument, and finally tailored to a 25-item instrument known as the NEI-VFQ-25 (the National Eye Institute Visual Functioning Questionnaire, 25-item), The NEI-VFQ-25 still contains primarily functional questions.[68,69] The NEI-VFQ-25 is shown in Table 7.10.

TABLE 7.10

National Eye Institute Visual Functioning Questionnaire, 25 Item (NEI-VFQ-25)*
The following is a survey with statements about problems that involve your vision or feelings that you have about your vision condition. After each question please choose the response that best describes your situation. Please answer all the questions as if you were wearing your glasses or contact lenses (if any).

PART 1: GENERAL HEALTH AND VISION

1. In general, would you say your overall health is: *(Circle one)*

   Excellent 1

   Very good 2

   Good .3

   Fair .4

   Poor .5

2. At the present time, would you say your eyesight using both eyes (with glasses or contact lenses, if you wear them) is excellent, good, fair, poor, or very poor, or are you completely blind? *(Circle one)*

   Excellent 1

   Good .2

   Fair 3

   Poor .4

   Very poor 5

   Completely blind 6

3. How much of the time do you worry about your eyesight? *(Circle one)*

   None of the time 1

   A little of the time 2

   Some of the time 3

   Most of the time 4

   All of the time 5

4. How much pain or discomfort have you had in and around your eyes (for example, burning, itching, or aching)? *(Circle one)*

   None 1

   Mild 2

   Moderate 3

   Severe 4

   Very severe 5

PART 2: DIFFICULTY WITH ACTIVITIES

The next questions are about how much difficulty, if any, you have doing certain activities wearing your glasses or contact lenses if you use them for that activity.

5. How much difficulty do you have reading ordinary print in newspapers? *(Circle one)*

   No difficulty at all 1

   A little difficulty 2

   Moderate difficulty 3

   Extreme difficulty 4

   Stopped doing this because of your eyesight 5

   Stopped doing this for other reasons or not interested in doing this 6

6. How much difficulty do you have doing work or hobbies that require you to see well up close, such as cooking, sewing, fixing things around the house, or using hand tools? *(Circle one)*

   No difficulty at all 1

   A little difficulty 2

   Moderate difficulty 3

   Extreme difficulty 4

   Stopped doing this because of your eyesight 5

   Stopped doing this for other reasons or not interested in doing this 6

7. Because of your eyesight, how much difficulty do you have finding something on a crowded shelf? *(Circle one)*

   No difficulty at all 1

   A little difficulty 2

   Moderate difficulty 3

T A B L E   7.10 continued

National Eye Institute Visual Functioning Questionnaire, 25 Item (NEI-VFQ-25)*

Extreme difficulty 4

Stopped doing this because of
your eyesight 5

Stopped doing this for other
reasons or not interested in
doing this 6

8. How much difficulty do you have
reading street signs or the names of
stores? *(Circle one)*

No difficulty at all 1

A little difficulty 2

Moderate difficulty 3

Extreme difficulty 4

Stopped doing this because of
your eyesight 5

Stopped doing this for other
reasons or not interested in
doing this 6

9. Because of your eyesight, how
much difficulty do you have going
down steps, stairs, or curbs in dim
light or at night? *(Circle one)*

No difficulty at all 1

A little difficulty 2

Moderate difficulty 3

Extreme difficulty 4

Stopped doing this because of
your eyesight 5

Stopped doing this for other
reasons or not interested in
doing this 6

10. Because of your eyesight, how
much difficulty do you have noticing
objects off to the side while you are
walking along? *(Circle one)*

No difficulty at all 1

A little difficulty 2

Moderate difficulty 3

Extreme difficulty 4

Stopped doing this because of
your eyesight 5

Stopped doing this for other
reasons or not interested in
doing this 6

11. Because of your eyesight, how
much difficulty do you have seeing
how people react to things you say?
(Circle one)

No difficulty at all 1

A little difficulty 2

Moderate difficulty 3

Extreme difficulty 4

Stopped doing this because of
your eyesight 5

Stopped doing this for other
reasons or not interested in
doing this 6

12. Because of your eyesight, how
much difficulty do you have picking
out and matching your own clothes?
(Circle one)

No difficulty at all 1

A little difficult 2

Moderate difficulty 3

Extreme difficulty 4

Stopped doing this because of
your eyesight 5

Stopped doing this for other
reasons or not interested in
doing this 6

13. Because of your eyesight, how
much difficulty do you have visiting
with people in their homes, at par-
ties, or in restaurants? *(Circle one)*

No difficulty at all 1

A little difficulty 2

Moderate difficulty 3

Extreme difficulty 4

Stopped doing this because of
your eyesight 5

Stopped doing this for other
reasons or not interested in
doing this 6

continued

TABLE 7.10 continued

National Eye Institute Visual Functioning Questionnaire, 25 Item (NEI-VFQ-25)*

14. Because of your eyesight, how much difficulty do you have going out to see movies, plays, or sports events? *(Circle one)*

No difficulty at all 1

A little difficulty 2

Moderate difficulty 3

Extreme difficulty 4

Stopped doing this because of your eyesight 5

Stopped doing this for other reasons or not interested in doing this 6

15. Are you currently driving, at least once in a while? *(Circle one)*

Yes 1

Skip to Question 15c

No 2

15a. IF NO: have you never driven a car or have you given up driving? (Circle one)

Never drove 1

Skip to Part 3, Question 17

Gave up 2

15b. IF YOU GAVE UP DRIVING: was that mainly because of your eyesight, mainly for some other reason, or because of both your eyesight and other reasons? *(Circle one)*

Mainly eyesight 1

Skip to Part 3, Question 17

Mainly other reasons 2

Skip to Part 3, Question 17

Both eyesight and other reasons .3

Skip to Part 3, Question 17

15c. IF CURRENTLY DRIVING: how much difficulty do you have driving during the daytime in familiar places? *(Circle one)*

No difficulty at all 1

A little difficulty 2

Moderate difficulty 3

Extreme difficulty 4

16a. How much difficulty do you have driving at night? *(Circle one)*

No difficulty at all 1

A little difficulty 2

Moderate difficulty 3

Extreme difficulty 4

Stopped doing this because of your eyesight 5

Stopped doing this for other reasons or not interested in doing this 6

16b. How much difficulty do you have driving in difficult conditions, such as in bad weather, during rush hour, on the freeway, or in city traffic? *(Circle one)*

No difficulty at all 1

A little difficulty 2

Moderate difficulty 3

Extreme difficulty 4

Stopped doing this because of your eyesight 5

Stopped doing this for other reasons or not interested in doing this 6

PART 3: RESPONSES TO VISION PROBLEMS

The next questions are about how things you do may be affected by your vision. For each one, please circle the number to indicate whether for you the statement is true for you all, most, some, a little, or none of the time.

Read Categories

For each of the following statements, please circle one.

17. Do you accomplish less than you would like because of your vision?

TABLE 7.10 continued

National Eye Institute Visual Functioning Questionnaire, 25 Item (NEI-VFQ-25)*

1 = All of the time
2 = Most of the time
3 = Some of the time
4 = A little of the time
5 = None of the time

18. Are you limited in how long you can work or do other activities because of your vision?

1 = All of the time
2 = Most of the time
3 = Some of the time
4 = A little of the time
5 = None of the time

19. How much does pain or discomfort in or around your eyes, for example, burning, itching, or aching, keep you from doing what you'd like to be doing?

1 = All of the time
2 = Most of the time
3 = Some of the time
4 = A little of the time
5 = None of the time

For each of the following statements, please circle the number to indicate whether for you the statement is definitely true, mostly true, mostly false, or definitely false, or you are not sure.

20. I stay home most of the time because of my eyesight.

1 = Definitely true
2 = Mostly true
3 = Mostly false
4 = Definitely false
5 = Not sure

21. I feel frustrated a lot of the time because of my eyesight.

1 = Definitely true
2 = Mostly true
3 = Mostly false
4 = Definitely false
5 = Not sure

22. I have much less control over what I do because of my eyesight.

1 = Definitely true
2 = Mostly true
3 = Mostly false
4 = Definitely false
5 = Not sure

23. Because of my eyesight, I have to rely too much on what other people tell me.

1 = Definitely true
2 = Mostly true
3 = Mostly false
4 = Definitely false
5 = Not sure

24. I need a lot of help from others because of my eyesight.

1 = Definitely true
2 = Mostly true
3 = Mostly false
4 = Definitely false
5 = Not sure

25. I worry about doing things that will embarrass myself or others, because of my eyesight.

1 = Definitely true
2 = Mostly true
3 = Mostly false
4 = Definitely false
5 = Not sure

* Reprinted courtesy of the National Eye Institute.

In a cohort of 323 consecutive ophthalmic patients previously described, we calculated a 0.75 correlation between the VF-14 and visual acuity in the better-seeing eye and an r^2 of 0.56, meaning that the visual acuity in the better-seeing eye explains 56% of the variance in the VF-14.[59] Accordingly, visual acuity measurement in the better-seeing eye appears to be a reasonable measure of the quality of life associated with diseases that affect vision.

The ophthalmic quality-of-life instruments are not generally applicable to systemic health states or comparable with the results obtained from more generic quality-of-life instruments such as the SIP, the SF-36, and the QWB Scale. This inapplicability and incomparability outside ophthalmology, as well as the inability to use the data in healthcare economic analyses, limits the usefulness of the VF-14 and the NEI-VFQ-25 for making resource allocation decisions.

CORE CONCEPTS

- Function-based quality-of-life instruments assess function associated with:
  - vocation
  - avocation
  - physical activity
  - cognitive activity
  - social interaction
  - psychological well-being
  - reaction to pain
- Function-based quality-of-life instruments can be
  - generic: applicable across all specialties
  - Specialty-specific: applicable to one disease or a relatively small number of diseases
- Categorical rating instruments (American Heart Association Functional Capacity Classification, American College of Rheumatology Classification of Global Functional Status in Rheumatoid Arthritis, Modified Rankin Scale for stroke, and so on) can be considered as elementary health-related quality-of-life instruments.
- These elementary categorical rating instruments can be correlated with data from many clinical trials and also with utility values, thus acting as intermediaries to allow clinical trial data to be converted to utility value (value-based) format.
- The Medical Outcomes Study (RAND) 36-Item Short-Form Health Survey (SF-36) is among the most commonly used function-based quality-of-life instruments. It has not been used in cost-utility analysis.
- Among the function-based quality-of-life instruments, the Quality-of-Well-Being Scale is one that generates values that can be used in place of utility values in cost-utility analysis.

REFERENCES

1. Ware JE, Sherbourne CD. The MOS 36-item short-form health survey (SF-36), I: conceptual framework and item selection. *Med Care.* 1992;30:473–483.

2. Andresen EM, Bowley N, Rothenberg BM, Panzer R, Katz P. Test-retest performance of a mailed version of the Medical Outcomes Study 36-Item Short-Form Health Survey among older adults. *Med Care.* 1996;34:1165–1170.

3. RAND Corporation. RAND 36-Item Health Survey 1.0. Available at: www.rand.org/health/surveys/sf36item. Accessed March 27, 2004.

4. Edelman D, Williams GR, Rothman M, Samsa GP. A comparison of three health status measures in primary care patients. *J Gen Intern Med.* 1999;14:759–762.

5. University of Oxford, Oxford, England. The UK SF-36 health survey questionnaire. Available at: www.hsru.ox.uk/shortfrm.htm. Accessed December 20, 2002.

6. Hobart JC, Williams LS, Moran K, Thompson AJ. Quality of life measurement after stroke: uses and abuses of the SF-36. *Stroke.* 2002;33:1176–1177.

7. O'Mahony PF, Ridgers H, Thomson RG, et al. Is the SF-36 suitable for assessing health status of older stroke patients? *Age Ageing.* 1998;27:19-22.

8. Parker SG, Peet SM, Jagger C, et al. Measuring health status in older patients: the SF-36 in practice. *Age Ageing.* 1998;27:13–18.

9. Fryback DG, Dasbach DJ, Klein R, et al. The Beaver Dam Outcomes Study: initial catalog of health-state quality factors. *Med Decis Making.* 1993;13:89–102.

10. Meletiche DM, Doshi D, Lofland JH. Medical Outcomes Study Short Form 36: a possible source of utilities? *Clin Ther.* 1999;21:2016–2026.

11. Gandek B, Ware JE, Aaronson NK, et al. Cross-validation of item selection and scoring for the SF-12 Health Survey in nine countries: results from the IQOLA Project. International Quality of Life Assessment. *J Clin Epidemiol.* 1998;51:1171–1178.

12. Ware J Jr, Kosinski M, Keller SD. A 12-Item Short-Form Health Survey: construction of scales and preliminary tests of reliability and validity. *Med Care.* 1996;34:220–233.

13. Gandhi SK, Salmon JW, Zhao SZ, Lambert BL, Gore PR, Conrad K. Psychometric evaluation of the 12-item short-form health survey (SF-12) in osteoarthritis and rheumatoid arthritis in clinical trials. *Clin Ther.* 2001;23:1080–1098.

14. Pickard AS, Johnson JA, Penn A, Lau F, Noseworthy T. Replicability of SF-36 summary scores by the SF-12 in stroke patients. *Stroke.* 1999;30:1213–1217.

15. Bergner M, Bobbitt RA, Carter WB, Gilson BS. The Sickness Impact Profile: development and final revision of a health status measure. *Med Care.* 1981;119:787–805.

16. Weinberger M, Samsa GP, Tierney WM. Generic versus disease specific health status measures: comparing the Sickness Impact Profile and the Arthritis Impact measurement scales. *J Rheumatol.* 1992;19:543–546.

17. Visser MC, Fletcher AE, Parr G, et al. A comparison of three quality of life instruments in subjects with angina pectoris: the Sickness Impact Profile, the Nottingham

Health Profile, and the Quality of Well Being Scale. *J Clin Epidemiol.* 1994;47:157–163.

18. Kaplan RM, Anderson JP. The general health policy model: an integrated approach. In: Spikler B, ed. *Quality of Life and Pharmacoeconomics in Clinical Trials.* 2nd ed. Philadelphia, Pa: Lippincott-Raven; 1996:309–322.

19. Kaplan RM, Ganiats TG, Sieber WJ, Anderson JP. The Quality of Well-Being Scale: critical similarities and differences with the SF-36. *Int J Qual Health Care.* 1998;10:509–520.

20. Andresen EM, Patrick DL, Carter WB, Malmgren JA. Comparing the performance of health status measures for healthy older adults. *J Am Geriatr Soc.* 1995;43:1030–1034.

21. Katz S, Ford AB, Moskowitz RW, Jackson BA, Jaffe MW. Studies of illnesses in the aged: the index of ADL: a standardized measure of biological and psychosocial function. *JAMA.* 1963;185:914–919.

22. Lawton MP, Brody EM. Assessment of older people: self-maintaining and instrumental activities of daily living. Gerontologist. 1969;9:179–186.

23. Gill TM, Williams CS, Tinetti ME. Assessing risk for the onset of functional dependence among older adults: the role of physical performance. *J Am Geriatr Soc.* 1995;43:603–609.

24. Karnofsky DA, Abelmann WH, Craver LF, Burchenal JH. The use of nitrogen mustards in the palliative treatment of cancer. *Cancer.* 1948;1:634–656.

25. Brezinski D, Stone PH, Muller JE, et al. Prognostic significance of the Karnofsky Performance Status score in patients with acute myocardial infarction: comparison with the left ventricular ejection fraction and the exercise treadmill performance. *Am Heart J.* 1991;121:1374–1381.

26. Liem BJ, Holland JM, Kang MY, Hoffelt SC, Marques CM. Karnofsky Performance Status Assessment: resident versus attending. *J Cancer Educ.* 2002;17:138–141.

27. Roila F, Lupattelli M, Sassi M, et al. Intra and interobserver variablity in cancer patients' performance status assessed according to Karnofsky and ECOG scales. *Ann Oncol.* 1991;2:437–439.

28. Rosner B. *Fundamentals of Biostatistics.* 5th ed. Pacific Grove, Calif: Duxbury Thomson Learning; 2000:451–453, 562–565.

29. Oken MM, Creech RH, Toomey DC, et al. Toxicity and response criteria of the Eastern Cooperative Oncology Group. *Am J Clin Oncol.* 1982;5:649–655.

30. Buccheri G, Ferrigno D, Tamburini M. Karnofsky and ECOG performance status scoring in lung cancer: a prospective, longitudinal study of 536 patients from a single institution. *Eur J Cancer.* 1996;32:1135–1141.

31. Verger G, Salamero M, Conill C. Can Karnofsky performance status be transformed to the Eastern Cooperative Oncology Group scoring scale and vice versa. *Eur J Cancer.* 1992;28:1328–1330.

32. Ahmed A. American College of Cardiology/American Heart Association chronic heart failure evaluation and management guidelines: relevance to the geriatric practice. *J Am Geriatr Soc.* 2003;51:123–126.

33. American Heart Association. Classification of functional capacity and objective assessment. Available at: www.americanheart.org. Accessed April 29, 2003.

34. Hochberg MC, Chang RW, Dwosh I, Lindsey S, Pincus Y, Wolfe F. The American College of Rheumatology 1991 revised criteria for the classification of global functional status in rheumatoid arthritis. *Arthritis Rheum.* 1992;35:498–502.

35. Stucki G, Stoll T, Bruhlmann P, Michel BA. Construct validation of the ACR 1991 revised criteria for global functional status in rheumatoid arthritis. *Clin Exp Rheumatol.* 1995;13:349–352.

36. Chang RW, Pellisier JM, Hazen GB. A cost-effectiveness analysis of total hip arthroplasty for osteoarthritis of the hip. *JAMA.* 1996;275:858–865.

37. Bonita R, Beaglehole R. Recovery of motor function after stroke. *Stroke.* 1988;19:1497–1500.

38. Rankin J. Cerebral vascular accidents in patients over the age of 60. *Scott Med J.* 1957;2:200–215.

39. Van Swieten JC, Koudstaal PJ, Visser MC, Shouten HJ, van Gijn J. Interobserver agreement for the assessment of handicap in stroke patients. *Stroke.* 1988;19:604–607.

40. Goldstein B, Samsa GP. Reliability of the National Institutes of Health Stroke Scale: extension to non-neurologists in the context of a clinical trial. *Stroke.* 1997;28:307–310.

41. National Institute of Neurological Disorders and Stroke rt-PA Stroke Study Group. *N Engl J Med.* 1995;333:1581–1587.

42. Duncan PW, Lai SM, Keighley J. Defining post-stroke recovery: implications for design and interpretation of drug trials. *Neuropharmacology.* 2000;39:835–841.

43. Tengs TO, Yu M, Luistro E. Health-related quality of life after stroke: a comprehensive review. *Stroke.* 2001;32:964–972.

44. Dewey HM, Donnan GA, Freeman EJ, et al. Interrater reliability of the National Institutes of Health Stroke Scale: rating by neurologists and nurses in a community-based stroke incidence study. *Cerebrovasc Dis.* 1999;9:323–327.

45. Kasner SE, Cucchiara LB, McGarvery ML, Luciano JM, Liebeskind DS, Chalela JA. Modified National Institutes of Health Stroke Scale can be estimated from medical records. *Stroke.* 2003;34:568–570.

46. Moller HJ. Methodological aspects in the assessment of severity of depression by the Hamilton Depression Scale. *Eur Arch Psychiatry Clin Neurisci.* 2001;251(suppl 2):13–20.

47. Ross LE, Evans SE, Sellers EM, Romach MK. Measurement issues in postpartum depression, part 2: assessment of somatic symptoms using the Hamilton Rating Scale for Depression. *Arch Women Ment Health.* 2003;6:59–64.

48. Hamilton M. Development of a rating scale for primary depressive illness. *Br J Soc Clin Psychol.* 1967;6:278–296.

49. Hedlund JL, Vieweg BW. The Hamilton rating scale for depression: a comprehensive review. *J Operational Psychol.* 1979;10:149–165.

50. Caracciolo B, Giaquinto S. Criterion validity of the Center for Epidemiological Studies Depression (CES-D) Scale in a sample of rehabilitation patients. *J Rehabil Med.* 2002;34:221–225.

51. Irwin M, Artin KH, Oxman MN. Screening for depression in the older adult: criterion validity of the 10-item Center for Epidemiological Studies Depression Scale (CES-D). *Arch Intern Med.* 1999;159:1701–1704.

52. Rouch-Leroyer I, Sourgen C, Barberger-Gateau P, Fuhrer R, Dartigues JF. Detection of depressive symptomatology in elderly people: a short version of the CES-D scale. *Ageing.* 2000;12:228–233.

53. Lewinsohn PM, Seeley JR, Roberts RE, Allen NB. Center for Epidemiologic Studies Depression Scale (CES-D) as a screening instrument for depression among community-residing older adults. *Psychol Aging.* 1997;12:227–287.

54. Lee AG, Beaver HA, Jogerst G, Daly JM. Screening elderly patients in an outpatient ophthalmology clinic for dementia, depression, and functional impairment. *Ophthalmology.* 2003;110:651–657.

55. Brown GC, Brown MM, Sharma S, Brown H, Gozum M, Denton P. Quality-of-life associated with diabetes mellitus in an adult population. *J Diabetes Complications.* 2000;14:18–24.

56. Bennett KJ, Torrance GW, Boyle MH, Guscott R. Cost-utility analysis in depression: the McSad utility measure for depression health states. *Psychiatr Serv.* 2000;51:1171-1176.

57. Bennett KJ, Torrance GW, Boyle MH, Guscott R, Moran LA. Development and testing of a utility measure for major, unipolar depression (McSad). *Qual Life Res.* 2000;9:109-120.

58. Thall EH, Miller KM, Rosenthal P, Schecter RJ, Steinert RF, Beardsley TL. *Basic and Clinical Science Course: Optics, Refraction and Contact Lenses.* San Francisco, Calif: American Academy of Ophthalmology; 1999.

59. Brown GC. Vision and quality of life. *Trans Am Ophthalmol Soc.* 1999;97:473–512.

60. Brown MM, Brown GC, Sharma S, Shah G. Utility values and diabetic retinopathy. *Am J Ophthalmol.* 1999;128:324–330.

61. Brown GC, Brown MM, Sharma S. Health care in the 21st century: evidence-based medicine, patient preference-based quality and cost-effectiveness. *Qual Manage Health Care.* 2000;19:23–31

62. Brown GC, Brown MM, Sharma S, Kistler J. Utility values associated with age-related macular degeneration. *Arch Ophthalmol.* 2000;118:47–51.

63. Brown GC, Brown MM, Sharma S. Difference between ophthalmologist and patient perceptions of quality-of-life associated with age-related macular degeneration. *Can J Ophthalmol.* 2000;35:27–32.

64. Brown MM, Brown GC, Sharma S, Smith AF, Landy J. A utility analysis correlation with visual acuity: methodologies and vision in the better and poorer eyes. *Int Ophthalmol.* 2001;24:123–127.

65. Sharma S, Brown GC, Brown MM, Hollands H, Robbins R, Shah G. Validity of the time trade-off and standard gamble methods of utility assessment in retinal patients. *Br J Ophthalmol.* 2002;86:493–496.

66. Brown MM, Brown GC, Sharma S, Landy J. Quality of life with visual acuity loss from diabetic retinopathy and age-related macular degeneration. *Arch Ophthalmol.* 2002;120:481-484.

67. Steinberg EP, Tielsch JM, Schein OD, et al. The VF-14: an index of functional impairment in patients with cataract. *Arch Ophthalmol.* 1994;112:630–638.

68. Mangione CM, Lee PP, Gutierrez PR, et al. Psychometric properties of the National Eye Institute Visual Function Questionnaire (NEI-VFQ). *Arch Ophthalmol.* 1998;116:1496–1504.

69. Mangione CM, Lee PP, Gutierrez PR, et al. Development of the 25-item National Eye Institute Visual Function Questionnaire. *Arch Ophthalmol.* 2001;119:1050–1058.

8

Preference-Based Quality-of-Life Instruments

Preference-based quality-of-life instruments elicit the desirability or undesirability of a patient or surrogate respondent for a given health state or disease. A list of preference-based quality-of-life instruments is shown in Table 8.1.[1] There are three basic groups of preference-based instruments:

- utility analysis,
- rating scale, and
- multiattribute utility analysis.

Preference-based instruments evaluate health states according to their desirability (or undesirability).

Utility analysis instruments compose a subgroup of preference-based instruments that require subjects to decide which health state they prefer:

1. their present health state, or
2. a normal health state for which they take a risk or give up (trade) something of value in return.

The risk can include immediate death (standard-gamble utility analysis), and the object of value they trade can be time of life (time-tradeoff utility analysis) or monetary resources (willingness-to-pay utility analysis). Some have limited the category of utility analysis to only the standard gamble variant, as it requires risk-taking behavior in the face of uncertainty, whereas the time-tradeoff and willingness-to-pay methodologies deal with trading known entities, and thus have a known outcome.[1] We believe the differentiation is academic and confusing, especially because the time-tradeoff and willingness-to-pay methods are often referred to in the literature as *utility instruments*.[2]

Rating scale instruments, also referred to as continuous rating scales, require a patient or surrogate respondent to select a preference for a value point estimate correlating with his or her perceived health along a continuum scale ranging from

0.0 to 1.0 or 0 to 100. Rating instruments are not typically referred to as utility values but, as is the case with utility values, are preference-based instruments.

Multiattribute instruments, such as the EuroQol 5D and the Health Utilities Index, are preference-based quality-of-life instruments that assess several parameters (mobility, pain, anxiety, and so on) and subtract disutilities (quality-of-life impairments) from the utility value associated with perfect health (1.0). The disutilities are typically already derived from a population-based study of a community, either by using time-tradeoff utility analysis or a rating scale.

In contrast to function-based quality-of-life instruments, preference-based quality-of-life instruments are all generic, meaning that they are theoretically applicable across all specialties, and all are applicable to cost-utility analysis. Nevertheless, the different preference-based instruments are not directly comparable with each other. Cost-utility analyses must therefore utilize one consistent measure of patient preferences to be comparable.

> The three forms of utility analysis are:
> 1. standard gamble,
> 2. willingness to pay, and
> 3. time tradeoff.
> Continuous rating scales and multiattribute instruments can also be used in cost-utility analysis.

TABLE 8.1

Preference-Based, Health-Related Quality-of-Life Instruments

Instrument	Category	Preference-Based	Use in CUA
1. Utility Analysis			
Standard gamble	Generic	Yes	Yes
Willingness to pay	Generic	Yes	Yes
Time tradeoff	Generic	Yes	Yes
2. Rating Scale Instruments			
Continuous scales	Generic	Yes	Yes
3. Multiattribute Instruments*			
EuroQol 5D	Generic	Yes	Yes
HUI	Generic	Yes	Yes

CUA indicates cost-utility analysis; HUI, Health Utilities Index.

* The Quality-of-Well-Being Scale, an instrument with many function-based questions, has also been considered by some to be a multiattribute instrument.[1] It has four dimensions: (1) a mobility scale, (2) a physical activity scale, (3) a social activity scale, and (4) a general health scale utilizing symptom-problem complexes (gastrointestinal upset, pain, headache, respiratory difficulty, and so on). A rating scale from 0.0 (death) to 1.0 (normal health) is used to measure each and disutilities are subtracted from 1.0, similar to the EuroQol 5D and the Health Utilities Index. When more than one condition is present, the most serious is studied.

> All preference-based quality-of-life instruments are *generic.* They are theoretically applicable across all specialties.

We agree with the United States Panel on Cost-Effectiveness in Health and Medicine[3,4] that cost-utility analyses should be performed with data obtained using preference-based instruments. A discussion of the positive and negative aspects of preference-based instruments for use in cost-utility analysis follows in Chapter 9. Four major advantages of all preference-based instruments over function-based instruments, however, is that they:

1. are all-encompassing
2. are applicable across all specialties,
3. have a low burden of administration, and
4. can be used in cost-utility analysis.

> Cost-utility analyses should be performed using *preference-based* quality-of-life instruments.

> All preference-based instruments can be used in cost-utility analysis but not interchangeably.

A good preference-based assessment tool must have reasonable responsiveness or the ability to detect change. If utility values are being elicited from patients who have the disease in question, then responsiveness refers to whether the utility score changes appropriately when a disease improves or worsens. If utilities are being elicited from people who are not suffering from the disease, then responsiveness refers to whether the utility score changes appropriately when their framing of the disease or health state in question is changed.

> *Useful caveat:* The reimbursement system in the United States requires that a diagnosis code and a procedure code be listed for payment. It is therefore helpful from the point of resource allocation if the score from a health-related quality-of-life instrument can be correlated with a disease in the International Classification of Diseases[5] used for payment, rather than a health state consisting of multiple diseases.

UTILITY ANALYSIS

In this section we discuss utility analysis in more detail. Some of the material is repetitive, but sufficiently important to be repeated, especially considering the difficulty of select concepts.

Background

The term *utility* has been bandied about for centuries, often with related, but differing, meanings.[1,6,7] In 1944, John von Neumann, a Hungarian mathematician, and Oscar Morgenstern, an economist, published their classic text, *The Theory of Games and Economic Behavior,* on their theory of rational decision making in the presence of uncertainty.[8] Their model included axioms describing how a rational individual ought to make decisions when uncertainty exists. They described a method of decision making under conditions of *uncertainty,* using a set of logical axioms that must be adhered to. This approach enables a reasonable decision maker to make the best decision in accordance with his or her fundamental preferences. Further work regarding uncertainty, risk theory, and preference measurements proliferated and was applied to healthcare in the late 1960s and 1970s.[9–11]

"A day in perfect health is not the same as a day in poor or mediocre health."[12] Therein lies the belief by which quality enters into our medical decision making. Currently, measuring preferences in health states has enjoyed a plethora of researcher interest, yet it still remains a study of varying opinions on usage and accuracy. Earlier, students tended to be economists. With an educational and occupational history steeped in economic theory, the literature tended to be theoretical and not particularly easy to apply to clinical medicine. In the past decade, however, those practicing the healthcare sciences have begun to apply cost-effectiveness analysis, more specifically cost-utility analysis, to healthcare.[13] We believe this is a sign that cost-utility analysis and value-based medicine (VBM) will play a much larger role in the healthcare system in the near future.

Rationale

Utility analysis gives a quantitative measure of subjects' preferences regarding the quality of life associated with a particular health state. Simply, it quantifies how valuable their level of health is to them. The word *preference* is relevant because subjects can prefer either their current health state or a better health state that can only be achieved by risking or trading something of value. Utility analysis recognizes an individual's personal attitude toward illness, rather than rote evaluation of the functional state of such individuals as defined by the majority of quality-of-life instruments.

Utility analysis assesses the preference for a health state. In essence, it measures the quality of life associated with a health state.

An All-Encompassing Instrument

We agree with Redelmeier and Detsky[14] that utility analysis is among the most all-encompassing quality-of-life instruments in that it theoretically takes into account all possible variables associated with a health state.[2,15,16] Its perspective is broad and one that is less likely to miss critical aspects of illness altogether. While many function-based quality-of-life instruments take into account multiple function variables, utility analysis takes all functions into account, as well as fear of the future, the multiple economic parameters associated with illness, sensory deprivation, caregiver support, worry about dependents, and others.

Whether directly or indirectly in the thought process, utility analysis takes into account all of the variables listed in Table 5.2 and more.

Utility analysis is an all-encompassing quality-of-life instrument.

Methods of Utility Analysis

There are three methods of utility analysis:

1. standard-gamble utility analysis,
2. willingness-to-pay utility analysis, and
3. time-tradeoff utility analysis.

Each of the three methods asks participants to make a sacrifice or take a risk theoretically to return to a normal health state.[1,14] Exactly what is being sacrificed or risked is the basis for the difference among the methodologies.

Which ones are utilities?   Some purists have suggested that only the standard-gamble method is a true utility measurement as per the original von Neumann and Morgenstern criterion of assuming risk in the face of uncertainty.[1] The standard-gamble methodology is considered a true preference because of the uncertainty of the outcome of the gamble (whether it will be sudden death or a cure), while the time-tradeoff and willingness-to-pay methodologies lack this uncertainty in that the subject knows with certainty the outcomes (trading a set amount of remaining time of life or money, or remaining in the same health state). Thus, only the standard-gamble method theoretically yields real utility values.[1]

The authors of this text believe that such a strict classification excluding time-tradeoff and willing-to-pay values as utility measures only causes further confusion with an already difficult literature that often treats them both as utility values.[2] Although such an approach is theoretically sound, we believe too much theory reduces the usefulness of the methodology and complicates the issues for very little gain in return. They all measure on a scale from 0.0 to 1.0 and are all preference-based.

In this book, we consider time-tradeoff values, standard-gamble values, and willingness-to-pay values as utility variants[17,18] and record the difference as accepted, but not relevant, in the attempt to make utility theory understandable and usable to clinicians and noneconomists.[2] What is most important is that the reader understands the methodology of derivation and applicability of each variant.

How Do We Measure Utility Values?

By convention, a utility value is ranked on a continuum ranging from an anchor of 0.0 (death) to an anchor of 1.0 (perfect health). These numbers are referred to as *utility values*, although in practice they are commonly referred to as just *utilities.* The closer the value is to 1.0, the better the quality of life associated with a health state or disease, while the closer the value is to 0.0, the poorer the quality of life associated with a health state or disease. As examples, the time-tradeoff utility value associated with treated systemic arterial hypertension is 0.98,[19] while that associated with a Rankin grade 5 stroke is 0.34.[20]

Utility Value Anchors:
   Perfect health = 1.0
   Death = 0.0

A *utility value* is also commonly referred to as a *utility.*

Can there be upper utility value anchors other than perfect health?   Yes. As an example, when asking about cardiac disease, the anchor is perfect heart health. With deafness, the upper anchor is perfect hearing and for vision loss the upper anchor is perfect vision. Theoretically, the upper anchor should be the best possible health state. Therefore, for each of the three diseases mentioned, a utility value of 1.0, respectively, refers to permanent perfect heart health, permanent perfect hearing, and permanent perfect vision. An upper anchor of return to normal health without a guarantee of permanency is not the best possible health state, since the concern about future disease typically precludes a perfect utility value of 1.0.

An upper anchor of return to perfect health without a guarantee of permanency is not the best possible health state, as concern about the uncertainty of future disease often precludes a perfect utility value of 1.0.

Can there be lower utility value anchors less than zero?   Theoretically, a person can have a utility less than 0.0, indicating that death is preferred over the health state that has an associated utility value of less than 0.0. An example of a health state associated with a utility value of less than 0.0 might be that of a globally paralyzed person on a respirator with the "locked-in" syndrome, but with the five senses and thought processes still intact.

Most often, utility values less than 0.0 are assigned by researchers—not actual patients—who have never experienced the health state in question. In practicality, very few people are alive who have experienced health states worse than death. Since primary utilities from such affected patients are extraordinarily uncommon and politically controversial (preferring death as an alternative, thereby suggesting euthanasia is preferred), we do not advocate the incorporation of utility values less than zero into cost-utility analyses.

Generally the use of utility values less than zero is not a problem encountered with the three straightforward forms of utility analysis (time-tradeoff, standard-gamble, and willingness-to-pay), but is a drawback encountered with the use of multiattribute instruments.

> The use of utility values less than 0.0 (indicating that death is preferable to a health state) in cost-utility analyses is highly questionable.

Standard-Gamble Utility Analysis

From a healthcare perspective, the first von Neumann fundamental axiom states that a person can quantify a probability (p) of indifference between the following two outcomes:

1. a sure outcome of remaining in the health state under evaluation, and
2. a gamble with two additional possible outcomes (perfect health and death) (Figure 8.1).

Thus, a person can elect one of two choices: remain in the same health state, or select a gamble in which the only possible outcomes are perfect health and death. Probability p corresponds to the probability of obtaining best possible outcome (perfect health, or a utility value of 1.0) for the person who has selected the gamble. Probability $1 - p$ corresponds to the probability of receiving

FIGURE 8.1

Standard-Gamble Utility Analysis Options. The rectangular box represents a *decision node*, a point at which a subject must make a decision between a gamble and remaining in the same health state. The oval node is a *chance node* corresponding to the gamble, a point at which the subject has the possible outcomes of returning to perfect health and dying. The probability of returning to the outcome of perfect health (p) is the standard-gamble utility value and the probability of the outcome of death ($1 - p$) is the percent risk of death a subject is willing to assume in undertaking the gamble. The triangular nodes are *terminal nodes*, endpoints at which a utility (located to the right of each triangle) is assigned to each the outcomes described just above the respective branch on the right side of the tree. A utility of 1.0 corresponds to perfect health, a utility of 0.0 corresponds to death.

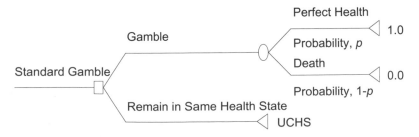

UCHS indicates utility of the current health state.

the worst possible outcome (death, or a utility value of 0.0). Probability p is defined as the standard-gamble utility for a particular outcome. A utility elicited through the standard-gamble method is often referred to as a von Neumann-Morgenstern (vN-M) utility in the literature.[21] The standard gamble is said to measure utilities under *risky*, or *uncertain*, conditions because an individual is forced to quantify a probability but is not assured of any particular outcome (that is, the individual is playing a game of chance).

Sample wording of a standard-gamble utility analysis question to measure the utility value associated with systemic arterial hypertension is presented below.

Sample Standard-Gamble Utility Analysis Question

Suppose there is a technology that permanently eradicates your systemic arterial hypertension. However, it doesn't always work. When it works, patients respond perfectly and are free from hypertension for the rest of their lives. When it doesn't work, however, the technology fails and patients do not survive. Thus, it either cures your hypertension or results in immediate death.

What is the highest percent risk of death—if any—you would be willing to accept before refusing the technology to treat your hypertension?

This percent risk a respondent is willing to accept is subtracted from 1.0 to yield the utility value. Consequently, if the respondent is willing to accept a 2% chance of immediate death to otherwise ensure permanent freedom from hypertension, the corresponding standard gamble utility value for that patient is $1.0 - 0.02 = 0.98$. In this case, probability p corresponds to the standard-gamble utility value (0.98), which is also the probability of obtaining a perfect outcome (utility value = 1.0), while $1 - p$ ($1.00 - 0.98 = 0.02$) is the probability of experiencing death (utility value = 0.0) as a result of the gamble. As is also the case for time-tradeoff utility analysis, visual instruments have been developed by some researchers to help explain standard-gamble utility analysis to respondents.

To ensure maximal reproducibility, the following variables must be considered (for all forms of utility analysis and other health-related quality-of-life instruments as well). Does the question imply that just the hypertension will be cured or that hypertension-associated comorbidities such as myocardial infarction, stroke, and nephropathy will be cured as well? In addition, is the question referring to treated hypertension or untreated hypertension? If treated, is it with current treatment, or can another treatment be substituted? In asking the question about return to normal health, the health state in question must be clearly defined and delineated. For example, in the case of hypertension, we tell the respondent that in return for time traded, the hypertension as it currently exists (treated, untreated, treated with multiple therapies, and so on) will be eradicated, as well as possible further complications from the hypertension. Any complications from the hypertension—such as myocardial infarction, stroke, and nephropathy—that already exist, however, will not be eradicated. Asking what proportion of remaining time of life a person will trade to be rid of hypertension and what proportion of remaining time a person will trade to be rid of hypertension and its associated comorbidities are very different questions.

> The health state or disease assessed with utility analysis must be defined very strictly in regard to:
> 1. diagnosis,
> 2. severity,
> 3. whether treated or untreated, and
> 4. whether it includes or does not include disease-releated comorbidities or future disease-related comorbidities.

While standard-gamble methodology is well grounded in economic theory[1] and believed to be a valid response scale for eliciting utilities, the technique has been criticized for being more risk-aversive than acceptable.[22] In other words, the aversion to the prospect of sudden death falsely elevates the utility that, if measured another way, might more accurately reflect the health state of interest. Some have stated that the standard-gamble method is a thought process familiar to patients because they are required to sign written permits before undertaking many interventions. They argue that patients are used to dealing with the terminology of the risk of sudden death to obtain a health intervention that will

TABLE 8.2

Advantages and Drawbacks of Standard-Gamble Utility Analysis*

Advantages

1. It is applicable to all health states.
2. It has good to excellent reproducibility but not as good as time-tradeoff utility analysis.
3. It can be directly correlated with ICD-9-CM and CPT® diagnostic and procedure codes.
4. There is a low burden of administration.

Disadvantages

1. It is insensitive to milder health states and diseases.
2. It may be difficult for some patients to comprehend.
3. Risk aversion to death biases utilities toward higher values.[22]
4. Many patients take no risk (and thus there is a skew toward a utility value of 1.0) because of the chance of immediate death.

CPT indicates Current Procedural Terminology; ICD-9-CM, *International Classification of Diseases, Ninth Revision, Clinical Modification.*
* Refer also to Table 8.6.

improve their health state. As many people have difficulty relating to probabilities and gambles, an adaptable visual aid symbolizing the varying gambles and health situations has been used to theoretically improve clarity.[10]

Standard gamble methodology does not have good sensitivity for milder health problems, as many people are not willing to risk death for a milder affliction. The advantages and drawbacks of standard-gamble utility analysis are listed in Table 8.2.

Willingness-to-Pay Utility Analysis

Schelling[23] is credited with being the first to propose, in 1966, a willingness-to-pay methodology for valuing changes in health status. Since then, multiple variants of willingness-to-pay utility analysis have evolved.

Willingness-to-pay utility analysis utilizes the basic principle of paying money for an improvement in health or return to normal health.[24,25] Thus, there are two commonly used alternatives when presented with a willingness-to-pay strategy: remain in the same health state, or pay money to return to a perfect health state (Figure 8.2). The money paid can take the form of a single sum, a percentage of family monthly income, a percentage of total wealth, or another variant.[1,26] The outcomes can be variable as well; they can be temporary, such as a reduction of angina for a three-month period,[25] or permanent, as with a definitive surgical procedure such as cholecystectomy.[24] A specific payment for each quality-adjusted life-year (QALY) gained can also be undertaken.

Sample wording of a willingness-to-pay utility analysis question for systemic arterial hypertension is presented here.

Sample Willingness-to-Pay Utility Analysis Question

Please imagine that by permanently paying a percentage of your monthly income you could permanently eradicate your systemic arterial hypertension. What is the maximum percentage of your monthly salary—if any—you would be willing to pay to be rid of your hypertension?

When the answer to the question is a proportion of wealth or of salary paid, this proportion can be subtracted from 1.0 to yield a utility value. Thus, a person who is willing to pay 20% of his or her monthly income to be permanently rid of diabetes has a utility value of $1.00 - 0.20 = 0.80$. It is difficult to calculate a utility value when a sum of money alone, unrelated to overall wealth, total income, or salary, is solicited.

The willingness-to-pay methodology has been shown to be responsive to small changes in health status,[27] but it has a sufficient number of shortcomings that we have elected not to use it at the present time. The major drawback is that it is influenced by income, and is thus linked to the ability to pay.[28,29] It is also influenced by gender and age.[28] Furthermore, people are willing to pay more for a health outcome if the cost is paid by an insurance company rather than with their personal funds.[30] The advantages and drawbacks of willingness-to-pay utility analysis are listed in Table 8.3.

FIGURE 8.2

Willingness-to-Pay Utility Analysis Options. Respondents can decide whether they prefer to remain in the same health state or pay money in return for a cure or amelioration of their health state. The rectangle represents a *decision node*, a point at which subjects must chose between two possible outcomes: paying money for improvement in their health state (usually to the utility of 1.0 associated with perfect health), and remaining in the same health state. The triangular nodes are terminal nodes, endpoints at which a utility is assigned to each outcome described just above each branch on the right side of the tree. A utility of 1.0 corresponds to perfect health.

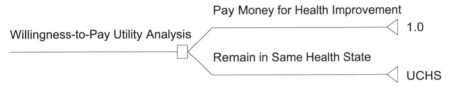

UCHS indicates utility of the current health state.

TABLE 8.3

Advantages and Drawbacks of Willingness-to-Pay Utility Analysis

Advantages

1. It is applicable to all health states.
2. It is sensitive to milder health states.
3. It is readily understood by patients.
4. It can be directly correlated with ICD-9-CM and CPT® diagnostic and procedure codes.[5]
5. There is a low burden of administration.

Disadvantages

1. It has poor reproducibility.
2. The results are affected by overall wealth and earnings, a very serious drawback.

CPT indicates Current Procedural Terminology; ICD-9-CM, *International Classification of Diseases, Ninth Revision, Clinical Modification.*

Time-Tradeoff Utility Analysis

The time-tradeoff method of utility value measurement was developed specifically for use in healthcare by Torrance and colleagues in 1972.[10,11] There are a number of variants, but essentially the methodology is based upon asking, in units of time, what is the maximum proportion of remaining time of life a respondent is willing to trade in return for a guaranteed improvement in his or her health condition. For instance, the investigator can ask respondents to identify what proportion of their remaining time of life they would be willing to trade for perfect health instead of their current health state. Thus, there are two choices: remaining in the same health state, or trading theoretical remaining time of life in return for perfect health (Figure 8.3). The utility value is calculated by subtracting the proportion of the remaining time of life a person is willing to trade from 1.0.

Sample wording of two time-tradeoff utility analysis questions is presented in the following sidebar, again using the example of systemic arterial hypertension.

Sample Time-Tradeoff Utility Analysis Questions

1. How many additional years do you expect to live?
2. Suppose there was a treatment that could eradicate your hypertension for as long as you live. The treatment always works but decreases your survival. It increases your quality of life, but decreases your length of life. What is the maximum amount of time—if any—you would be willing to give up if you could receive this treatment and have no hypertension for those years that are left?

For example, if a man with hypertension believes he will live for another 20 years and is willing to trade three of those 20 years to be cured of hypertension, his utility value for hypertension is $1.0 - (3/20) = 0.85$. If he trades seven of 20 remaining years to be rid of the hypertension, the resultant utility value is $1.0 - (7/20) = 0.65$. The actual time-tradeoff utility value for the average person with treated hypertension has been shown to be 0.98.[19]

There is no good tool to convert values obtained from one form of utility analysis to other forms of utility analysis or to a rating scale. The advantages and drawbacks of time-tradeoff utility analysis are listed in Table 8.4. From data on a large, previously described cohort, we found the correlation coefficient (r) between standard-gamble and time-tradeoff utility values to be 0.662, while the r^2 was 0.438.[15] This suggests that just interchanging the values is not desirable.

FIGURE　8.3

Time-Tradeoff Utility Analysis Options. The rectangular *decision node* is a point at which a subject must decide between two possible outcomes: trading time of his or her theoretical remaining life in return for a cure, and remaining in the same health state. The utility associated with each outcome is located to the right of each triangular *terminal node*. A utility of 1.0 is associated with a cure.

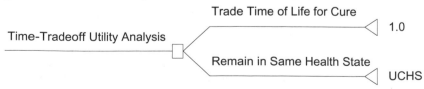

UCHS indicates utility of the current health state.

TABLE 8.4

Advantages and Drawbacks of Time-Tradeoff Utility Analysis

Advantages

1. It is applicable to all health states.
2. It has good to excellent reproducibility.
3. It is readily understood by patients.
4. It can be directly correlated with ICD-9-CM and CPT® diagnostic and procedure codes.[5]
5. There is a low burden of administration.
6. It is generally unaffected by age, gender, ethnicity, level of education, or income.
7. It has good construct validity.

Disadvantages

1. It has good, but not excellent, sensitivity to milder health states.
2. It is skewed toward 1.0 but less so than standard gamble utility values.

CPT indicates Current Procedural Terminology; ICD-9-CM, *International Classification of Diseases, Ninth Revision, Clinical Modification.*

CONTINUOUS RATING SCALE INSTRUMENTS

In our analysis of the multiple quality-of-life instruments, we have made the commitment to work with time-tradeoff utility analysis after comparing its reliability (reproducibility) and construct validity with those of other instruments (Chapter 9). Nonetheless, we agree with the Panel on Cost-Effectiveness in Health and Medicine[31] that the rating scales also have considerable potential for use in cost-utility analysis. To date, there has been insufficient study in this area. More is certainly indicated.

Rating-scale instruments have also been referred to as *rating instruments, analog scales,* or *scaling instruments.* The scales are *continuous,* meaning that a point estimate can be made by a subject anywhere along the scale to estimate the quality of life associated with a particular health state or disease.[11] "Feeling thermometers" have been used as visual aids in performing the task. With visual analog scales, participants are asked to assess their quality of life by selecting a position on an unmarked or marked linear scale with anchors of 0 (death) and 100 (perfect health). These are, of course, completely interchangeable with scale anchors of 0.0 to 1.0. Alternatively, the upper anchor can be permanent normal health, perfect health, best possible health, or the best imaginable health state, the last of which is used in the EuroQol 5D. The lower anchor can be death, the worst possible health, or the worst imaginable health state, the last again used with the EuroQol 5D. We believe permanent normal health and death are the most appropriate.

It is unclear how to interchange the numerical results obtained from scaling with utility values obtained by standard-gamble or time-tradeoff methodologies, but measures for the same health state typically note the standard-gamble utility value as the highest, the time-tradeoff value in the middle, and scaling methods with the lowest values.[31,32] Thus, moderate osteoarthritis of the hip might be associated with a standard-gamble value of 0.90, a time-tradeoff value of 0.80, and a rating-scale value of 0.70. A correlation coefficient (r) of 0.56 to 0.65 has been noted between standard-gamble methodology and time-tradeoff and scaling methodologies.[33] This is almost identical to the above-mentioned correlation of 0.66 we noted between time tradeoff and standard-gamble values.[15]

In our experience, rating scales can effectively be used in specialties with diseases that have death as a lower anchor (for example, cardiac, pulmonary, neurologic, and so on), but the concept is difficult in specialties with diseases in which death is not typically the lower anchor (dermatology, otolaryngology, ophthalmology, plastic surgery, and so on). For example, there is often conceptual difficulty when patients are asked to evaluate their psoriasis or their hearing deficit on a scale ranging from death (0) to perfect health (100), or from death (0) to normal skin (100), or death (0) to normal vision (100). This may account for the fact that previous authors[34] have found scaling methods to have poorer test-retest reliability, both short-term and long-term, than either the standard-gamble or time-tradeoff methodologies. A scale with anchors, such as permanently normal skin (1.0) and the worst possible skin (0.0), can be used, but then the difficulty arises as to how to correlate this scale with a scale using death (0.0) as an anchor.

Rating scale values can be used in cost-utility analysis. While not typically the case, some authors[32] have included rating scales within the realm of utility analysis. In the strictest sense, they are preference-based instruments, but they do not require that a person risk a gamble with the possible outcome of death in return for a better health state, as is the case with standard-gamble utility analysis. We consider the differentiation, however, to be minor and agree with others[31] that further research on scaling methodologies as substitutes for utility values could be very productive. The advantages and drawbacks of rating scales are listed in Table 8.5.

How Do the Preference-Based Instruments Compare?

Table 8.6 lists parameters evaluating the three utility instruments and the rating scale methodology for the measurement of health-related quality of life. Time-tradeoff utility analysis is the most reproducible on a short-term (one week) and long-term (one year) basis. As per Froberg and Kane,[34] the use of utility analysis generally requires more thoughtful consideration than the use of rating scale instruments.

MULTIATTRIBUTE INSTRUMENTS

Multiattribute instruments are generic and applicable across all diseases. They were developed to simplify the evaluation of all variants and combinations of different health states.

TABLE 8.5

Advantages and Drawbacks of Rating Scales*

Advantages

1. They are applicable to all health states.

2. They are sensitive to less serious health states.

3. They have a low burden of administration.

4. They can be directly correlated with ICD-9-CM and CPT® diagnostic and procedure codes.[5]

Drawbacks

1. They may be conceptually difficult for patients, especially when the lower anchor is death and diseases not associated with death are evaluated.

2. The results are not as reproducible on a short-term or long-term basis as those obtained with time-tradeoff or standard-gamble utility analysis.[34]

3. They require less thoughtful reflection than time-tradeoff or standard-gamble utility analysis.

CPT indicates Current Procedural Terminology; ICD-9-CM, *International Classification of Diseases, Ninth Revision, Clinical Modification*.

* Refer also to Table 8.6.

Overview

An alternative to measuring utilities directly from individuals is to use a prescored, multiattribute, health status classification system obtained from a cross section of the community. Examples of such systems include the EuroQol 5D and the Health Utilities Index. The original work on utility theory by von Neumann and Morgenstern[8] was expanded to cover multiple attributes by Keeney and Raiffa[35] by extending the assumptions used in the original mathematical proof. Essentially, Keeney and Raiffa demonstrated how the utility of a multiattribute outcome could be expressed as a function of the utilities of the individual attributes. The theory demonstrates several multiattribute functions (additive, multiplicative, and multilinear) along with independence conditions that are more or less rigorous depending on the multiattribute function being employed.

Rather than ask patients about one utility value they assign to their health state or disease, subjects are asked five (EuroQol 5D) or six or more (Health Utilities Index) questions about dimensions, or attributes, of their health state or disease. Each combination of scores is assigned a weight according to a formula derived from multiattribute utility theory and results obtained from a community-based utility survey. These community-derived utilities are elicited using time-tradeoff, standard-gamble, or rating-scale techniques; consequently, multiattribute instruments are all preference-based. If there is less than a perfect value in one or more of the five or more dimensions, the disutility from each dimension is subtracted from 1.0.

TABLE 8.6

Test-Retest Reliability (Reproducibility) and Other Features of Instruments Used for Cost-Utility Analysis*

	Instrument			
	TTO	**SG**	**RS**	**WTP**
Reliability (Test-Retest Reproducibility)				
≤ 1 Week	0.87	0.80	0.77	NA
One Year	0.62	0.53	0.49	0.25
Intrarater Reliability	0.77 – 0.88	0.77	NA	0.70 – 0.94
Interrater Reliability	0.86†	NA	NA	NA
Sensitivity to Milder Health States	Good	Fair	Excellent	Excellent
Effective Use for Health State in Which Death Is Not a Usual Anchor	Excellent	Excellent	Poor	Excellent
Patient Comprehension	Good	Fair	Good	Good
Correlation Coefficient With TTO‡	1.00	0.66	Visual Analog: 0.47	NA
Thoughtful Consideration Required	Substantial	Substantial	Minimal	Moderate

NA indicates not available; RS, rating scale; SG, standard-gamble utility analysis; TTO, time-tradeoff utility analysis; WTP, willingness-to-pay utility analysis.

* Adapted from Froberg and Kane.[34] Each number shown represents a correlation coefficient (r). The correlation coefficient provides a quantitative measure of the dependence between two variables. The closer the value is to 1.00, the greater the chance that one variable can be predicted from another. If $r = 1.00$, one variable will be predicted exactly from another. A correlation coefficient (r) of greater than 0.75 indicates excellent reproducibility, a coefficient between 0.40 and 0.75 indicates good reproducibility, and a coefficient less than 0.40 indicates poor reproducibility.[36]

† Center for Value-Based Medicine data.

‡ Data from 323 consecutive patients from the Center for Value-Based Medicine.

What Are Holistic and Decomposed Strategies?

Multiattribute instruments are also known as *decomposed* instruments since they utilize premeasured dimensions that contribute to quality of life, vs *holistic* instruments, which apply to one specific disease or health state.[37] The EuroQol 5D and the Health Utilities Index are both decomposed instruments, while time-tradeoff, standard-gamble, and willingness-to-pay utility analysis, as well as rating scales, are all holistic instruments.

A *holistic strategy* is one that considers a single disease (or a health state), such as stroke or osteoarthritis of the knee, and correlates utility values specifically with that disease and the levels of severity of the disease. For example, a stroke with no sequelae (Rankin Grade 0)[38] is associated with a time-tradeoff utility value of 0.93, while a moderate stroke (Rankin Grade 2, able to look after own affairs, but unable to carry out all previous activities) is associated with a utility value of 0.73, and a severe stroke (Rankin Grade 5, bedridden and incontinent) is associated with a utility value of 0.34.[20] The holistic strategy is most compatible with the healthcare compensation system in the United States since this strategy is disease-specific and the reimbursement for healthcare services is also disease-specific.[5]

> A *holistic* strategy is disease-specific or health state-specific. It compares one disease, or one health state, with one utility value.

A decomposed strategy, also know as a *multiattribute strategy*, designates values previously obtained from the community for various dimensions (mobility, self-care, anxiety, pain, performing usual activities, and so on) believed to compose quality of life. Abnormalities in these quality-of-life parameters are equated with disutilities that are then subtracted from 1.0 with both the EuroQol 5D and the Health Utilities Index. This result can be correlated with a specific disease, but the disutilities have previously been gathered from the general population, which may or may not include patients with a disease under investigation.

> A decomposed strategy assesses multiple dimensions believed to compose quality of life and subtracts the disutilities associated with them from 1.0.

EuroQol 5D (Five Dimensions)

The EuroQol 5D was initiated by a group of European investigators in 1990[39] and has been used across many specialties. The most recent version consists of five dimensions, which arc listed in Table 8.7.

TABLE 8.7

EuroQol 5D Health Measurement Dimensions

Dimension	Degree of Difficulty		
1. Mobility (Walking)	No Problem	Some Problems	Confined to Bed
2. Self-Care	No Problem	Some Problems	Unable to Wash or Dress
3. Usual Activity*	No Problem	Some Problems	Unable to Perform
4. Pain/Discomfort	None	Moderate	Extreme
5. Anxiety/Depression	None	Moderate	Extreme

* Usual activity indicates work, study, housework, or family or leisure activities, courtesy of the EuroQol Group.

With the addition of two states of dead and unconscious, there are a total of 245 possible combinations of health states. Preferences for each dimension and its severity have been determined in a number of European countries using time-tradeoff utility analysis, as is the case using the responses of 3,000 randomly chosen adults in the United Kingdom.[40,41] The result for each of the dimensions can differ for each country, causing the final outcomes to vary in different European countries.

The EuroQol was developed with the intention of measuring quality of life in a timely manner with greater simplicity than the utility analysis variants. Scoring of the EuroQol is performed by subtracting disutilities associated with each of the five dimensions from 1.0. If a person is normal for each of the dimensions, the utility value is 1.0. However, if a person with moderate osteoarthritis of the hip has moderate pain (−0.15 in utility value) and some difficulty walking (−0.12 in utility value), the resultant score is 1.0 − 0.27 = 0.73. The scores theoretically range between 0.0 (dead) and 1.0 (perfect health), allowing this preference-based tool to be used for cost-utility analyses. Nonetheless, for severe, adverse health states, the utility value can be substantially less than 0.0 (for example, −0.50), a limiting factor for use in cost-utility analysis since the new scale should be reconfigured on a 0.0 to 1.0 scale.

A second part of the EuroQol is a rating scale with a range from 0 to 100 and a feeling thermometer with the appearance of a linear outdoor thermometer. The anchors are 100 (best imaginable health state) and 0 (worst imaginable health state).

In addition to the problem with not fitting within the 0.0 to 1.0 scale, the EuroQol has been found to be insensitive for milder health states—such as moderate hearing loss[42]—and also for the evaluation of very severe health states.[43] The treating of anxiety and depression as a single unit is also problematic due to the marked clinical difference between the two diagnoses.

Although it was created to simplify quality-of-life measures, we believe the EuroQol in the United States will still require correlation with each individual disease and the severity of each disease. This is especially true since reimbursement in the United States is disease-specific and dependent upon the *International Classification of Diseases.*[5] Thus, for stroke, the five dimensions of the EuroQol must be evaluated for each of the levels of severity, as compared to a single answer required for each of the levels of severity when using time-tradeoff utility analysis. The capacity of the instrument to save a step in the evaluation of diseases is therefore negated. The ability to match previous evidence-based medicine data directly with the EuroQol health states is also open to much interpretation.

We have found that some respondents have difficulty conceptualizing the quality of life associated with one disease since the instrument takes overall health into account and more patients have multiple diseases as opposed to a single disease.[44] For example, a person with depression associated with concomitant kidney transplant, hypertension, and Guillain-Barré syndrome may find it difficult to separate how much of the depression occurs secondary to the kidney transplant, the hypertension, the Guillain Barré syndrome, or a primary cause. The advantages and the drawbacks of the EuroQol 5D are shown in Table 8.8.

We believe that using time-tradeoff utility analysis is actually a more simplistic way to obtain utility values than using multiattribute instruments. Anything that can simplify the relatively difficult process of cost-utility analysis should be welcomed.

Health Utilities Index

Three forms of the Health Utilities Index (HUI1, HUI2, and HUI3) have been developed.[1] It is scored in a manner similar to the EuroQol 5D. The HUI1, based in part on the Quality-of-Well-Being Scale, utilized community-based time-tradeoff utilities, while the HUI2 and the HUI3 utilizes standard-gamble utilities. A visual analog scale is also employed. They are based upon a health states classification system and one or more scoring formulas. The most recent, the HUI3, uses complex multiplicative and multilinear models to calculate the disutilities in eight domains:

1. vision,
2. hearing,
3. speech,
4. dexterity,
5. mobility,
6. emotion,
7. cognition, and
8. pain.

TABLE 8.8

Advantages and Drawbacks of the EuroQol 5D

Advantages
1. It is applicable to all health states.
2. It uses prescored utility values.
3. Theoretically it permits the rapid evaluation of any health state.

Drawbacks
1. Its range is not between 0.0 and 1.0, and thus must be adjusted.
2. It is insensitive to milder health states.[42]
3. It is insensitive to severe health states.[43]
4. It is not compatible with ICD-9-CM and CPT® diagnostic and procedure codes[5]; thus, values must be correlated to ICD-9 and CPT format in the United States for use in cost-utility analysis.
5. It is difficult to separate out the contribution of individual diseases when multiple diseases are present.
6. Its underlying utility values are community-based, not patient-based.
7. It treats depression and anxiety, two markedly different diseases, synonymously.

CPT indicates Current Procedural Terminology; ICD-9-CM, *International Classification of Diseases, Ninth Revision, Clinical Modification.*

The HUI3 takes approximately ten minutes for self-administration, but only two to three minutes for interviewer-administration. In essence, it is a multiattribute combination of utility values for the eight parameters previously mentioned. The score ranges essentially between 0.0 and 1.0, allowing the methodology to be used for cost-utility analyses.

We believe that, while useful at times, this multiattribute utility value derived from the general population has shortcomings similar to those of the EuroQol 5D. It is no more applicable to the disease-specific, United States reimbursement system than the simpler time-tradeoff utility analysis. Advantages and drawbacks of the Health Utilities Index are listed in Table 8.9.

WHICH METHOD IS BEST?

Different preference-based instruments and different elicitation techniques are both known to produce different utility values for use in cost-utility analysis.[15,33,45] Because these values are not comparable, the decision about which instrument to use in a cost-utility analysis is critically important. In 1996, the Panel on Cost-Effectiveness in Health and Medicine did not to come to a conclusion about which was the best preference-based assessment technique for use in cost-utility analysis.[4]

Several facts deserve note in this regard. First, there is no perfect method to measure health-related quality of life. But of equal importance is the fact that

TABLE 8.9

Advantages and Drawbacks of the Health Utilities Index

Advantages

1. It is applicable to all health states.
2. It uses prescored utility values.
3. Theoretically it permits the rapid evaluation of any health state (ten minutes when self-administered and two to three minutes when interviewer-administered).[1]

Drawbacks

1. It is not compatible with ICD-9-CM and CPT® diagnostic and procedure codes[5]; thus, values must be converted to ICD-9 format in the United States for use in cost-utility analysis.
2. It is difficult to separate out the contribution of individual diseases when multiple diseases are present.
3. Its underlying utility values are community-based, not patient-based.
4. It is insensitive to health states such as organ transplantation.

CPT indicates Current Procedural Terminology; ICD-9-CM, *International Classification of Diseases, Ninth Revision, Clinical Modification.*

the lack of widespread acceptance of any quality-of-life measure prevents the establishment of a meaningful system of value-based medicine (VBM) for use in healthcare policy decisions. This indecisiveness over a methodology will continue to hinder the development of standardized cost-utility analyses unless someone or some group chooses a methodology and stays with it. This latter aspect of selecting a quality-of-life instrument and staying with it is as important as which quality-of-life instrument is used.

> The indecisiveness over use of a quality-of-life instrument for cost-utility analysis is a major reason this form of healthcare economic analysis has not yet been incorporated into public policy.

> Selecting a quality-of-life instrument for the development of VBM quality standards and staying with it is as important as the instrument chosen.

At this time, we believe time-tradeoff utility analysis is the most suitable health-related quality-of-life measure to use in cost-utility analysis to create a database for VBM. Ideally, the quality-of-life values obtained should come from a population-based sample of patients with diseases under study, meaning that a representative cross section of the public should be utilized. While the time-tradeoff method may not be perfect, we believe a value-based system incorporating it would be far superior to the haphazard systems of healthcare practice in the United States at the present time.

> Currently, the peer-reviewed literature and our experience at the Center for Value-Based Medicine suggest that time-tradeoff utility analysis is best suited to quantify the quality-of-life improvement used in cost-utility analysis.

Will time-tradeoff utility analysis always be the best method to measure value and use in cost-utility analysis? Not necessarily. Scaling instruments have potential and more research is indicated in this area. But at this point, time-tradeoff utility analysis appears to the most reliable preference-based instrument, is well understood by patients, and the results are compatible with the diagnostic and billing system in the United States. Thus, we emphasize the use of time-tradeoff utility analysis in this text. The most critical factor for establishing comparable cost-utility analyses and a VBM database to create healthcare quality standards is to pick the health-related quality-of-life instrument deemed most fitting and use it for cost-utility analyses across all interventions in healthcare. At the current time, time-tradeoff utility analysis best fits that description.

> The most critical factor for the establishment of a VBM database is to pick the health-related quality-of-life instrument deemed best and use it for cost-utility analyses across all interventions in health-care. In essence—pick it and run with it!

CORE CONCEPTS

- Preference-based instruments measure the quality of life associated with a health state.
- Included among preference-based health-related quality-of-life instruments are:
  - utility values (standard gamble, willingness to pay, and time tradeoff),
  - rating scales, and
  - multiattribute utility value instruments.
- All preference-based quality-of-life instruments are *generic.*
- All preference-based quality-of-life instruments can be used in cost-utility analysis.
- Utility instruments require patients to choose between their current health or the alternative of normal health for which they must risk or trade some-thing of value in return.
- Utility values generally vary from a lower anchor of death (0.0) to an upper anchor of permanent normal health (1.0).
- The closer the utility value is to 0.0, the poorer the quality of life associated with a health state, while the closer the utility value is to 1.0, the better the quality of life associated with a health state.
- Standard-gamble utility analysis is performed by asking patients what per-cent risk of immediate death, if any, they would be willing to assume if the alternative is permanent normal health. The percent risk assumed is sub-tracted from 1.0 to arrive at the utility value.
- Willingness-to-pay utility analysis is performed by asking patients what pro-portion of their monthly wage (or some other amount), if any, they would be willing to pay in return for permanent normal health. The proportion paid is subtracted from 1.0 to arrive at the utility value.
- Time-tradeoff utility analysis is performed by asking patients what propor-tion of their theoretically remaining time of life, if any, they would trade in return for permanent normal health. This proportion is subtracted from 1.0 to arrive at the utility value.
- Continuous scaling (rating) instruments ask patients to choose a point esti-mate from 0 to 100 (or 0.00 to 1.00) which they believe correlates with the quality of life associated with their health state or disease.
- While only the standard gamble utility is believed to be a true *von Neumann Morgenstern utility* because it deals with uncertainty, we and others believe it

is reasonable to include time-tradeoff values, willingness-to-pay values, and rating-scale values as utilities for use in cost-utility analysis.

■ It is important that a health-related quality-of-life instrument have the capability to be correlated with the International Classification of Diseases and Current Procedural Terminology (CPT®) codes, both of which are utilized for healthcare intervention payment in the United States.

■ Multiattribute instruments (EuroQol and the Health Utilities Index) ask questions about quality-of-life dimensions (mobility, self-care, usual activity, pain/discomfort, anxiety/discomfort) and subtract disutility values associated with each dimension from 1.0 to arrive at a final utility value.

■ Time-tradeoff utility analysis currently appears to the health-related quality-of-life instrument best suited for use in cost-utility analysis to create VBM standards.

■ Among the preference-based quality-of-life instruments, time-tradeoff utility analysis appears to be the most reproducible.

■ Continuous scaling (rating) instruments merit additional study for use in cost-utility analysis.

REFERENCES

1. Drummond MF, O'Brien B, Stoddart GL, Torrance GW. *Methods for the Economic Evaluation of Health Care Programmes.* 2nd ed. Oxford, England: Oxford University Press; 2000:139–199.

2. Brown GC, Brown MM, Sharma S. Cost-utility analysis. *Ann Intern Med.* 2001;134:625–626.

3. Siegel JE, Weinstein MC, Russell LB, Gold MR. Recommendations for reporting cost-effectiveness analyses: Panel on Cost-Effectiveness in Health and Medicine. *JAMA.* 1996;276:1339–1341.

4. Weinstein MC, Siegel JE, Gold MR, Kamlet MS, Russell LB. Recommendations of the Panel on Cost-Effectiveness in Health and Medicine. *JAMA.* 1996;276:1253–1258.

5. Hart AC, Hopkins CA, eds. *International Classification of Diseases, Ninth Revision, Clinical Modification.* Salt Lake City, Utah: Ingenix; 2003.

6. Cooper R, Rappoport P. Were the ordinalists wrong about welfare economics? *J Economic Literature.* 1984;22:507–530.

7. Miyamoto JM. Generic utility theory: measurement foundations and applications in multi-attribute utility theory. *J Mathematics Psychol.* 1988;32:357–404.

8. Von Neumann J, Morgensterno. *The Theory of Games and Economic Behavior.* London, England: Princeton University Press; 1944:647.

9. Klarman H, Francis J, Rosenthal G. Cost-effectiveness applied to the treatment of chronic renal disease. *Med Care.* 1968;6:48–55.

10. Torrance GW, Thomas W, Sackett D. A utility maximization model for evaluation of health care programs. *Health Serv Res.* 1972;7:118–133.

11. Torrance GW. Social preference for health states: an empirical evaluation of three measurement techniques. *Socioecon Planning Sci.* 1976;10:129–136.

12. Kassirer JP. Incorporating patient's preferences into medical decisions. *N Engl J Med.* 1994;330:1895–1896.

13. Chapman RH, Stone PW, Sandberg EA, Bell C, Neumann PJ. A comprehensive league table of cost-utility ratios and a sub-table of "panel-worthy" studies. *Med Decis Making.* 2000;20:451–467.

14. Redelmeier DA, Detsky AS. A clinician's guide to utility measurement. *Med Decis Making.* 1995;22:271–280.

15. Brown GC. Vision and quality of life. *Trans Am Ophthalmol Soc.* 1999;97:473–512.

16. Tsevat J, Cook EF, Green ML, et al. Health values of the seriously ill. *Ann Intern Med.* 1995;122:514–520.

17. Donaldson C, Shackley P. Does "process utility" exist? A case study of willingness to pay for laparoscopic cholecystectomy. *Soc Sci Med.* 1997;44:699–707.

18. Ethgen O, Tancredi A, Lejeune E, Kvasz A, Zegels B, Reginster JY. Do utility values and willingness-to-pay suitably reflect health outcome in hip and knee osteoarthritis? A comparative analysis with the WOMAC Index. *J Rheumatol.* 2003;30:2452–2459.

19. Stein J, Brown GC, Brown MM, Sharma S, Hollandsh, Stein HD. The quality of life of patients with hypertension. *J Clin Hypertens.* 2002;4:181–188.

20. Duncan PW, Lai SM, Keighley J. Defining post-stroke recovery: implications for design and interpretation of drug trials. *Neuropharmacology.* 2000;39:835–841.

21. Sox HC, Blatt MA, Higgins MC, Marton KI. *Medical Decision Making.* Toronto, Ontario: Butterworth; 1988:406.

22. Wakker P, Stiggelbout A. Explaining distortions in utility elicitation through the rank-dependent model for risky choices. *Med Decis Making.* 1995;15:180–186.

23. Schelling TC. The life you save may be your own. In: Chase SB, ed. *Problems in Public Expenditure Analysis.* Washington, DC: Brookings Institution; 1966.

24. Cuningham SJ, Hunt NP. Relationship between utility values and willingness to pay in patients undergoing orthognathic treatment. *Community Dent Health.* 2000;17:92–96.

25. Kartman B, Andersson F, Johannesson M. Willingness to pay in angina pectoris attacks. *Med Decis Making.* 1996;16:248–253.

26. Petitti DB. *Meta-Analysis, Decision Analysis and Cost-Effectiveness Analysis.* 2nd ed. New York, NY: Oxford University Press; 2000:169–181.

27. Smith RD. The relative sensitivity of willingness-to-pay and time-tradeoff to changes in health status: an empirical investigation. *Health Econ.* 2001;10:487–497.

28. Frew E, Wolstenholme JL, Whynes DK. Willingness-to-pay for colorectal cancer screening. *Eur J Cancer.* 2001;37:1746–1751.

29. O'Brien B, Viramontes JL. Willingness-to-pay: a valid and reliable measure of health state preference? *Med Decis Making.* 1994;14:289–297.

30. Gan TJ, Ing RJ, de L Dear G, Wright D, E-Moalem HE, Lubarsky DA. How much are patients willing to pay to avoid intraoperative awareness? *J Clin Anesth.* 2003;15:108–112.

31. Gold MR, Patrick DL, Torrance GW, et al. Identifying and valuing outcomes. In: Gold MR, Siegel JE, Russel LB, Weinstein MC, eds. *Effectiveness in Health and Medicine.* New York, NY: Oxford University Press; 1996:82–134.

32. Jampel HD, Friedman DS, Quigley H, Miller R. Correlation of the binocular visual field with patient assessment of vision. *Invest Ophthalmol Vis Sci.* 2002;43:1059–1067.

33. Read JL, Quinn DM, Berwick DM, Fineberg HV, Weinstein MC. Preferences for health outcomes: comparisons of assessment methods. *Med Decis Making.* 1984;4:215–329.

34. Froberg DG, Kane RL. Methodology for measuring health state preferences, II: scaling methods. *J Clin Epidemiol.* 1989;42:459–471.

35. Keeney R, Raiffa H. *Decisions With Multiple Objectives: Preferences and Value Tradeoffs.* New York, NY: John Wiley & Sons; 1976.

36. Rosner B. *Fundamentals of Biostatistics.* 5th ed. Pacific Grove, Calif: Duxbury Thomson Learning; 2000:451–453, 562–565.

37. Froberg DG, Kane RL. Methodology for measuring health-state preferences, I: measurement strategies. *J Clin Epidemiol.* 1989;42:345–354.

38. Bonita R, Beaglehole R. Modification of Rankin Scale: recovery of motor function after stroke. *Stroke.* 1988;19:1497–1500.

39. EuroQol Group. EuroQol: a new facility for the measurement of health-related quality of life. *Health Policy.* 1990;16:199–208.

40. Dolan P, Gudex C. Time preference, duration and health state valuations. *Health Econ.* 1995;4:289-299.

41. Dloan P, Gudex C, Kind P, Williams A. The time tradeoff method: results from a general population study. *Health Econ.* 1996;5:141-154.

42. Joore MA, Van Der Stel H, Peters HJ, Boas GM, Anteunis LJ. The cost-effectiveness of hearing-aid fitting in the Netherlands. *Arch Otolaryngol Head Neck Surg.* 2003;129:297–304.

43. Granja C, Teixeira-Pinto A, Costa-Pereira A. Quality of life after intensive care— evaluation with EQ-5D questionnaire. *Intensive Care Med.* 2002;28:898–907.

44. Brown MM, Brown GC, Sharma S, Hollands H. Quality-of-life and systemic comorbidities in patients with ophthalmic disease. *Br J Ophthalmol.* 2002;86:8–11.

45. Bakker C, van der Linden S. Health related utility measurement: an introduction. *J Rheumatol.* 1995;22:1197–1199.

c h a p t e r

9

Time-Tradeoff
Utility Analysis

No quality-of-life instrument is or ever will be perfect. But the absence of a universal model has been a major factor responsible for the lack of acceptance of cost-utility analysis for healthcare policy-making decisions. While we are waiting for the perfect model, healthcare costs continue to rise well above general inflation, care is inaccessible to more than 40 million people, and quality is substandard compared to what it could be. Thus, selecting the best instrument available and using it to standardize cost-utility analyses to create a value-based medicine (VBM) database is of paramount importance.

> While we are waiting for the perfect cost-utility model, healthcare costs continue to rise well above general inflation, care is inaccessible to more than 40 million people, and quality is substandard compared to what it could be.

THE PREFERRED
QUALITY-OF-LIFE INSTRUMENT

We agree with the Panel on Cost-Effectiveness in Health and Medicine that a preference-based instrument should be used in cost-utility analysis.[1,2] Preference-based instruments theoretically encompass all aspects of health-related quality of life, have a minimal burden of administration, and require a patient to devote considerable heedful thought, especially the time-tradeoff and standard-gamble utility analysis variants.

After extensive use of the time-tradeoff utility analysis method, the standard-gamble method, and other preference-based and non–preference-based quality-of-life instruments, we believe at this time that time-tradeoff utility analysis

> Time-tradeoff utility analysis using patient preferences is a most suitable quality-of-life measurement instrument for use in cost-utility analysis.

using patient preferences is a most suitable instrument for use in cost-utility analyses for healthcare policy-making decisions.[3–7]

Time-tradeoff utility analysis has the following advantageous features for use as a quality-of-life instrument in cost-utility analysis. The advantages include:

1. excellent short-term and good long-term reliability (reproducibility) (see Table 8.6 in Chapter 8),[8–11]
2. excellent intraobserver and interobserver reliability (see Table 8.6 in Chapter 8),
3. excellent construct validity (see Chapter 10),
4. applicability across all specialties,
5. good patient comprehension,
6. a low burden of administration,
7. facility of incorporation into clinical trials (when correlated with other quality-of-life instruments used in the trials),
8. facility of correlating with the *International Classification of Diseases,*
9. good sensitivity with most health states including milder and more severe health states, and
10. consistency across gender, level of education, age, ethnicity, income, national borders, and the presence of comorbidities.[3,7,12–15]

> The time-tradeoff method is the most reliable (reproducible) form of utility analysis.

> Throughout the remainder of this book we consider *preferences* and *utilities* to be synonymous with *time-tradeoff utility analysis values.*

Willingness-to-Pay Utility Analysis

The fact that those with more financial resources are willing to pay more for return to a normal health state[16,17] is a serious drawback of the willingness-to-pay methodology. It also demonstrates very poor long-term reproducibility (correlation coefficient $[r] = 0.25$ at one year).[18] We therefore do not recommend that it be employed in developing a standardized quality-of-life database for use in cost-utility analysis.

Standard-Gamble Utility Analysis

Many respondents do not understand the standard-gamble question. In addition, there is risk aversion to the concept of immediate death.[19] Therefore, the standard-gamble method tends to be insensitive to the measurement of less serious health states, such as treated systemic arterial hypertension, that have a minimal effect on quality of life. Of critical importance also is the fact that the test-retest reliability (reproducibility) for the time-tradeoff methodology is superior to that of the standard-gamble methodology on both a short-term basis (respective correlation coefficients of 0.87 vs 0.80) and a long-term basis (respective correlation coefficients of 0.62 vs 0.53).[18,20] (See Table 8.6 in Chapter 8.)

In a study of 323 consecutive patients evaluated with both time-tradeoff and standard-gamble instruments, we found the Pearson correlation between standard-gamble and time-tradeoff utility values to be 0.662. The r^2 was 0.438, indicating that the standard-gamble utility scores explained 43.8% of the variance of time-tradeoff utility scores and vice versa. These data support the data of Read and associates,[10] who noted that standard-gamble and time-tradeoff methods are not interchangeable.

Rating Scales

While there is a reasonable rationale for using rating scales in cost-utility analysis, more research on this instrument is needed. Rating scales have good sensitivity to milder health states, but the reproducibility of rating scale values is not as good as the reproducibility of time-tradeoff values and standard-gamble values.[18] However, the greatest drawback to rating scales occurs when a scale is used to evaluate diseases in which death is not generally encountered. For example, patients with onychomycosis (fungal infection of the nails) often have a difficult time conceptualizing where the quality of life associated with their disease lies on a scale from 0 (death) to 100 (perfect health). If a scale with anchors of 0.00 (poorest nail health) to 1.00 (normal nail health) is used, the difficulty then arises on how to integrate this scale with one that ranges from 0.00 (death) to 1.00 (normal permanent health).

Multiattribute Utility Instruments

Both the EuroQol 5D and the Health Utilities Index provide valuable information and deserve further study. However, the lack sensitivity for select diseases and the fact that they are generally based upon values previously obtained from the general public, rather than from patients with a disease under study, are drawbacks to their use.

Are the Instruments Interchangeable?

Unfortunately, time-tradeoff values, standard-gamble values, rating-scale values, and multiattribute values are not interchangeable.[10] Therefore, cost-utility analyses performed with one of these preference-based quality-of-life instruments are

> The values obtained from standard-gamble utility analysis, time-tradeoff utility analysis, willingness-to-pay utility analysis, rating scales, and multiattribute instruments are not interchangeable.

> The same quality-of-life measurement instrument must be used for cost-utility analyses to be comparable.

comparable only with cost-utility analyses that use the same quality-of-life instrument.

Studies that have compared time-tradeoff and standard-gamble methodologies have typically found standard-gamble utility values to be higher than time-tradeoff utility values, which in turn are higher than rating scales for the same health state.[1,3,5,8,10,14,21,22] As an example, one of our subjects with moderate to severe lower limb neuropathy had a standard-gamble utility value of 0.90, a time-tradeoff utility value of 0.80, and rating scale value of 0.70 associated with the neuropathy.

> **Preferences for the same health state:**
> SG > TTO > RS
> in which SG indicates standard-gamble utility analysis; TTO, time tradeoff utility analysis; and RS, rating scale.

COMPLIANCE AND TIME-TRADEOFF UTILITY VALUES

When patients with obvious dementia from Alzheimer disease or other causes are excluded, approximately 97% of consecutive adult patients are able to successfully answer time-tradeoff utility questions.[5,8,12,23] Those who cannot typically have difficulty conceptualizing the theory or may not wish to answer for what they term as religious reasons. Trust in the interviewer is a critical aspect for obtaining reliable and valid utility values, especially because utility instruments require asking a person to trade time of life or risk life itself. Our experiences with many interviewers suggest that the empathetic interviewer will be considerably more successful than the dispassionate interviewer in obtaining valid, reproducible utility values.

> The empathetic utility value interviewer will be considerably more successful in obtaining reliable and valid utility values than the dispassionate interviewer.

UTILITY VALUES IN THE LITERATURE

The most comprehensive list of utility values in publication is probably that of Tengs and Wallace,[24] in which 1,000 health-related quality-of-life estimates are reported using various quality-of-life instruments and various respondents. The report demonstrates the great need for a quality-of-life database that is standardized according to the type of instrument and the respondent population. Because of the lack of standardization of the quality-of-life instruments used and the respondents solicited, most utility values in the literature are incomparable. Due to the large number of utility values reported, however, some can be compared.

Utility values can be ascertained from the peer-reviewed literature database of the National Library of Medicine, which contains the abstracts of more than

15 million articles and can be accessed via the Internet at www.ncbi.nlm.nih.gov. There is also variation in the literature among utility values with the same disease and severity of disease, as values obtained span the work of many researchers. For cost-utility analyses for which utility values are not available in the literature, the researcher may have to obtain utility values from a cohort of patients with the health state to be analyzed using the methodology described in Chapter 8.

Examples of time-tradeoff utility values obtained from patients are shown in Tables 9.1 and 9.2. Those from the Beaver Dam Health Outcomes Study (Table 9.2) are useful for some analyses, but they are limited in that they do not take into account the severity of the majority of the conditions studied.

TABLE 9.1

Patient-Derived Time-Tradeoff Utility Values Associated With Systemic Health States*

Health State	Utility Value	Reference
AIDS	0.70	Tengs and Lin[25]
HIV, Symptomatic	0.82	Tengs and Lin[25]
HIV, Asymptomatic	0.94	Tengs and Lin[25]
Angina, Mild	0.88	Phillips et al[26]
Angina, Moderate	0.83	Phillips et al[26]
Angina, Severe	0.53	Phillips et al[26]
Atrial Fibrillation (Use of Warfarin)	0.99	Gage et al[27]
Breast Cancer, Early Stage, Lumpectomy or Mastectomy	0.94	Hayman et al[28]
Breast Cancer, Radiotherapy	0.89	Hayman et al[28]
Breast Cancer, Chemotherapy	0.74	Hayman et al[28]
Diabetes Mellitus	0.88	Brown et al[12]
Impotence and Incontinence After TURP	0.60	Krummins et al[29]
Myocardial Infarction, Mild	0.91	Tsevat et al[30]
Myocardial Infarction, Moderate	0.80	Tsevat et al[30]
Myocardial Infarction, Severe	0.30	Tsevat et al[30]
Osteoarthritis, Hip, Mild	0.69	Laupacis et al[31]
Osteoarthritis, Hip, Six Months After Surgery	0.82	Laupacis et al[31]
Prostate Cancer, No Symptoms	0.78	Chapman et al[32]
Prostate Cancer, Moderate Symptoms	0.72	Chapman et al[32]
Prostate Cancer, Severe Symptoms	0.35	Chapman et al[32]
Renal Disease, Hemodialysis	0.57	Laupacis et al[33]
Renal Disease, Kidney Transplant, 12 Months After Surgery		Laupacis et al[33]
Stroke, Minor Residual Effects	0.89	Tengs et al[34]

continued

TABLE   9.1 continued

Patient-Derived, Time-Tradeoff Utility Values Associated with Systemic Health States*

Health State	Utility Value	Reference
Stroke, Major	0.30	Tengs et al[34]
Ulcerative Colitis, Preoperative	0.58	McLeod et al[35]
Ulcerative Colitis, One Year After Surgery	0.98	McLeod et al[35]
Visual Loss, 20/40 Better Eye	0.80	Brown[3]
Visual Loss, 20/200 Better Eye	0.66	Brown[3]

TURP indicates transurethral resection of the prostate.

* Adapted from Brown et al.[36]

DEFINING THE HEALTH STATE

The exact health state or disease measured by time-tradeoff utility analysis or another quality-of-life instrument must be well defined. With time-tradeoff analysis subjects are asked what proportion of their remaining time of life they are willing to trade in return for normal health. The important question in defining the health state is, what exactly is the time traded for? If a person is guaranteed an immediate cure for systemic arterial hypertension, including the complications it has caused (stroke, nephropathy, cardiomyopathy, and so on), the answer will be different than if the person is guaranteed a cure for the hypertension, but with no effect (other than lack of further progression) upon the complications that have already occurred secondary to the hypertension. Furthermore, is the patient trading time for treated hypertension or untreated hypertension? And for what level of hypertension? Is it mild or malignant hypertension?

Researchers have used various methods to describe health states associated with utility values. Many researchers utilize a disease-specific or holistic classification system, in which utility values are assigned to health states defined in well-known disease diagnosis format, with explicit definitions of levels of severity of affliction.[20] We see the use of a disease-specific classification system as a logical format given its current use for billing purposes by the public and private sectors. Since the Medicare Catastrophic Coverage Act of 1988 was instituted in April 1989, providers have been required to include diagnosis codes when providing services to Medicare beneficiaries.[37] The Centers for Medicare and Medicaid Services currently require providers to submit bills using the *International Classification of Diseases, Ninth Revision, Clinical Modification* (ICD-9-CM).[37] Cost-utility analyses used for policy decisions in the United States should therefore utilize the same standardized diagnostic nomenclature to facilitate their incorporation into public policy decisions.

Using decomposed or multiattribute measures[20] such as the EuroQol 5D,[38] which are not specific for any disease, requires additional steps to apply these

TABLE 9.2

Time-Tradeoff Utility Values of Patients Currently Affected (or Affected in the Past) With 28 Common Conditions*

Disease	Incidence (n = 1,358)	TTO Utility Value
Arthritis	44%	0.815
Gout	4%	0.859
Severe Back Pain	18%	0.786
Severe Neck Pain	7%	0.765
Migraine	5%	0.817
Angina	5%	0.786
Congestive Heart Failure	2%	0.710
Myocardial Infarction	1%	0.729
Stroke	1%	0.903
Hypertension	35%	0.830
Hyperlipidemia	8%	0.902
Cataract	23%	0.821
Glaucoma	5%	0.824
Macular Degeneration	3%	0.754
Diabetes, Insulin-Dependent	3%	0.627
Diabetes, Non–Insulin-Dependent	6%	0.761
Asthma	3%	0.706
Emphysema	3%	0.751
Chronic Bronchitis	3%	0.724
Chronic Sinusitis	7%	0.874
Depression	4%	0.703
Anxiety	4%	0.774
Ulcer	6%	0.790
Colitis	4%	0.815
Hiatal Hernia	3%	0.845
Sleep Disorder	10%	0.790
Thyroid Disorder	6%	0.882
Miscellaneous Allergies	2%	0.844

TTO indicates time tradeoff.

* Source: 1,356 interviewees in the Beaver Dam Health Outcomes Study.[23]

tools to each individual disease (health state). Instead of asking the two-part time-tradeoff utility analysis question, the researcher must ask five questions related to the dimensions of the disease. (See Chapter 8.)

W e see the use of a disease-specific (holistic) classification system as a logical format, given the current acceptance by the Centers for Medicare and Medicaid Services, as well as private payers, of the *International Classification of Diseases, Ninth Revision, Clinical Modification.*[37]

Because of the importance of defining and strictly delineating the disease in question, we prefer an *interviewer-administered* time-tradeoff instrument, as an astute subject often has questions and/or makes individually unique assumptions. These include "gaming" the system to avoid taking risk. In regard to treated hypertension, questions might include:

1. Do we assume that only the hypertension is cured for the trade, or are all associated hypertension-related complications (stroke, nephropathy, cardiomyopathy, and so on) cured as well?

2. Do we assume that the hypertension is being treated or is not treated? Also, how is it treated?

3. Can another therapy, such as switching from a beta-blocker to an angiotensin-converting enzyme inhibitor, be substituted without trading time?

If the disease under study is osteoarthritis of the hip, one patient might assume that the question refers to untreated osteoarthritis, while another might assume it refers to osteoarthritis treated with an over-the-counter nonsteroidal anti-inflammatory agent (NSAID), and a third might think, "Why not just obtain a total hip replacement and trade no time?" The utility value would be expected to be different for each of the three scenarios. In regard to defining the utility value associated with the primary untreated disease, the clarification should be made that the only way to receive a cure is to trade time, rather than simply institute a pharmaceutical and/or surgical intervention and not trade time.

Utility analysis studies must very specifically define:
1. the disease or health state,
2. the severity of the disease,
3. whether the disease is untreated or treated,
4. how comorbidities related to the primary disease are handled, and
5. the fact that the only way to obtain a guaranteed cure is to trade theoretical time of remaining life.

THE SEVERITY OF DISEASE

Some investigators[23] have evaluated time-tradeoff utility values in patients by inquiring about general conditions such as arthritis, congestive heart failure, stroke, and other common diseases. Unfortunately, much of this information cannot be used in cost-utility analysis because the severity of these diseases is not specified. For example, in the Beaver Dam Study, Fryback et al[23] noted that the mean time-tradeoff utility value associated with stroke was 0.90. However, Tengs and associates[34] noted in an extensive literature review that time-tradeoff utility values range from 0.89 for mild stroke to 0.30 for severe stroke. Obviously, the utility value associated with stroke varies dramatically depending upon the severity of the stroke. For the greatest reliability and validity in the performance of utility value analysis, it is critical to quantify the severity of a disease associated with a utility value.

The utility analysis researcher must therefore decide beforehand exactly the healthcare condition he or she is investigating, usually one specific disease of a specific severity. The severity, or stage when referring to many cancers, must be defined in some categorical way, such as using the American College of Rheumatology (ACR) Classification of Global Functional Status in Rheumatoid Arthritis[39,40] or using the Karnofsky Performance Status Scale.[41] Obviously, the answers can be very different depending upon the possible circumstances outlined. We have noted the utility value associated with untreated ACR Class III osteoarthritis (limited in performing vocational and avocational activities) to be 0.79, while conversion of Class III to Class II disease (limited in performing avocational activities) by the use of an over-the-counter, nonsteroidal anti-inflammatory agent raises the utility value to 0.95. In some instances, the definitions of *mild, moderate,* and *severe disease* can be correlated with utility values, but we have not found these categories as useful as the categorical scales such as the ACR Classification or the Karnofsky Performance Status Scale.

Can Multiple Utility Values for the Same Disease Be Obtained From One Patient?

Yes. Some patients can provide a wealth of utility values regarding one disease depending upon the disease severity at different times. For example, a patient with American Heart Association Functional Capacity Class IV angina (angina at rest) will readily appreciate the degree to which this severe disease affects quality of life.[42–44] If the angina is treated with a beta blocker and improves to Class II (angina with ordinary activity), then improves to Class I (no angina with ordinary activity) after coronary artery bypass graft, the patient is typically able to express a preference (number of years traded for time-tradeoff utility analysis) for each of the three health states.

Can Multiple Utility Values for Different Diseases Be Obtained From One Patient?

Yes. Utility analysis can assess the quality-of-life loss attributable to an individual disease even if a patient has multiple diseases. For example, in a person with congestive heart failure, osteoarthritis, and benign prostatic hypertrophy, utility values can be obtained for each of these individual entities by asking what proportion of remaining years of life a person would be willing to trade in return for eradication of the heart failure, eradication of the arthritis, and eradication of the prostate hypertrophy, respectively.

We have observed the lowest utility value associated with the most severe disease is generally the value patients would trade to be rid of their multiple diseases. Rather than demonstrating additive properties, the most severe disease typically dominates less severe diseases in contributing to an overall health utility value. Consequently, if the utility value for heart failure is 0.65, that for arthritis is 0.80, and that for prostatic hypertrophy is 0.95, the patient most often relates a utility value of 0.65 for overall total health rather than a total disutility of –0.60. The same patient would typically trade seven of 20 years (utility = 0.65) to be rid of the heart failure and seven of 20 years (utility = 0.65) to eradicate the heart failure, arthritis, and prostatic hypertrophy.

The lowest utility value among those associated with multiple diseases in a respondent is often similar to a person's overall health utility value.

The reason VBM should be incorporated into public policy: *value-based medicine greatly benefits patients.*

Does Utility Analysis Have an Advantage When Multiple Diseases Are Present in the Same Patient?

Yes. While utility analysis can select out individual diseases very effectively, other quality-of-life instruments have difficulty differentiating between multiple diseases. For example, with time-tradeoff utility analysis it is possible to separate out disease entities by asking a patient with diabetes, diabetic neuropathy, and diabetic nephropathy what proportion of remaining years he or she is willing to trade to be rid of the diabetes, the neuropathy, the nephropathy, or all three conditions. Most patients can very readily visualize and conceptually grasp the thought of the time they would trade for a cure of each condition.

Patients can readily differentiate the proportion of life's time traded for the eradication of each disease when multiple diseases are present.

This type of disease-specific measure in which the diseases are separated out is more difficult to perform with an instrument such as the 36-Item Short-Form Health Survey (SF-36)[45] or a multiattribute instrument such as the EuroQol 5D.[38] The SF-36 would require 36 questions for each disease, and there would likely be overlap among the diseases contributing to the inability to perform certain tasks or the adverse effects experienced. The EuroQol 5D requires five dimension questions for each disease, with the overlap of diseases again theoretically posing a differentiation problem.

HOW DEMOGRAPHIC VARIABLES AFFECT TIME-TRADEOFF UTILITY VALUES

Demographic variables describe a population of patients and include adult age, ethnicity, gender, level of education, and income bracket. These variables have been shown repeatedly to not affect, or negligibly affect, time-tradeoff utility values.[3,5,12,46–50] We have found time-tradeoff variables are similar across state borders and even across national borders.[11] Time-tradeoff utility values appear to be innate to human nature rather than affected by demographics.

> Time-tradeoff utility values are generally unaffected by age, ethnicity, gender, level of education, and income bracket.

Despite the lack of a confounding effect of demographic variables upon utility values, we believe a utility value database used to perform cost-utility analyses for healthcare resource allocation should be population-based for the United States, thereby reflecting the general ethnic, educational, and income strata encountered across the entire US population. Values obtained without diversity of these variables, such as the case with those obtained in the Beaver Dam Health Outcomes Study (99.6% of subjects were white),[23] would likely meet stiff sociopolitical resistance if proposed for use for public policy purposes, especially for resource allocation decisions.

> Time-tradeoff utility values appear to be innate to human nature.

HOW SHOULD WE HANDLE COMORBIDITIES?

Comorbidities are additional, or secondary, health conditions that accompany a primary disease under study. For example, if diabetic neuropathy is the primary disease of interest, possible comorbidities would likely include the diabetic-related problems of nephropathy, neuropathy, retinopathy, peripheral vascular disease, and gastroparesis. If someone has comorbidities, should these affect a reference case cost-utility analysis for an intervention? The question is important and has been handled in different ways by different researchers.

What Is the Prevalence of Comorbidities in the Adult Population?

The Beaver Dam Health Outcomes Study is a longitudinal cohort study that enrolled adults between the ages of 43 and 84 years living in Beaver Dam,

Wisconsin.[23] Among 1,356 interviews completed over an 18-month period in 1991 and 1992, people were asked whether they were affected by 28 common conditions (Tables 9.2 and 9.3). Just over 18% of the subjects had none of these conditions and 20% had one, but 61.4% had more than one condition. Approximately one fourth were affected with at least four conditions and 13% were affected with five or more conditions. Extrapolating from this study to the overall population of the United States suggests that the most of middle-aged adults and senior citizens have at least one major condition that adversely affects health, while the majority have at least one comorbidity as well.

Over 60% of adults aged 43 to 84 years have at least one comorbidity in addition to a primary disease.

Time-tradeoff utility values for some diseases are unaffected by comorbidities, while with other diseases the utility values are affected by comorbidities.[12,13] Thus, comorbidities may or may not influence the utility value associated with a health state. Certainly, more research is needed in this area. The important question that arises, however, is how should comorbidities influence a cost-utility analysis? Should the value of the intervention of carotid endarterectomy for atherosclerotic obstruction be measured differently in a diabetic patient, than in a person with no comorbidities? Or should it be valued the same in each case?

TABLE 9.3

Number of Medical Conditions Affecting People in the Past Year*

Number of Conditions	Number of People (%) (n = 1,356)
0	248 (18.3%)
1	274 (20.2%)
2	274 (20.2%)
3	228 (16.8%)
4	159 (11.7%)
5	86 (6.3%)
6	45 (3.3%)
7	23 (1.7%)
8	11 (0.8%)
9	4 (0.3%)
10	4 (0.3%)

* Source: The Beaver Dam Health Outcomes Study.[23]

How Do We Handle Comorbidities in Assessing the Value Conferred by Interventions?

There is controversy in this area, but we believe that comorbidities associated with a health state under study should not generally influence the utility values used in cost-utility analyses. Why? Because this practice can discriminate against those who are handicapped or disadvantaged. Assessing a total hip arthroplasty as more valuable in someone who is otherwise in good systemic health than in someone who has had a kidney transplant and painful polyneuropathy is an example of discrimination against a person who is disabled by comorbidities.

Another clinical example readily illustrates the methodology some authors adhere to when measuring the value of an intervention in a person with no comorbidities vs someone with one or more comorbidities. Let us assume that a completely healthy group (other than for osteoarthritis of the hip) undergoes total hip arthroplasty that improves the mean utility value from 0.79 to 1.00. With no comorbidities present, there is a utility value improvement of 0.21 (1.00 − 0.79) conferred by the procedure.

Select researchers,[51,52] however, measure the *overall health utility* of a group and attribute the decreased utility from a specific abnormality, such as osteoarthritis of the hip, only to the additional decrement below the overall health utility value of the group. For example, if the overall health utility value for a population is 0.90 and patients associate a utility value of 0.79 with their osteoarthritis of the hip, these researchers attribute the utility loss due to the hip disease as 0.11 (0.90 − 0.79). The other 0.10 loss is attributed to the overall systemic diminution in quality of life. Thus, total hip arthroplasty with a perfect result in this group would therefore only yield an improvement of 0.11 in a patient cohort with comorbidities, substantially less than the 0.21 (1.00 − 0.79) value obtained when no utility loss from comorbidities is factored in.

Specific interventions can therefore be assigned greater value in patients with better systemic health compared to a population with more comorbidities. The implication follows that if healthcare resources are allocated, the intervention with greater value (in the healthier patient) would be given preference over the exact same intervention in the sicker patient because the intervention for the sicker patient confers lesser value.

While some researchers[51] believe failure to consider comorbidities falsely increases the value of an intervention, we believe just the opposite—integrating comorbidities is flawed and inappropriate because it diminishes the value of an intervention in a cohort with comorbidities compared to a cohort with otherwise perfect systemic health.[12,13,52–55] Furthermore, since an older population has more comorbidities than a younger population, the use of comorbidities would bias the value of interventions against older individuals, a concept we believe is unacceptable in a country with the resources of the US.

It is doubtful that the US public, the courts, or policy makers would accept any form of discrimination that values interventions more highly in patients with good health than in patients with poorer health. Even more importantly, however, the Americans With Disabilities Act of 1990 specifically prohibits discrimination against those with disabilities (Table 9.4).[56]

The Title III regulation of the Americans With Disabilities Act expressly states that *public accommodations must eliminate unnecessary eligibility standards that deny individuals with disabilities an equal opportunity to enjoy the goods and services of a place of public accommodation.*[57] Perfect health other than for the health condition of interest can certainly be considered as an eligibility standard. Included among places of public accommodations are doctors' offices and hospitals, and included among the goods and services of a place of public accommodation are healthcare interventions.

> The Title III regulation of the Americans With Disabilities Act of 1990 specifically states that *public accommodations [doctors' offices and hospitals] must eliminate unnecessary eligibility standards that deny individuals with disabilities an opportunity to enjoy the goods and services [healthcare interventions] of a place of public accommodation.*

Consequently, for public policy to adopt cost-utility analyses employing any methodology that denies individuals with disabilities an equal opportunity to enjoy the same healthcare interventions as a person with no disabilities would violate current written law. Diminishing the value conferred by an intervention because of comorbidities is exactly the type of violation prohibited by the Americans With Disabilities Act, especially when more systemically healthy patients are given preference over more disabled patients in receiving the same intervention.

Needless to say, a cost-utility analysis database developed using discriminatory methodology against a person or a population would not and should not be allowed to play a role in public policy. A VBM database developed for the allocation of healthcare resources should therefore be based upon calculations of quality-of-life estimates not influenced by comorbidities in a fashion that would

TABLE 9.4

Examples of Disabilities as per the Americans With Disabilities Act of 1990*

A disability is a physical or mental impairment that substantially affects one or more of life's major activities, including:

Walking	Speaking	Breathing
Performing manual tasks	Sitting	Lifting
Seeing	Hearing	Learning
Caring for oneself	Working	Reading

* Adapted from Gomez-Mejia et al.[56]

decrease the quality-of-life improvement conferred by interventions for those with comorbidities compared to otherwise healthy individuals.

> Generally, a cost-utility database developed for the allocation of healthcare resources should not be based upon quality-of-life estimates influenced by comorbidities in a fashion that would diminish the value conferred by an intervention for those with comorbidities as compared to those without comorbidities.

Comorbidities and More Comorbidities

The introduction of comorbidities into cost-utility analyses also increases the number of utility values and cost-utility analyses needed for a comprehensive VBM database by factorial amounts. For example, coronary artery angioplasty administered for ischemic heart disease occurs in primarily an older population. Factoring in the innumerable possible comorbidities of hypertension and/or arthritis and/or diabetes and/or emphysema, and so on, and their variant combinations would exponentially increase the number of required analyses for just one intervention for ischemic heart disease.

Just how many health state variations are possible by adding in variations in comorbidities? There are approximately 4,000 diagnoses in the *International Classification of Diseases, Ninth Revision.*[37] The factorial number—4,000!—yields a number beyond imagination, literally trillions times trillions of combinations. To calculate utility values associated for each of these possible variants, or cost-utility analyses for interventions to treat limitless diagnostic variants, is a virtual impossibility. Thus, the facts that there are strong legal precedents and political ramifications preventing the use of comorbidities for cost-utility analysis obviates the problem of the necessity of calculating utility values for an almost infinite number of health states when evaluating an intervention.

> Shortcomings of the use of comorbidities in assessing value conferred by interventions for use in cost-utility analysis include:
> 1. discrimination against the disabled,
> 2. violation of the Americans With Disabilities Act of 1990, and
> 3. an almost infinite number of cost-utility analyses required for just one intervention.

A major problem encountered by the Panel on Cost-Effectiveness in Health and Medicine was the inability to arrive at a clear-cut policy concerning the treatment of comorbidities. We have presented compelling reasons not to take comorbidities into account when quantifying the value conferred by healthcare interventions for public policy, thus overcoming at least one major hurdle standing in the path of the development of VBM quality standards.

UTILITY VALUE RESPONDENTS

A fundamental question surrounding utility theory concerns the most appropriate source of respondents for utility elicitation.[58] There are two general groups to choose from:

1. those who have personally experienced the health state under study, and
2. those who have not, also known as *surrogate respondents.*

Examples of people from the first group are patients with active disease or persons who have been afflicted with the disease in the past. The surrogate respondent group that has not experienced the disease firsthand might consist of the general public (community), people who are sick but who do not have the health state in question, a group of healthcare professionals, a group of experts (researchers and/or physicians), administrators, proxy respondents (relatives or others who live with a patient), or others (Table 9.5).[48,58]

While some may debate the pros and cons of one instrument or another, we believe there is no leeway in choosing the respondents from whom to obtain quality-of-life values—*they must be patients who live or have lived with a disease of interest.* We rigidly adhere to the fact that only those who have lived with a disease or in a health state firsthand are qualified to appreciate the quality of life associated with it. The affected patient can also most appropriately determine the improvement in quality of life conferred by a medical intervention. Using patient preferences limits the biases of healthy participants or clinicians attempting to indirectly infer how patients will likely react to illness. Others have also indicated their belief that the preferences of patients with a health state should be the criterion or gold standard for scientific use.[59–61] The use of patient prefer-

TABLE 9.5

Possible Sources of Utility Values*

---

1. Patients with the health state under study
2. Patients in another health state
3. The general community (a population-based sample)
4. Experts (healthcare providers and/or researchers)
5. Administrators
6. Authors of a manuscript
7. Proxy respondents (relatives or caregivers acting on a patient's behalf)
8. Others

---

* Adapted from Tengs and Wallace.[24]

ences to calculate the value gained from interventions and the cost-utility of interventions is an essential tenet of VBM.

> Patients who live or have lived in a health state are most able to assess the quality of life associated with that health state. The use of patient preferences to calculate value gained from interventions and the cost-utility of interventions is an essential tenet of VBM.

Some believe that if quality-of-life data are to be used for healthcare resource allocation decisions, then population-based (from a representative sample) community values are the appropriate source of utilities.[2] We respectfully, but firmly, disagree with this supposition. We believe that patient-based utility values obtained in a population-based fashion are the most appropriate to use.

Cost-utility analysis based upon a solid compilation of individual patient utilities does not preclude the opportunity for the community or society to evaluate how healthcare resources should be used once VBM data become available; it only keeps the various influencing factors separate and therefore inherently accountable for their impact on decisions.

> Cost-utility analysis performed using patient-based utility values *does not* preclude the opportunity for society to decide how healthcare resources will be allocated.

A common practice is to use the preferences of study researchers or clinicians (experts). This notion is based on the idea that information gathered from persons with experience caring for those with particular health states is reliable because healthcare providers have an appreciation for the prognosis, complications, and other parameters associated with disease. Additionally, utility values are easier to obtain from this group of surrogate respondents. But again, we hold patient-derived values to be the criterion.

Are Surrogate Respondent Utilities Ever Acceptable?

Yes. In groups such as children and persons who lack mental capacity, utility values obtained from surrogate respondents are absolutely necessary. Included in the latter group are those with congenital psychomotor retardation, schizophrenia, other psychoses, Alzheimer's disease, and so on.

HOW DO UTILITY VALUES FROM DIFFERENT GROUPS COMPARE?

Utility values for the same health state can differ dramatically, depending upon whether the respondents are patients with that health state, healthcare providers (experts), the general community (representative sample of the population),[48,53,54] or others. This is not surprising, since disparities concerning quality of life measured with instruments other than utility analysis have been noted between physicians and patients in multiple specialties in medicine.[62–64]

> Utility values obtained from patients who live in a health state and physicians who treat that health state can differ dramatically.

Community Underestimation of Patient Quality-of-Life Loss

Utility values obtained from the general community are typically higher for a disease than those obtained from patients who actually have the disease. Accordingly, community utility values often *underestimate* the quality-of-life impairment associated with a disease or health state as compared to people who have that disease or health state.[23,65] A list of several examples is shown in Table 9.6.

> Community respondents most often *underestimate* the burden of a disease upon a patient's quality of life.

The Beaver Dam Health Outcomes Study[23] published time-tradeoff utility values for 28 diseases. When the mean values obtained from patients with specific diseases were compared to those without the disease, the utility values were noted to be 8.5% higher in respondents without a disease than in those with a disease ($p = 0.00003$). Only for stroke (patient utility value = 0.90, non-patient utility value = 0.86) and chronic sinusitis (patient utility value = 0.87,

TABLE 9.6

Community Underestimation of Quality-of-Life Loss Compared to Patients With the Actual Disease

Condition	Actual Patient TTO Utility Values	Community TTO Utility Values	Reference
Arthritis	0.81	0.90	Fryback et al[23]
Asthma	0.71	0.87	Fryback et al[23]
Depression	0.70	0.87	Fryback et al[23]
Macular Degeneration, Severe	0.40*	0.86†	*Brown et al[5] †Stein et al[55]

TTO indicates time tradeoff.

nonpatient utility value = 0.86) did the patients with diseases have a higher utility value than nonpatients. Overall, patients had lower utility values than nonpatients for 93% (26/28) of diseases. We have noted the same phenomenon for multiple other diseases as well. People without a disease or health state generally perceive less impairment of the quality of life associated with the condition than do those who live with that disease or health state on a daily basis. The use of community-based utility values would therefore likely result in a diminution of the value conferred by interventions as compared to the use of patient-based utility values.

> The use of community-based utility values generally results in an underestimation of the value conferred by healthcare interventions as compared to patient-based utility values.

Sometimes the disparity between patient-based and community-based utility values is marked, as is also the difference between patient-based and physician-based utilities (Table 9.7). A good example is the remarkable difference noted among patient-based, physician-based, and community-based time-tradeoff utility values for age-related macular degeneration. The average time-tradeoff utility value for patients with severe macular degeneration was 0.40, while it was 0.67 for treating ophthalmologists asked to assume they had severe macular degeneration.[42] Needless to say, the ophthalmologists were not anywhere close in appreciating the severity of quality-of-life diminution caused by the disease since their mean estimate of quality-of-life loss was about half that of patients. The general community, however, was even further distanced from patients, with an average utility value of 0.86.[55] In this instance, the maximum possible improvement in utility value that an intervention could confer using community-based utility values is 0.14 (1.00 − 0.86), while the maximum possible improvement using patient-based values is 0.60 (1.00 − 0.40), or 329% greater. Using community-based utility values in a cost-utility analysis for the treatment of

TABLE 9.7

Lack of Comparability of Mean Utility Values for Severe
Macular Degeneration*

Group	TTO Utility Value
Patients	0.40
Physicians	0.67
Community	0.86

TTO indicates time tradeoff.
* Adapted from Brown et al[18] and Stein et al.[55]

age-related macular degeneration would cause a treatment to appear considerably less cost-effective than using patient-based utility values.

Community Overestimation of Loss of Quality of Life

The utility value discrepancy can go in the other direction as well—although less commonly—with surrogate respondents overestimating the effect of a health state upon quality of life. Sackett and Torrance[50] found the mean community utility value associated with hospital-based dialysis to be 0.52, while the mean dialysis patient utility value was 0.64 (Table 9.8). Stein and colleagues[54] also noted this phenomenon for treated systemic arterial hypertension. The average treated hypertensive patient had a time-tradeoff utility value of 0.98, while the average community member estimated a mean value of 0.95. The average healthcare provider who treated hypertensive patients estimated a mean utility value of 0.94, similar to that of the average person in the community and significantly different from the average affected person.

The Criterion or Gold Standard

We teach in the healthcare professions from day one that the patient is the most important person in the system and should always come first. When there is the potential for a large disparity between the preferences of patients and surrogate respondents, we believe that the preferences of patients should take precedence. *In fact, we cannot overemphasize how important it is to use utility values obtained from patients with the health state or disease of interest in cost-utility analysis.* These values may not be readily available for a particular study under consideration, but every effort should be made by researchers performing a cost-utility analysis to obtain them from the literature or directly from a patient cohort. Societal (community) input is reasonable to use for resource allocation once value-based quality standards have been established, but it is not reasonable to use to calculate the total patient value conferred by interventions.

TABLE 9.8

Community Overestimation of Quality-of-Life Loss Compared to Patients With the Actual Disease

Disease	Patient Values	Community Values	Reference
Home Dialysis	0.64	0.54	Sackett and Torrance[50]
Hospital Dialysis	0.64	0.52	Sackett and Torrance[50]
Stroke	0.90	0.86	Fryback et al[23]
Hypertension	0.98	0.95	Stein et al[54]

Utility values obtained from those patients *with the health state* under study are the *criterion*, or gold standard, for use in cost-utility analysis.

ARE TIME-TRADEOFF UTILITY VALUES WIDELY APPLICABLE?

Yes. Time-tradeoff utility values have been shown to be unaffected by:

1. gender,[3,12,13]
2. level of education,[3,5–8,12,13,36,53,54]
3. income,[3,5–8,12,36,53,54]
4. ethnicity,[49] and
5. international borders.[15]

Instead, they appear to be innate to human nature and widely applicable across demographic groups.

Time-tradeoff utility values are generally unaffected by gender, age, ethnicity, level of education, or level of income.

As is the case with other quality-of-life measures,[66] time-tradeoff utility values appear be to be consistent among different age groups, meaning that generally, people are willing to trade the same proportion of remaining time despite different ages.[3] For example, we have observed that diabetics in their 30s, 50s, and 70s are willing to trade a similar proportion of their remaining time left to be permanently rid of their diabetes.

Time-tradeoff utility values have shown consistency across international borders.[15]

UTILITY VALUE ANCHORS

The anchors, or the lowest possible value and highest possible value, associated with time-tradeoff utility value analysis can vary. This is undesirable since utility value databases with different anchors typically produce different utility values for the same health state. We agree with Gold et al[1] that utility value anchors should be *death* on the lower end and *optimal health* (*permanent normal* health) on the upper end.

Lower Anchor

Lower and upper anchors are values that define the lowest and highest possible utility values, respectively. The lower anchor of 0.0 can be death, the worst possible health, or the worst imaginable health state, the last used with the EuroQol 5D.[33] In our endeavor to standardize value-based variables, we recommend that death be used as the lower anchor for time-tradeoff utility analysis. The worst imaginable health state or worst possible health state can raise a large number of variable images, but death has a finality that virtually all lucid people recognize and that all have contemplated seriously many times during their lives.

Even when measuring time-tradeoff utility values associated with nonlethal entities such as dermatologic disorders, arthritis, loss of hearing, or loss or vision, we still recommend the use of death as the lower anchor. Unlike the case with rating scales, respondents can readily appreciate death as part of the scale. For example, if a person is willing to trade all of his or her remaining time of life, he or she fully realizes that this is equated with death.

Using death as the lower anchor with ophthalmic utility values, the worst possible vision (no perception of light in both eyes) is associated with a utility value of 0.26.[6] Needless to say, ophthalmic utility values on a scale ranging from 0.26 to 1.00 (using death as the lower anchor of 0.00 and 1.00 as permanent perfect vision) are quite different from utility values on a scale ranging from 0.00 to 1.00 (using an anchor of 0.00 to connote worst possible vision and 1.00 as perfect vision permanently). The critical factor again is to put all diseases and their varying levels of severity on the same scale. Using death as the lower anchor helps to facilitate this goal.

The suggestion has been made that some health states are worse than death, and therefore have a utility value less than 0.00. The researchers who suggest that this is the case, however, have not lived in such a state themselves or obtained utility values from cohorts of patients who have lived in "health states worse than death." For this reason, as well as the fact that euthanasia is most controversial, we recommend that utility values less than 0.00 not be used in cost-utility analysis.

We recommend the use of death as the lower utility value anchor of 0.00.

Upper Anchor

We recommend that the time-tradeoff utility value scale go from the lower anchor of death (utility value = 0.00) to the upper anchor of a permanent optimal health state (utility value = 1.00) for the condition under study. When overall health is undertaken, the upper anchor refers to all organ systems collectively. For congestive heart failure this means a permanent return to normal cardiac health, while for arthritis it means a permanent return to normal joint status, and for severe psoriasis it means a permanent return to normal skin health. If the upper anchor is a return to optimal health with no guarantee that it will remain, this parameter should be specified. Return to an optimal health state and return to an optimal health state *permanently* are two different outcomes.

> We recommend use of a *permanent optimal (normal) health state for the condition under study* to equate with the upper utility value anchor of 1.00.

It is also critical to inform patients whether their time of life traded is for a return to permanent normal health using their current treatment, or whether it means returning to permanent normal health with no treatment; in the latter instance, the only way to return to permanent normal health is by trading time. In a case of cardiac angina, the time-tradeoff utility value associated with chest pain treated with sublingual nitroglycerin is very different than the utility value associated with chest pain for which no treatment is given.

THE EFFECT OF TIME ON DISEASE

Utility values can change for the same health state with time, although they have been shown, for the most part, to be independent of the length of time of disease beyond the first year after onset.[3, 5, 12] For example, Laupacis et al[33] found the kidney-related time-tradeoff utility value of patients just prior to renal transplantion to be 0.57. At one year after transplant, the patient-based value was 0.74, while at 18 months it was 0.70 and at 24 months it was 0.70, exactly the same as six months previously.

When measuring long-term utility values, however, researchers must be certain that the severity of the symptoms and signs of the disease are unchanged. A change in the manifestations of the disease itself will cause a variation in utility value.

> Long-term utility values are typically stable unless the severity of the disease or health state has changed.

SHORT-TERM UTILITY VALUES

In general, time-tradeoff utility values are used for the measure of chronic health states. Nonetheless, utility values can also be used to measure short-term health states, as is the case with acute trauma and hospitalization (utility value = 0.08).[67, 68] In addition, we have been able to evaluate short-term health conditions, such as acute diarrhea or nausea that might occur secondary to a pharmaceutical agent or surgical intervention. This is accomplished by asking respondents who have had moderate to severe diarrhea or moderate to severe nausea what proportion of their remaining time of life they would trade, respectively, if the alternative was to live with moderate or severe diarrhea or moderate to severe nausea for the remainder of their lives. Other researchers[67] have measured short-term, or temporary, time-tradeoff utility values for varied time scenarios

FIGURE   9.1

Decision Analysis With the Options of No Drug Treatment or Drug Treatment for Arthritis. The numbers beneath the arms to the right are the incidences of *no complications* (92%) and *moderate to severe diarrhea* (8%). The utility value associated with the outcome of no complications is the 0.95 utility value just to the right of the upper triangular terminal node. Factoring in the utility value for moderate to severe diarrhea (0.82 just to the right of the lower triangular terminal node) yields an overall arthritis-related utility value outcome of 0.94 for the average drug-treated patient. The preferred strategy is use of the drug since it yields a higher utility value than no drug.

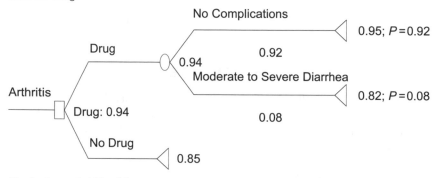

P indicates probability of the outcome.

(weeks, months, or years, the last of which is the case with our methodology) and have noted no effect of duration upon the scores.

As an example of the use of a short-term utility, we have found the time-tradeoff utility value associated with moderate to severe diarrhea to be 0.82. Thus, if a drug improves an arthritis-related utility value from 0.85 to 0.95 when it is associated with no adverse effects, but has the adverse effect of moderate to severe diarrhea in 8% of those who take it, the diarrhea must be factored into the therapeutic equation using decision analysis. If the drug is used for one month, the average person's treated arthritis-related utility value is 0.94 during that time since the diarrhea in 8% of treated patients decreases the mean utility value from 0.95 to 0.94 for the reference case (average patient) (Figure 9.1).

In regard to a surgical operation, we have noted the utility value associated with a six-inch skin incision to be 0.64. Let us assume that a femoral artery to popliteal artery bypass operation to ameliorate claudication improves a patient's utility value from 0.74 to 0.95 for exactly one year due to lessening of the calf pain with walking. The total gain in value for one year after surgery initially appears to be $0.95 - 0.74 = 0.21 \times 1$ year $= 0.21$ quality-adjusted life-year (QALY). For the first month after the surgery, however, the short-term disutility (an adverse effect that causes loss of value) due to the incision must be subtracted from the total value gained from the surgery. This resultant final QALY gain during the first year after the bypass surgery is therefore 0.1842 (Table 9.9).

TABLE 9.9

Value Gained From Surgery Over a One-Year Period Following Surgery*

Time	Utility Value	Utility (Gain or Loss) From Preoperative Health State)	QALY (Gain or Loss Compared to Preoperative Health State)
Month 1	0.64	0.64 − 0.74 = −0.10	−0.0083
Months 2–12	0.95	0.95 − 0.74 = +0.21	+0.1925
		Total Value Gained	+0.1842 QALYs

* Preoperative utility value = 0.74; postoperative utility value = 0.95; utility value associated with six-inch incision = 0.64.

As is apparent, utility values can be applied to conditions that are short-term in nature. These types of utility values are very helpful in assessing the overall value conferred by short-term treatments, especially pharmaceutical interventions. Thus, the value of a drug such as an antiviral agent that shortens the course of an upper respiratory infection by even one day can be measured.

UTILITY VALUES IN CHILDREN

Very few utility values have been obtained in children, although Yi and colleagues[46] acquired values from adolescents aged 12 to 15 years with cystic fibrosis. We are uncertain about the construct validity of such values.

Cost-utility analyses involving diseases in children have typically employed the utility values of surrogate respondents. We agree that parents have the best appreciation among surrogate respondents for the health state of their children, especially younger ones, and its effect upon their daily activities of living.[69] Living with their children on a 24-hour-a-day basis usually provides parents with a much greater appreciation of the adverse effects of a child's disease upon daily function and psychosocial aspects than physicians who might see the children for only ten minutes each month. Nonetheless, differences between the primary quality-of-life values of patients and proxy values (values proffered for a patient by a surrogate) of their primary caregivers can differ substantially.[70] Adult proxy surrogates for other adults typically underestimate morbidity, particularly in response to pain and emotions.[71] As we have discussed, adult surrogate respondents can overestimate or underestimate the quality of life associated with a health state, although underestimation of the quality of life lost that patients experience is more common.

A good example of a childhood disease that requires parental responses is croup, an upper respiratory infection that occurs within the first decade of life and usually does not occur in adults. In a disease such as asthma, which can start in childhood and remain throughout adult life, we believe the utility values of adult asthmatics are reasonable to use in cost-utility analysis. Researcher discretion in regard to which utilities to use is important in such instances. Again, whenever possible, utilities obtained from patients who have experienced the disease under study should be utilized.

CORE CONCEPTS

- Quality-of-life values obtained with a preference-based instrument should be used in cost-utility analysis.

- We recommend time-tradeoff utility analysis as the preference-based quality-of-life instrument currently best suited to create VBM standards.

- Utility values obtained from patients with a disease under study should be the gold standard, or *criterion*, for use in cost-utility analysis. The use of patient-based preferences is an essential tenet of VBM.

- Time-tradeoff utility values range from a lower anchor of death (utility = 0.00) to an upper anchor of permanent optimal (normal) health (utility = 1.00).

- Time-tradeoff utility values demonstrate applicability across all diseases, good reliability (reproducibility), good construct validity (see Chapter 10), good patient comprehension, and a low burden of administration.

- When obtaining time-tradeoff utility values, the exact disease under study, the severity of the disease and whether or not it is treated must be clearly defined.

- Time-tradeoff utility values are generally unaffected by age, ethnicity, gender, level of education, or income bracket.

- Time-tradeoff utility values are applicable across virtually all segments of the population.

- Interventions should not be valued greater for patients with a primary disease who are otherwise healthy, than for patients who have comorbidities in addition to their primary disease. To value them greater violates the Americans With Disabilities Act of 1990.

- Community respondents and physicians generally underestimate the decrease in quality of life caused by a disease as compared to patients who live or have lived with that disease.

- The validity of utility values obtained from children is uncertain. For diseases that affect children and adults, we recommend the use of utility values obtained from the adults.

- For diseases that affect only children, proxy utility values from parents are best able to ascertain the effect of the disease upon the quality of life of their children.

- The bottom line: *time-tradeoff utility values obtained from patients who have the disease under study should be used in cost-utility analysis calculation whenever possible.*

REFERENCES

1. Gold MR, Patrick DL, Torrance GW, et al. Identifying and valuing outcomes. In: Gold MR, Siegel JE, Russell LB, Weinstein MC, eds. *Cost-Effectiveness in Health and Medicine.* New York, NY: Oxford University Press; 1996:82–134.

2. Weinstein MC, Siegel JE, Gold MR, Kamlet MS, Russell LB. Recommendations of the Panel on Cost-Effectiveness in Health and Medicine. *JAMA.* 1996;276:1253–1258.

3. Brown GC. Vision and quality of life. *Trans Am Ophthalmol Soc.* 1999;97:473–512.

4. Brown GC, Brown MM, Sharma S. Cost-utility analysis. *Ann Intern Med.* 2001;134:625–626.

5. Brown GC, Brown MM, Sharma S, Kistler J. Utility values associated with age-related macular degeneration. *Arch Ophthalmol.* 2000;118:47–51.

6. Brown MM, Brown GC, Sharma S, Kistler J, Brown H. Utility values associated with blindness in an adult population. *Br J Ophthalmol.* 2001;85:327–331.

7. Brown MM, Brown GC, Sharma S, Shah G. Utility values and diabetic retinopathy. *Am J Ophthalmol.* 1999;128:324–330.

8. Brown GC, Brown MM, Sharma S, Beauchamp G, Hollands H. The reproducibility of ophthalmic utility values. *Trans Am Ophthalmol Soc.* 2001;99:71–76.

9. Hollands H, Lam M, Pater J, et al. Reliability of the time trade-off technique of utility assessment in patients with retinal disease. *Can J Ophthalmol.* 2001;36:202–209.

10. Read JL, Quinn DM, Berwick DM, Fineberg HV, Weinstein MC. Preferences for health outcomes: comparisons of assessment methods. *Med Decis Making.* 1984;4:215–329.

11. Tijhuis GJ, Jansen SJ, Stiggelbout AM, Zwinderman AH, Hazes JM, Vlieland TP. Value of the time trade-off method for measuring utilities in patients with rheumatoid arthritis. *Ann Rheum Dis.* 2000;59:852–897.

12. Brown GC, Brown MM, Sharma S, Brown H, Gozum M, Denton P. Quality-of-life associated with diabetes mellitus in an adult population. *Diabetes Complications.* 2000;14:18–24.

13. Brown MM, Brown GC, Sharma S, Hollands H. Quality-of-life and systemic comorbidities in patients with ophthalmic disease. *Br J Ophthalmol.* 2002;86:8–11.

14. Sharma S, Brown GC, Brown MM, Hollands H, Robbins R, Shah G. Validity of the time trade-off and standard gamble methods of utility assessment in retinal patients. *Br J Ophthalmol.* 2002;86:493–496.

15. Sharma S, Oliver A, Bakal J, Hollands H, Brown GC, Brown MM. Utilities associated with diabetic retinopathy: results from a Canadian sample. *Br J Ophthalmol.* 2003;87:259–261.

16. Frew E, Wolstenholme JL, Whynes DK. Willingness-to-pay for colorectal cancer screening. *Eur J Cancer.* 2001;37:1746–1751.

17. O'Brien B, Viramontes JL. Willingness-to-pay: a valid and reliable measure of health state preference? *Med Decis Making.* 1994;14:289–297.

18. Froberg DG, Kane RL. Methodology for measuring health state preferences, II: scaling methods. *J Clin Epidemiol.* 1989;42:459–471.

19. Wakker P, Stiggelbout A. Explaining distortions in utility elicitation through the rank-dependent model for risky choices. *Med Decis Making.* 1995;15:180–186.

20. Froberg DG, Kane RL. Methodology for measuring health-state preferences, I: measurement strategies. *J Clin Epidemiol.* 1989;42:345–354.

21. Brown GC, Brown MM, Sharma S. Cost-effectiveness of therapy for threshold retinopathy of prematurity. *Pediatrics.* 1999;104:47.

22. Post PN, Stiggelbout AM, Wakker PP. The utility of health states after stroke: a systematic review of the literature. *Stroke.* 2001;32:1425–1429.

23. Fryback DG, Dasbach EJ, Klein R, et al. The Beaver Dam Outcomes Study: initial catalog of health-state quality factors. *Med Decis Making.* 1993;13:89–102.

24. Tengs TO, Wallace MA. One thousand health-related quality-of-life estimates. *Med Care.* 2000;38:583–637.

25. Tengs TO, Lin TH. A meta-analysis of utility estimates for HIV/AIDS. *Med Decis Making.* 2002;22:475–481.

26. Phillips KA, Shlipak MG, Coxson P, et al. Health and economic benefits of increased beta blocker use following myocardial infarction. *JAMA.* 2000;284:2748–2754.

27. Gage BF, Cardinalli AB, Albers GW, Owens DK. Cost-effectiveness of warfarin and aspirin for prophylaxis of stroke in patients with nonvalvular atrial fibrillation. *JAMA.* 1995;274:1839–1845.

28. Hayman JA, Hillner BE, Harris JR, Weeks JC. Cost-effectiveness of routine radiation therapy following conservative surgery for early-stage breast cancer. *J Clin Oncol.* 1998;16:1022–1029.

29. Krummins PE, Fihn SD, Kent DL. Symptom severity and patients' values in the decision to perform a transurethral resection of the prostate. *Med Decis Making.* 1988;8:1–8.

30. Tsevat J, Goldman L, Lamas GA, et al. Functional status versus utilities in survivors of myocardial infarction. *Med Care.* 1991;29:1153–1159.

31. Laupacis A, Bourne R, Rorabeck C, et al. The effect of elective total hip replacement on health-related quality of life. *J Bone Joint Surg Am.* 1993;75:1619–1626.

32. Chapman GB, Elstwin AS, Kuzel TM, et al. Prostate cancer patients' utilities for health states: how it looks depends on where you stand. *Med Decis Making.* 1998;18:278–286.

33. Laupacis A, Keown P, Pus N, et al. A study of the quality of life and cost-utility of renal transplantation. *Kidney Int.* 1996;50:235–242.

34. Tengs TO, Yu M, Luistro E. Health-related quality of life after stroke: a comprehensive review. *Stroke.* 2001;32:964–972.

35. McLeod RS, Churchill DN, Lock AM, et al. Quality of life of patients with ulcerative colitis preoperatively and postoperatively. *Gastroenterology.* 1991;101:1307–1313.

36. Brown MM, Brown GC, Sharma S, Landy J. Health care economic analyses and value-based medicine. *Surv Ophthalmol.* 2003;48:204–223.

37. Hart AC, Hopkins CA, eds. *International Classification of Diseases, Ninth Revision, Clinical Modification.* Salt Lake City, Utah: Ingenix; 2003.

38. EuroQol Group. EuroQol: a new facility for the measurement of health-related quality of life. *Health Policy.* 1990;16:199–208.

39. Hochberg MC, Chang RW, Dwosh I, Lindsey S, Pincus Y, Wolfe F. The American College of Rheumatology 1991 revised criteria for the classification of global functional status in rheumatoid arthritis. *Arthritis Rheum.* 1992;35:498–502.

40. Trucki G, Stoll T, Bruhlmann P, Michel B. Construct validation of the ACR 1991 criteria for global functional status in rheumatoid arthritis. *Clin Exp Rheumatol.* 1995;13:349–352.

41. Karnofsky DA, Abelmann WH, Craver LF, Burchenal JH. The use of nitrogen mustards in the palliative treatment of carcinoma: with particular reference to bronchogenic carcinoma. *Cancer.* 1948;1:634–638.

42. Ahmed A. American College of Cardiology/American Heart Association chronic heart failure evaluation and management guidelines: relevance to the geriatric practice. *J Am Geriatr Soc.* 2003;51:123–126.

43. AHA medical/scientific statement: 1994 revisions to classification of functional capacity and objective assessment of patients with diseases of the heart. *Circulation.* 1994;90:644–645.

44. Chacko KA. AHA Medical/Scientific Statement: 1994 revisions to classification of functional capacity and objective assessment of patients with diseases of the heart. *Circulation.* 1995;92:2003–2005.

45. Ware JE, Sherbourne CD. The MOS 36-item short-form health survey (SF-36), I: conceptual framework and item selection. *Med Care.* 1992;30:473–483.

46. Yi MS, Britto MT, Wilmott RW, et al. Health values of adolescents with cystic fibrosis. *J Pediatr.* 2003;142:133–140.

47. Brown GC, Brown MM, Sharma S. Health care in the 21st century: evidence-based medicine, patient preference-based quality and cost-effectiveness. *Qual Management Health Care.* 2000;19:23–31.

48. Brown GC, Brown MM, Sharma S. Difference between ophthalmologist and patient perceptions of quality-of-life associated with age-related macular degeneration. *Can J Ophthalmol.* 2000;35:27–32.

49. Brown GC, Brown MM, Sharma S, Landy J. Ethnic preferences and quality of life in patients with diabetes mellitus. Submitted for publication.

50. Sackett DL, Torrance GW. The utilities of different health states as perceived by the general public. *J Chronic Dis.* 1978;31:697–704.

51. Harris RA, Nease RF Jr. The importance of patient preferences for comorbidities in cost-effectiveness analyses. *J Health Econ.* 1997;16:113–119.

52. Schiffman RM, Walt JG, Jacobsen G, Doyle JJ, Lebovics G, Sumner W. Utility assessment among patients with dry eye disease. *Ophthalmology.* 2003;110:1412–1419.

53. Landy J, Stein JD, Brown GC, Brown MM, Sharma S. Patient, community and clinician perceptions of the quality of life associated with diabetes mellitus. *Med Sci Monitor.* 2002;8:543–548.

54. Stein JD, Brown GC, Brown MM, Sharma S, Hollands H, Stein HD. The quality of life of patients with hypertension. *J Clin Hypertens.* 2002;4:181–188.

55. Stein JD, Brown MM, Brown GC, Sharma S, Hollands H. Quality of life with macular degeneration: perceptions of patients, clinicians and community members. *Br J Ophthalmol.* 2003;87:8–12.

56. Gomez-Mejia LR, Balkin DB, Cardy RL. *Managing Human Resources.* Englewood Cliffs, NJ: Prentice Hall; 1995:134–136.

57. US Department of Justice, Civil Rights Division, Disability Rights Section. Title III highlights. Available at: www.usdoj.gov/crt/ada/t3hilght.htm. Accessed January 16, 2004.

58. Boyd NF, Sutherland HJ, Heasman KZ, Tritchler DL, Cummings BJ. Whose utilities for decision analysis? *Med Decis Making.* 1990;10:58–67.

59. Angell M. Patients' preferences in randomized clinical trials. *N Engl J Med.* 1984;310:1385–1387.

60. Kassirer JP. Incorporating patient's preferences into medical decisions. *N Engl J Med.* 1994;330:1895–1896.

61. Kassirer JP. Adding insult to injury: usurping patients' prerogatives. *N Engl J Med.* 1983;308:898–901.

62. Lunde IM. Patients' perceptions: a shift in medical perspective. *Scand J Prim Health Care.* 1993;11:98–104.

63. Rothwell PM, McDowell Z, Wong CK, Dorman PJ. Doctors and patients don't agree: cross sectional study of patients' and doctors' perceptions and assessments of disability in multiple sclerosis. *BMJ.* 1997;314:1580–1583.

64. Schrader GD. Subjective and objective assessments of medical comorbidity in chronic depression. *Psychother Psychosom.* 1997;666:258–260.

65. Clarke AE, Goldstein MK, Michelson D, Garber AM, Lenert LA. The effect of assessment method and respondent population on utilities elicited for Gaucher disease. *Qual Life Res.* 1997;6:169–184.

66. Jones CA, Voaklander DC, Johnston DW, Suarez-Almazor ME. The effect of age on pain, function and quality of life after total hip and knee arthroplasty. *Arch Intern Med.* 2001;161:454–460.

67. Cook J, Richardson J, Street A. A cost utility analysis of treatment options for gallstone disease: methodological issues and results. *Health Econ.* 1994;3:157–168.

68. Jansen SJT, Stiggelbout AM, Wakker PP, et al. Patients' utilities for cancer treatments: a study of the chained procedure for the standard gamble and time tradeoff. *Med Decis Making.* 1998;18:391–399.

69. Cheng AK, Rubin HR, Powe NR, et al. Cost-utility analysis of the cochlear implant in children. *JAMA*. 2000;284:850–856.

70. Tamim H, McCusker J, Dendukuri N. Proxy reporting of quality of life using the EQ-5D. *Med Care*. 2002;40:1186–1195.

71. Grootendorst PV, Fenny DH, Furlong W. Does it matter whom and how you ask? Inter-rater and intra-rater agreement in the Ontario Health Survey. *J Clin Epidemiol*. 1997;50:127–135.

Construct Validity

Construct validity is a measure of the degree to which a health-related quality-of-life instrument actually measures the quality of life it is constructed to measure. Unfortunately, there is no single assessment parameter to which we can compare quality-of-life instruments to ascertain their construct. Multiple approaches are therefore required.

The construct validity of a measure of health-related quality of life can be evaluated by demonstrating a high degree of correlation with objective measures of disease severity, the ability to perform certain tasks, or other measures of health-related quality of life.[1] In order to ensure that utilities are valid, they should be significantly correlated to constructs that are both intuitive and important to patients.

Torrence[1] suggested that construct validity is related to the ability of an instrument to predict events and/or behaviors. *Clinical events* that may be important include the development of severe pain, degree of visual impairment as determined through a reading chart, loss of bowel function, or the ability to feel sensation, while *behaviors* include the inability to perform work coherently, the inability to leave the vicinity of a toilet, or the avoidance of walking more than one block. The distinction between an event or behavior is at times indistinct and not worth elaborating.

In essence, the scores from a quality-of-life measure should correlate appropriately along the continuum of disease severity from milder to more severe stages as experienced and judged by patients with a disease and/or clinicians. Time-tradeoff utility analysis is similar to any other quality-of-life instrument in this regard.

The construct validity of time-tradeoff utility analysis is demonstrated by its strong correlation to certain *events* (such as severe pain, ischemic necrosis of the foot, loss of bowel function, and so on) and certain *behaviors* (such as the inability to perform work coherently, the inability to leave the vicinity of a toilet, and so on) that are associated with a disease or health state and are known to be germane to patients and society in general.

CONSTRUCT VALIDITY AND
TIME-TRADEOFF UTILITY ANALYSIS

We have shown construct validity with time-tradeoff utility values by comparing them with patient-reported categorical scales (from mild to severe) of clinical symptoms and signs associated with a disease, as well as with functional, categorical quality-of-life instruments such as the Karnofsky Performance Status Scale,[2] the Eastern Cooperative Oncology Group Performance Status Scale,[3] the American Heart Association Functional Capacity Classification,[4] the American College of Rheumatology Classification of Global Functional Status in Rheumatoid Arthritis,[5] the Modified Rankin Scale,[6] and both Snellen and logMAR visual acuity levels. Overall, time-tradeoff utility values have demonstrated excellent construct validity by predicting (correlating with) events and behaviors expected for diseases as they progress from their mildest forms to their most severe forms. In some instances, the subjective categorical rating of mild, moderate, and severe organ dysfunction correlates most closely with utility values. In some cases other instruments measuring behavioral functional impairment correlate more closely with it, and in yet other instances, utility values may correlate with the severity of a given symptom or sign associated with a health state.

Time-tradeoff utility values demonstrate excellent construct validity because they correlate well with the severity of clinical symptoms and signs that patients experience.

As the symptoms and signs associated with a health state worsen and other quality-of-life instruments associated with a health state demonstrate increasing degrees of impairment, the associated utility value should decrease correspondingly in order to demonstrate convergent construct validity. When unexplained utility values are obtained it is often because there is a clinical correlation that may not at first be apparent. For example, a person who is unfamiliar with peripheral neuropathy may not realize that severe cases of numbness are associated with lack of proprioception, and therefore a high incidence of falling. This reinforces the view that expert clinical acumen and a good firsthand appreciation of the patient-perceived symptoms and the clinical signs associated with diseases are necessary factors for developing a health-related quality-of-life database with good construct validity.

Expert clinical acumen and a good firsthand appreciation of the patient-perceived symptoms and the clinical signs associated with diseases are necessary factors for the development of a health-related quality-of-life database with good construct validity.

EXAMPLES OF CONSTRUCT VALIDITY

Examples that demonstrate the construct validity of time-tradeoff utility values are illustrated in various specialties.

Irritable Bowel Syndrome

Irritable bowel syndrome (IBS) is a gastrointestinal disorder that generally presents before the age of 45 years with abdominal pain in association with diarrhea and/or constipation. Karnofsky Performance Status Scale values[2] and their respective time-tradeoff utility values are shown in Table 10.1 for patients with IBS. There is a substantial time-tradeoff utility value loss with a drop from 80 to 70 with the Karnofsky Scale, as well as a large drop from 70 to 60.

For some diseases, utility values will decrease in intervals similar to the decrease in Karnofsky Scale numbers. In the case of IBS, however, there is an inordinately large decrease in utility value when the Karnofsky Scale Score changes from 80 to 70 and 70 to 60. A reasonable question is, why? Are the utility values amiss, or is there some clinical reason that can explain the apparent discrepancy?

As with any disease, clinical experience and listening to patients with the disease is critical. We, as clinicians, expected that patients with severe IBS would be most adversely affected due to the discomfort associated with the disease. This is a major contributing factor, but the problem that appears to also cause a great loss of quality of life—and therefore the large drops in utility value from Karnofsky scores of 80 to 70 and 70 to 60—is primarily related to the inability of a patient to travel anywhere without a toilet within the immediate proximity. In essence, patients with IBS and severe diarrhea are bound as prisoners to the toilet during acute phases of the disease. This causes the inability to work at an occupation effectively or travel outside their home without embarrassment,

TABLE 10.1

Time-Tradeoff Utility Values Associated With Irritable Bowel Syndrome

Karnofsky Scale[2]	TTO Value	Most Disturbing Symptom and Impact of Health-Related Function (Event or Behavior)
100 (No signs or symptoms of disease)	1.00	Nothing
90 (Minor signs and symptoms)	1.00	Abdominal discomfort
80 (Normal activity with effort)	0.95	Abdominal discomfort
70 (No normal activity or active work)	0.68	Moderately severe diarrhea and pain, unable to work
60 (Requires occasional assistance) leave home	0.54	Very severe diarrhea and pain, unable to assistance) leave home

Karnofsky indicates Karnofsky Performance Status Scale (refer to Table 7.2 in Chapter 7); TTO, time-tradeoff.

therefore producing a marked diminution in quality of life. Thus, utility values obtained from patients suffering from IBS are significantly correlated to both events as measured through the Karnofsky scale and critical behaviors such as the ability to function without immediate access to a toilet. These high degrees of correlation suggest that utilities are highly valid measures of quality of life as measured against events and behaviors that are of critical importance to patient functioning.

In cases in which variability in time-tradeoff utility values is unexplained by a functional score, exploring the degree of suffering from symptoms or the impact of the disease on important patient function often reveals the reason(s) underlying these unexpectedly low utility values.

Peripheral Neuropathy

Peripheral neuropathies can occur secondary to multiple causes, including ischemia, inflammation, infection, trauma, and others. The symptoms that occur secondary to peripheral neuropathy include numbness, pain (including paresthesias and dysesthesias), and lack of proprioception. Time-tradeoff utility values associated with peripheral neuropathy are shown in Table 10.2. They

TABLE 10.2

Time-Tradeoff Utility Values Associated With Peripheral Neuropathy

Karnofsky Scale	TTO Value	Most Disturbing Problem (Event or Behavior)
100 (No symptoms or signs of disease)	1.00	None
90 (Minor signs and symptoms)	1.00	Numbness
80 (Normal activity with effort)	0.95	Numbness and pain
70 (No normal activity or active work)	0.78	Pain and numbness, unable to work
60 (Requires occasional assistance and frequent medical care)	0.65	Pain and numbness
50 (Needs considerable assistance)	0.39	Pain and numbness, unable to walk due to lack of proprioception, foot ulcers, and bone damage

Karnofsky Scale indicates Karnofsky Performance Status Scale[2] (refer to Table 7.2 in Chapter 7); TTO, time-tradeoff.

decrease accordingly as the Karnofsky Performance Status Scale[2] demonstrates greater overall impairment. The substantial utility value decrease from a Karnofsky score of 80 to 70 appears to occur because there is difficulty maintaining employment, while the even larger utility drop from a Karnofsky score of 60 to 50 occurs because of marked pain and numbness.

The large utility value drop, however, is seen with neuropathy variants characterized predominantly by pain (which we would expect), as well as those characterized primarily by numbness. But why the numbness? Because when numbness reaches a certain level (Karnofsky score of 50), proprioception is markedly impaired and a patient has great difficulty walking without falling. In addition, foot ulcers and bone damage can result due to injury exacerbated by lack of sensation. Consequently, the clinical symptoms, signs, and quality-of-life impairment of patient cohorts at the utility levels shown support the construct validity concept that time-tradeoff utility values can predict behaviors and events that become more limiting as the utility values concomitantly decrease. In essence, the worsening utility numbers again show what we found with IBS—decreasing quality of life as specific impairment parameters associated with severity of the disease are realized. In this case, patients relate that numbness causes some decrease in quality of life, but the most disturbing problems are pain, the numbness-induced inability to walk, and injuries to the feet caused by lack of sensation.

Angina Associated With Coronary Artery Disease

Time-tradeoff utility values associated with a cohort of patients with cardiac angina demonstrate significant correlation with both the American Heart Association Functional Classification[4] score and patient self-assessment using a categorical scale administered at the same time as time-tradeoff evaluation (Table 10.3). The construct validity of time-tradeoff values is supported by the fact that the utility values are strongly correlated to both the American Heart Association Functional Capacity Classification levels and self-assessment scores. These strong correlations demonstrate a series of stepwise decrements in utility as patients

TABLE 10.3

Utility Values Associated With Angina From Coronary Artery Disease

AHA Classification	TTO Utility Value	Categorical Scale (Event or Behavior)
II	0.87	Mild Pain
III	0.73	Moderate Pain
IV	0.53	Severe Pain

AHA Classification indicates American Heart Association Functional Capacity Classification[7]; II, ordinary activity causes angina; III, less than ordinary activity causes angina; IV, angina with any activity or at rest; TTO, time-tradeoff.

progress through various degrees of disease severity as measured through the use of the American Heart Association Functional Capacity Classification.

As the chest pain increases with lesser activity, the associated utility values decrease, exactly as a clinician would expect. This prediction of events confirms the construct validity of time-tradeoff utility values for cardiac angina.

Visual Loss

Utility values associated with ophthalmic diseases have been correlated with the visual acuity in the better-seeing eye.[8] As the event of vision decreasing in the better-seeing eye occurs, the corresponding utility value decreases (Table 10.4). While there is a correlation with vision in the better-seeing eye using both the standard-gamble and time-tradeoff methodologies, the correlation is greater with the time-tradeoff method than with the standard-gamble method.[9,10]

A linear regression formula using vision in decimal form (20/20 = 1.0, 20/40 = 0.3, 20/200 = 0.10, etc) has been developed to measure the time-tradeoff utility value associated with ocular diseases that cause visual loss.[11] The formula is *time-tradeoff utility value = 0.374x + 0.514*, where x is the visual acuity in the better-seeing eye in decimal form. If the vision is 20/100, this formula predicts a utility value of 0.374 (0.2) + 0.514 = 0.59. While this expected utility value result is close to that obtained empirically, the association between utility values and

TABLE   10.4

Utility Values Associated With Visual Acuity in the Better-Seeing Eye*

Visual Acuity (Event or Behavior)	TTO Utility Value
20/20 OU (permanent)	1.00
20/20 OU (ocular disease)	0.97
20/20	0.92
20/25	0.87
20/30	0.84
20/40	0.80
20/70	0.74
20/100	0.67
20/200	0.66
20/400	0.54
20/800	0.52
20/1600	0.35
No Light Perception	0.26

OU indicates both eyes; TTO, time-tradeoff.

* Unless otherwise indicated.

Source: Brown et al.[12]

vision in the better-seeing eye is not strictly linear, and we believe the values in Table 10.4 more accurately depict the patient time-tradeoff utility values associated with visual loss.

There are several critical factors related to function, psychological distress, and well-being that we have noted in ophthalmology that strongly support the construct validity of time-tradeoff utility values predicting events and behaviors in people with ocular diseases. Listed here, some can be applied across other organ systems as well:

■ People with ocular disease and normal 20/20 vision in each eye have a mean ophthalmic utility value of 0.97, rather than 1.00, due to the worry about losing vision in the future. Thus, the absence of symptoms in a person with a known ocular disease (diabetic retinopathy, macular degeneration, glaucoma, and so on) should not imply that they have a perfect utility value of 1.00. *Concern about the future can cause symptomless diseases to have an associated utility value less than 1.00.*

> Concern about the future can cause symptomless diseases to have an associated utility value of less than 1.00.

■ People with 20/20 vision in one eye and impaired vision in the second eye have a mean utility value of 0.92 rather than 1.00, not because of lack of depth perception, but because their quality of life is decreased by persistent daily worry about the long-term status of their one good eye. *The loss of one organ of a paired organ system (eye, ear, kidney, lung, and so on) is often associated with a decrease in utility value, predominantly due to concern about the long-term welfare of the remaining organ.*

> The loss of one organ of a paired organ system (eye, ear, kidney, lung, and so on) is often associated with a decrease in utility value.

■ Large utility value decrements correlate with the following critically important functional losses, as shown in Table 10.5.

TABLE 10.5

Critically Important Functional Losses Associated With Utility Value Decrements

Vision Loss in Better Eye	Utility Value Loss	Loss of Function
20/40 to 20/70	−0.06	Driving
20/200 to 20/400	−0.08	Reading*
20/800 to 20/1600	−0.17	Unaided Navigation

* Loss of reading with a low vision aid.

Larger ocular utility value decrements are often associated with critical functional losses, reinforcing the construct validity of utility values to predict events (loss of driving, reading, or unaided navigation).

Ocular utility values correlate most highly with the visual acuity in the better-seeing eye rather than the underlying cause of visual loss.[13] There is lesser correlation with vision in the poorer-seeing eye, some of which occurs secondary to the fact that ocular diseases (cataract, glaucoma, age-related macular degeneration, and diabetic retinopathy) often affect both eyes.[9]

Again, as in every other specialty, asking patients what bothers them the most about their disease and how it impacts their function in the real world is critical. In our experience, patients suffering from a given disease can quite readily identify the primary factor responsible for their decision to trade theoretical time, as well as justify the quantity of time traded.

FINAL THOUGHTS ON CONSTRUCT VALIDITY

Construct validity is a difficult concept to demonstrate, particularly because there is no set method to elucidate it across all diseases and also because the relationship between utility values and other accepted methods of disease assessment is not always linear. Using the criteria of Torrance[1] that construct validity is demonstrated by the ability to predict events (chest pain at rest, loss of bowel control, the inability to walk) or behaviors (inability to leave the vicinity of a toilet, the avoidance of sporting activities, the avoidance of walking short distances, and so on) is a reasonable approach.

A patient can readily discern what symptoms or signs of a disease most adversely affect their quality of life and relate this to the researcher. While obvious worsening of the severity of disease, as characterized by increasing pain and increasing loss of function, should be associated with correspondingly diminishing utility values, there are instances in which a patient with a disease reveals other relevant parameters that may not be superficially apparent to the researcher. Again, the critical point should be emphasized that the utility values of patients with a disease under study are those that should be used in cost-utility analysis. The quality-of-life parameters most adversely affected by a disease can be ascertained only by patients who live or have lived with that disease.

Patients who live or have lived with a disease are those best able to assess the quality of life associated with that disease.

CORE CONCEPTS

- *Construct validity* quantifies how well a health-related quality-of-life instrument measures what it is intended to measure—the quality of life associated with a disease or health state.

- Construct validity can be demonstrated by the ability of an instrument to predict clinical events and important patient behaviors.

- Examples of clinical *events* include experiencing angina at rest in a person with coronary artery disease and the loss of bowel control in a person with severe irritable bowel syndrome.

- Examples of important patient *behaviors* include the inability to leave the vicinity of a toilet in a person with severe IBS and the avoidance of sporting activities in a person with moderate angina.

- Time-tradeoff utility values generally demonstrate excellent construct validity since they correlate well with the severity of the clinical symptoms, signs, and patient perceptions of diseases (including events and behaviors as demonstrated previously).

- Concern about the future often causes symptomless disease to have an associated utility value less than 1.00.

- The loss of one organ of a paired organ system (eye, ear, kidney, lung, and so forth) is therefore often associated with a decrease in utility value due to concern about the welfare of the remaining organ.

- Large utility value decrements correlate with critically important functional losses such as loss of occupation, loss of the ability to walk, loss of the ability to read, and so on.

REFERENCES

1. Torrance GW. Social preference for health states: an empirical evaluation of three measurement techniques. *Socioecon Planning Sci.* 1976;10:129–136.

2. Karnofsky DA, Abelmann WH, Craver LF, Burchenal JH. The use of nitrogen mustards in the palliative treatment of carcinoma: with particular reference to bronchogenic carcinoma. *Cancer.* 1948;1:634–638.

3. Buccheri G, Ferrigno D, Tamburini M. Karnofsky and ECOG performance status scoring in lung cancer: a prospective, longitudinal study of 536 patients from a single institution. *Eur J Cancer.* 1996;32:1135–1141.

4. AHA medical/scientific statement: 1994 revisions to classification of functional capacity and objective assessment of patients with diseases of the heart. *Circulation.* 1994;90:644–645.

5. Hochberg MC, Chang RW, Dwosh I, Lindsey S, Pincus T, Wolfe F. The American College of Rheumatology revised criteria for the classification of global functional status in rheumatoid arthritis. *Arthritis Rheum.* 1992;35:498–502.

6. Bonita R, Beaglehole R. Modification of Rankin Scale: recovery of motor function after stroke. *Stroke.* 1988;19:1497–1500.

7. American Heart Association. Classification of functional capacity and objective assessment. Available at: www.americanheart.org. Accessed April 29, 2003.

8. Brown GC. Vision and quality of life. *Trans Am Ophthalmol Soc.* 1999;97:473–512.

9. Brown MM, Brown GC, Sharma S, Smith AF, Landy J. A utility analysis correlation with visual acuity: methodologies and vision in the better and poorer eyes. *Int Ophthalmol.* 2001;24:123–127.

10. Sharma S, Brown GC, Brown MM, Hollands H, Robbins R, Shah G. Validity of the time trade-off and standard gamble methods of utility assessment in retinal patients. *Br J Ophthalmol.* 2002;86:493–496.

11. Sharma S, Brown GC, Brown MM, et al. Converting visual acuity to utilities. *Can J Ophthalmol.* 2000;35:267–272.

12. Brown MM, Brown GC, Sharma S, Landy J. Health care economic analyses and value-based medicine. *Surv Ophthalmol.* 2003;48:204–223.

13. Brown MM, Brown GC, Sharma S, Landy J. Quality of life with visual acuity loss from diabetic retinopathy and age-related macular degeneration. *Arch Ophthalmol.* 2002;120:481–484.

11

Where Is the Value?

The transition from one health state to a better health state, such as the improvement from severe angina (with an associated utility value of 0.53) to mild angina (with an associated utility value of 0.88) outlined in Table 9.1 in Chapter 9, can be objectively measured. In this instance, there is an improvement in utility value of $0.88 - 0.53 = 0.35$. The improvement in quality of life conferred by an intervention can be measured in this manner for virtually every intervention in healthcare.

> The improvement in quality of life conferred by virtually any healthcare intervention is measured by subtracting the preintervention utility value from the postintervention utility value.

The increase in utility value after an intervention allows a measure of the improvement in quality of life conferred by an intervention, but it does not give the total *value* conferred by the intervention. To measure the total value conferred we make use of the quality-adjusted life-year (QALY). The conversion of evidence-based data to value-based format comprises the second tier of the value-based medicine pyramid (Figure 11.1).

THE QUALITY-ADJUSTED LIFE-YEAR

The concept of the QALY, introduced by Klarman et al[1] in their study of renal failure patients in 1968, was a major breakthrough in quality-of-life research in that it allowed a measure of the total *value* of life accrued by a person over time, as well as the total value conferred by a healthcare intervention. The QALY is the most widely used method of capturing improvement in quality and quantity of life for use in cost-utility analysis.[2] Quality-adjusted life-years are attractive because, as is the case with utility values, they can be applied to interventions across all specialties in healthcare.

The quality-of-life improvement gained from an intervention can be incorporated with the years of life added by an intervention to yield the total number of QALYs conferred by the intervention. A QALY can be conceptualized by

FIGURE 11.1

The Value-Based Medicine Pyramid

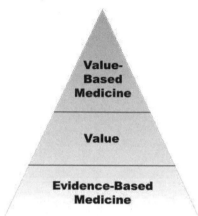

Figure courtesy Kathryn Brown.

examining Figure 11.2, where the *y*-axis represents health-related quality of life as measured on a utility scale from 0.0 to 1.0. The *x*-axis represents duration of life, and the curve represents various health states that a hypothetical person could go through within a specified period of time. Consequently, the area under the curve represents the QALYs associated with that particular set of health states over time.

By definition, the number of QALYs that a person accrues over time is calculated by multiplying the time (in years) lived in a health state by the utility value associated with that health state. Thus, if a person lives at a utility value of 1.0 for one year, one QALY is accrued. If a person lives at a utility value of 0.75 for a year, 0.75 QALY is accrued during that time.

One year spent in perfect health (utility = 1.0) = 1 QALY (quality-adjusted life year).

Quality-adjusted life years allow for inclusion of the measurement of improvement in both length of life and/or quality of life into a single measure. To calculate QALYs, the utility value for a specific health state is multiplied by the amount of time (in years) spent at that level of health.

FIGURE 11.2

Graphical Depiction of Quality-Adjusted Life-Years*

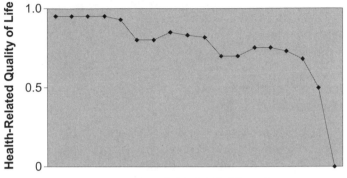

Duration of Life (Years)

* The area under the curve represents the quality-adjusted life-years (QALYs) gained over a specified period of time.

The total number of QALYs conferred from an intervention is therefore calculated by adding the following products:

(the utility value improvement conferred by the intervention) × *(the duration of treatment benefit during the pretreatment life expectancy)*

+

(the utility value of the postintervention health state) × *(the number of years of life added by the intervention)*

The time in each part of the equation is measured in years or fractions of years. For interventions in which length of life is unaffected, the total value gained is calculated by multiplying the improvement in utility value (improvement in quality of life) by the duration of the intervention benefit. For interventions in which length of life is improved and quality of life is unaffected, the total value gained is calculated by multiplying the utility value by the added years of life. The concept of the QALY is best illustrated by examples.

> The QALY (quality-adjusted life-year) is used to measure the total value conferred by a healthcare intervention. It takes into account the improvement in (1) length of life, and/or (2) quality of life.

Improvement in Quality of Life

Example: After total hip arthroplasty for osteoarthritis, a 75-year-old man improves from American College of Rheumatology Classification of Global Functional Status in Rheumatoid Arthritis Class III (able to perform usual self-care activities, but limited in vocational and avocational activities; utility value = 0.79) to Class I (completely able to perform usual activities of daily living such as self-care, vocational, and avocational activities; utility value = 0.99). The change in utility value after the intervention is 0.99 − 0.79 = 0.20. Assuming the duration of treatment benefit is ten years, the total *value* gained from the procedure is (0.20 in utility value) × (10 years) = 2.0 QALYs.

Improvement in Quality of Life and Length of Life

Example: A 50-year-old man with Marfan syndrome has aortic regurgitation and marked fatigue and dyspnea with less than ordinary activity (American Heart Association Functional Capacity Classification Class III, utility value = 0.74). After aortic valve replacement he becomes asymptomatic with normal activity (American Heart Association Functional Capacity Classification Class I, utility value = 0.94). In addition to improving the man's quality of life, data suggest his life expectancy will improve from five years to 20 years. The total *value gained* from the surgery is:

■ **In quality of life:** (0.20 utility points) × (5 years) = 1.0 QALY from improvement of quality of life conferred over the first five years following the intervention that raises the preintervention utility value of 0.74 to a post-intervention utility value of 0.94.

■ **In length of life:** (0.94 utility points) × 15 years = 14.1 QALYs from the gain of 15 years in length of life at a utility value of 0.94.

   Total value gained = 15.1 QALYs

The Benefit of Using QALYs

The benefit of using QALYs is easily seen. Quantifying the value of virtually all healthcare interventions with measures broad enough to include all major issues, and that are able to be compared across disparate health states, greatly facilitates the creation of a value-based medicine (VBM) database and quality standards.

Adverse Effects Measured by QALYs

The total value conferred by an intervention can also include adverse events, or disutilities that decrease quality of life, associated with the therapy. An example best demonstrates how adverse effects can be factored into the therapeutic equation. In the above case of aortic valve replacement in the patient with Marfan syndrome, let us assume the average patient is acutely hospitalized for two weeks at a utility value of 0.08 and undergoes rehabilitation for another 11 weeks at a utility value of 0.60. The total loss of life's value acutely associated with the surgery is calculated by subtracting the value lost from hospitalization and rehabilitation from the total value (15.1 QALYs) otherwise gained as shown in Table 11.1.

TABLE 11.1

Value Lost Due to Adverse Events Associated With Surgery

Condition	Utility Value	Expected Postoperative Utility Value	Difference	Time (Years)	QALYs Lost
Hospitalization	0.08	0.94	−0.86	0.038 (2 weeks)	−0.0327
Rehabilitation	0.60	0.94	−0.34	0.211 (11 weeks)	−0.0717
Remaining Life	0.94	0.94	0.00	19.75	0.0
				Total QALYs Lost =	**−0.1044**

The total value gained from the intervention includes that derived from all benefits, as well as the value lost due to adverse effects caused by the surgery. The total value conferred by the aortic value surgery is therefore (15.1 – value of the adverse effects) = (15.1 – 0.1044) = 14.9956 QALYs. (Remember that when the adverse effects are factored in, the first three months after the surgery are lived at the utility value level the patient has in the hospital for two weeks and in rehabilitation for 11 weeks.)

> The total value conferred by an intervention should take into account all value gains as well as the value lost due to adverse effects associated with the intervention.

The suggestion has been made that events that cause a minuscule change in the value conferred by a healthcare intervention do not have to be incorporated in a value calculation and cost-utility analysis.[3] We agree, but realize that the definition of *minuscule change* is vague. We consider discomfort for one to two days after surgery for an operation that confers a benefit for 20 years to be a minuscule, or negligible, change, but would consider postoperative discomfort that diminishes the utility value for a month to be a meaningful adverse effect that should be incorporated into value and cost-utility calculations.

WHOSE VALUE PERSPECTIVE?

The perspective of the total value gained from a healthcare intervention is critically important for public policy purposes. What do we mean by this? We mean that the total value of an intervention can be assessed from the perspective of:

1. an individual patient, or
2. the reference case (the average patient in a cohort).

The Panel on Cost-Effectiveness in Health and Medicine recommends the *reference case perspective*[3-5] to assess value, and we unreservedly agree.

> The total value conferred by an intervention can be calculated using the:
> 1. individual perspective, or
> 2. the reference case (average case) perspective.

The Individual Perspective

The individual perspective measures the value conferred from the viewpoint of one individual. For example, the total value conferred by total knee arthroplasty that improves the utility value of a 75-year-old person from 0.75 to 0.95 for his 12-year life expectancy is $(0.95 - 0.75) \times 12 = 2.4$ QALYs.

Assuming the same total knee arthroplasty lasts for the 26-year lifetime of a 55-year-old person, the total value gained is $(0.95 - 0.75) \times 26 = 5.2$ QALYs. With the individual perspective, the total value gained from an intervention is dependent upon the duration of benefit of the intervention, which is often related to the time of remaining life. Thus, the total value gained from the same intervention is greater for the 55-year-old with a longer life expectancy than for the 75-year-old patient. Needless to say, the individual perspective is often biased against older individuals because it attributes more value from the majority of interventions to younger individuals. In a society in which healthcare resources are very limited, the individual perspective might theoretically lead to greater resource allocation to younger individuals over older individuals.

While some might consider the individual perspective to be the most scientifically valid, there are strong arguments that prevent its implementation. Senior organizations would likely lobby very effectively in the political arena against this form of age discrimination. Moreover, the Age Discrimination in Employment Act (ADEA) of 1967 protects individuals 40 years of age or older from employment discrimination based upon age.[6] Under the ADEA, *it is unlawful to discriminate against a person because of his or her age with respect to any term, condition, or privilege of employment—including, but not limited to, hiring, firing, promotion, layoff, compensation, benefits, job assignments, and training.* The Older Workers Benefit Protection Act of 1990 (OWBPA) amended the ADEA specifically to prohibit employers from denying benefits to older employees.[6] This law can be interpreted to apply to the discriminatory denial of health benefits based upon age. Use of a reference case (average case) analysis precludes this form of bias against older individuals.

> The Older Workers Benefit Protection Act of 1990 specifically prohibits employers from denying health benefits to older employees on the basis of age.

Gender.   The individual perspective also biases treatment in favor of women, as compared to men, since the average woman in the United States has a mean life expectancy of 80.5 years and the average man has a mean life expectancy of 75.1.[7] The Civil Rights Act of 1964 specifically prohibits discrimination on the basis of gender in public accommodations, public facilities, and public educa-tion.[8] Public accommodations include healthcare facilities such as hospitals and healthcare providers' offices. Consequently, differentiation of treatment benefits according to gender should not be undertaken unless there is no other recourse, as is the case in gender-specific diseases. For example, the treatment of uterine fibroids can only be undertaken in women, while therapy for prostate cancer can only be undertaken in men.

> The Civil Rights Act of 1964 prohibits discrimination in public facilities (healthcare facilities) on the basis of gender or ethnicity.

Ethnicity. The average African-American in the United States has a mean life expectancy of 72.7 years, while the average Caucasian has a mean life expectancy of 78.4 years.[7] Every effort should be made to eradicate this disparity, an endeavor we believe VBM will facilitate.

Using ethnicity-specific longevity numbers to calculate the value conferred by interventions biases the value gained from many interventions against African-American patients since the decreased life expectancy of African-Americans decreases the duration of benefit for numerous interventions. As with gender, the Civil Rights Act of 1964 prohibits such discrimination.[8] The longevity esti-mates used in cost-utility analysis should therefore be those that ignore ethnicity and gender. The longevity of the average *person* in the US is the most appropri-ate value to use in most cost-utility analyses.

> The longevity estimates used in cost-utility analysis should be those for the *average person* in the US as this value ignores ethnicity and gender.

The Reference Case Value Perspective

The reference case value perspective is the case of the average patient who under-goes a healthcare intervention. For example, data from the Hip and Knee Registry, an observational database composed of data from the practices of orthopedic sur-geons in the United States during 1996 through 2001, reveal that the average per-son who undergoes a total knee arthroplasty is 69 years of age with a mean life expectancy of 16 additional years.[9] While to some it may seem counterintuitive, the conferred value of the intervention and the cost-utility of the intervention should be those associated with a person 69 years of age for comparison with the conferred value and cost-utility of other interventions. The value gained and the

> A reference case value perspective (case of the average patient) should be undertaken when employing cost-utility analysis for the comparability of dissimilar interventions.

cost-utility associated with other interventions also must be calculated using the average duration of benefit for the reference case for comparability.

> A reference case value perspective should not use longevity data influenced by gender and ethnicity unless the disease under study is gender-specific or ethnicity-specific.

WHY VALUE-BASED MEDICINE BEATS EVIDENCE-BASED MEDICINE

Value-based medicine gives a more accurate measure of the patient-perceived worth of a healthcare intervention than evidence-based medicine (EBM) alone. In doing so, VBM allows practitioners to deliver higher quality of care than EBM. The following sections illustrate why this is so.

> Value-based medicine allows a more accurate assessment of the patient-perceived worth of healthcare interventions than EBM alone.

Patient-Perceived Worth of Healthcare Interventions

How can VBM give a more accurate measure of the patient-perceived worth of healthcare interventions than EBM alone? This is a reasonable question that many have until they think about outcomes in a value-based fashion.

Evidence-based clinical trials to date have generally devoted scant attention to quality-of-life measures. Primary evidence-based outcomes are most often measured in terms of survival, number of heart attacks, number of strokes, lines of vision lost, gastroduodenal ulcers prevented, and so on. The quality-of-life parameters associated with these outcomes in a clinical trial are often not factored into the benefit equation. When they are factored in, the value of a treatment can change considerably. This can lead to a substantial *overestimation* or *underestimation* of the patient-perceived value conferred by an intervention.

> Value-based medicine identifies interventions that are harmful, neutral, or of superior value when this is not demonstrable by EBM data alone.

Overestimation of the Value of an Intervention With Evidence-Based Medicine

How can evidence-based data overestimate the value of an intervention? The following example sheds some light. The primary benefit outcome of chemotherapy for cancer is typically additional time of life gained from treatment. The adverse effects of chemotherapy upon quality of life are generally not quantitatively evaluated. In certain instances, however, the total value of remaining life may actually be decreased by treatment when quality-of-life variables are incorporated.

Consider the case of the average person (reference case) with breast cancer who undergoes chemotherapy, which adds a 13th month to her otherwise 12-month life expectancy (Table 11.2). In addition to the evidence-based data demonstrating the improvement in length of life, quality-of-life data reveal that her utility value associated with the chemotherapy is 0.70 due to moderate to severe vomiting from chemotherapy.

Evidence-Based Outcome. The primary evidence-based outcome of change in length of life shows that the patient lives for 13 months (1.083 years), one month longer than with no chemotherapy. Utility values are not considered and her evidence-based improvement in length of life from the treatment is therefore 8.3%.

Value-Based Outcome. The value-based outcome also shows that the patient lives for one extra month, an additional 8.3% in value. Nonetheless, her moderate to severe vomiting associated with the chemotherapy diminishes her utility value to 0.70. The total value gained during this time is therefore 1.083 years $\times$ 0.70 = 0.758 QALY, a 30% decrease in value compared to the evidence-based outcome of an 8.3% improvement in length of life, but in which quality of life is not considered. Needless to say, the evidence-based and value-based outcomes are dramatically different. In this instance, chemotherapy actually has a net negative effect upon the person's remaining value of life compared to no treatment.

Value-Based Outcome. Does the net harmful effect mean that treatment should be denied to this patient? No. Does it mean the patient should be fully informed of these outcomes before electing to undergo chemotherapy? Yes.

TABLE 11.2

Value of Remaining Life With Cancer Treated and Not Treated With Chemotherapy

Evidence-Based Medicine Perspective			
Treatment	Utility Value	Multiplied By Time	Value Accrued Over Remaining Life
No Chemotherapy	1.00	0.083	1.083 QALY
Value-Based Medicine Perspective			
Treatment	Utility Value	Multiplied By Time	Value Accrued Over Remaining Life
Chemotherapy	0.70	1.083	0.758 QALY

The value-based outcomes also indicate to the clinician that therapy should be modified in an attempt to yield a net positive benefit. Assuming that a potent antinausea and antiemetic agent such as dolasetron, a benzamide derivative that blocks serotonin uptake, eradicates the vomiting, the utility value rises back to 1.00. Thus, the patient will be able to live the 13 months at a utility value of 1.00, a net overall gain of 0.083 QALYs compared with no chemotherapy.

Underestimation of the Value of an Intervention With Evidence-Based Medicine

Just as evidence-based primary outcomes can overestimate the value of an intervention, they can also underestimate the value of an intervention. In this instance, the evidence-base outcome again includes only length of life.

Evidence-Based Outcome.　As an example, let us assume the primary evidence-based outcome of a study to evaluate a hydroxymethyl glutaryl coenzyme A reductase inhibitor, or "statin," shows that the drug increases life expectancy of the average person (reference case) with hyperlipidemia from four to five years. This evidence-based perspective thereby demonstrates a 25% (one year/four years) increase in the remaining value of the patient's life using length of life as the only outcome, as shown in Table 11.3. Quality-of-life variables are not considered in this EBM perspective.

Value-Based Outcome.　With the more accurate value-based perspective, both of the primary outcomes of quality of life and length of life change conferred by use of the statin are factored into the analysis. Let us assume the incidence of decreased quality of life from the disabling stroke (utility value = 0.50) in the

TABLE　11.3

Evidence-Based Medicine Perspective: The Improvement in Length of Life Is the Primary Outcome

	Utility Value*	Multiplied by Time	Value Accrued Over Remaining Life
No Treatment	1.00	4 years	4.0 QALYs
Evidence-Based Treatment	1.00	5 years	5.0 QALYs Outcome
		Gain =	1.0 QALY With Treatment

* The utility value, or quality of life, is insignificant in the evidence-based scenario, because only length of life is considered as the primary outcome.

value-based scenario is 20% of the untreated reference case cohort. This drops the overall utility value of the reference case to 0.90 with no treatment, a more accurate measure than the evidence-based scenario in which only survival is considered and the quality of life is ignored. (Remember that the reference case is the average person in a cohort of patients, thus representing the entire cohort.)

In addition to the statin increasing the length of life by 25%, we include with the VBM perspective the fact that the drug decreases the incidence of disabling stroke from 20% of the reference case cohort to 10% of the reference case cohort.

With no statin treatment, the average utility value of the reference case cohort is 0.90. This occurs because 80% of the theoretical cohort has a utility value of 1.00 and the 20% with a stroke has a utility value of 0.50. The resultant value of 0.90 is essentially a weighted average of the percent of the cohort without a stoke and the percent with a stroke (Table 11.4).

With statin treatment, the resulting utility value of the reference case is 0.95, because 90% of the theoretical cohort has a utility value of 1.00 and the 10% with a stroke has a utility value of 0.50.

In this case, the evidence-based treatment outcome of survival shows that the reference case gains 1.00 QALY with statin treatment, while the value-based treatment outcome, which includes quality-of-life changes with survival changes, more accurately shows that the reference case gains 1.15 QALYs. Hence, the EBM outcome shows a 25% gain in value over no treatment, while the VBM outcome shows a 32% (1.15 QALYs/3.6 QALYs) gain in value over no treatment.

> *Value-based medicine* allows the delivery of higher quality patient care than *evidence-based medicine* because it more accurately identifies the total value conferred by interventions.

These cases demonstrate the key concept that VBM allows the delivery of higher quality patient care than EBM because it more accurately identifies the

TABLE 11.4

Value-Based Medicine Perspective: The Improvement in Quality of Life and Length of Life Are the Primary Outcomes

	Utility Value	Multiplied by Time	Value Accrued Over Remaining Life
No Treatment	0.90	4 years	3.6 QALYs
Value-Based Treatment	0.95	5 years	4.75 QALYs Outcome
		Gain =	1.15 QALYs

total value that interventions deliver to patients. When providers appreciate which interventions are more valuable than others, they are able to provide patients with the interventions that confer greater value. A critical factor is that the value gained from these interventions is perceived from the patient point of view, that of the person who lives with a disease and experiences the effects of an intervention for that disease on a firsthand basis.

OTHER MEASURES OF VALUE

Other measures of the value of healthcare interventions, such as the health year equivalent (HYE)[10] and the disability-adjusted life-year (DALY), can be used theoretically to quantify the value conferred by an intervention for cost-utility analysis, but they have not gained favor to the extent of the QALY. The DALY was developed by the World Bank in 1993[11] to:

1. measure the burden of disease, and
2. increase the efficiency of resource allocation by identifying health interventions that, for a given budget, purchase the largest improvement in health, particularly in low-income countries.

The DALY takes into account both years of life lost and years lived with disability. As with the QALY, it weights different health states on a scale from 0.0 to 1.0 in regard to disability. A value of 0, however, indicates full health on the DALY scale, while 1.0 equates with death.

The DALY is more complex than the QALY in that it assigns different importance to a healthy life at different ages. Age weights rise from birth to age 25, then slowly decline. This reflects the increased productivity of healthy, middle-aged adults and the dependence of both the young and the elderly upon healthy, middle-aged adults. The DALY has been criticized for the following reasons[12]:

1. it discriminates against the elderly,
2. the calculation methodology is complex,
3. the manner in which the data are manipulated (25 years old is the most valuable age) is subjective, and
4. decisions have been made with little involvement of healthcare providers.

We believe the reader should be aware that the DALY exists, but we do not believe it will come into widespread use for cost-utility analysis and VBM because of the criticisms stated.

Since 2000, the World Health Organization has reported annually on the average health within its member countries using the health-adjusted life expectancy (HALE) in place of the DALY as a summary measure combining data on mortality and morbidity.[13,14] The HALE combines mortality with country-specific estimates of the prevalence of 135 conditions from the Global Burden of Disease 2000 Study[15] and an analysis of health surveys. While the HALE theoretically could be used for cost-utility analysis at some point in the future, the exact methodology is still under development.[13,16]

CORE CONCEPTS

- A quality-adjusted life-year (QALY) is a measure of life's value accrued over time.
- Living at a utility value of 1.00 for one year accrues one QALY. Living at a utility value of 0.50 for one year accrues 0.50 QALY.
- The QALY incorporates all improvements in length of life and/or quality of life conferred by a healthcare intervention.
- The QALYs conferred by a healthcare intervention objectively measure the total value gain from the intervention.
- The QALY can also integrate all adverse effects induced by a healthcare intervention.
- Events that cause a very small change in value (such as postoperative discomfort for one to two days after an operation that improves value for 20 years) do not have to be incorporated in interventional value and cost-utility calculations.
- QALYs are *comparable* across all interventions in healthcare.
- Cost-utility analyses used for public policy should be performed using a *reference-case analysis value perspective* (case of the average person undergoing a healthcare intervention).
- Value-based medicine provides a more accurate measure of the patient-perceived worth of a healthcare intervention than EBM because it incorporates quality-of-life variables that are often ignored in evidence-based clinical trial outcomes.
- Because VBM provides a more accurate measure of the patient-perceived worth of healthcare interventions, it allows clinicians to identify more valued interventions and thus deliver higher-quality care to patients.

REFERENCES

1. Klarman H, Francis J, Rosenthal G. Cost-effectiveness applied to the treatment of chronic renal disease. *Med Care.* 1968;6:48–55.

2. Drummond ME, O'Brien B, Stoddart GL, Torrance GW. *Methods for the Economic Evaluation of Health Care Programmes.* 2nd ed. New York, NY: Oxford University Press; 1999.

3. Gold MR, Patrick DL, Torrance GW, et al. Identifying and valuing outcomes. In: Gold MR, Siegel JE, Russell LB, Weinstein MC, eds. *Cost-Effectiveness in Health and Medicine.* New York, NY: Oxford University Press; 1996:82–134.

4. Siegel JE, Weinstein MC, Russell LB, Gold MR. Recommendations for reporting cost-effectiveness analyses. Panel on Cost-Effectiveness in Health and Medicine. *JAMA.* 1996;276:1339–1341.

5. Weinstein MC, Siegel JE, Gold MR, Kamlet MS, Russell LB. Recommendations of the Panel on Cost-Effectiveness in Health and Medicine. *JAMA.* 1996;276:1253–1258.

6. Equal Employment Opportunity Commission. Facts about age discrimination. Available at: www.eeoc.gov/facts/age.html. Accessed January 17, 2004.

7. Arias E. United States life tables, 2000. *Natl Vital Stat Rep.* 2002;51:1–39.

8. Gomez-Mejia LR, Balkin DB, Cardy RL. *Managing Human Resources.* Englewood Cliffs, NJ: Prentice Hall; 1995:126–133.

9. Anderson FA Jr, Hirsh J, White K, Fitzgerald RH Jr, Hip and Knee Registry Investigators. Temporal trends in prevention of venous thromboembolism following primary total hip or knee arthroplasty 1996-2001: findings from the Hip and Knee Registry. *Chest.* 2003;124(6 suppl):349S–356S.

10. Gafni A, Birch S. Economics, health and health economics: HYEs versus QALYs. *J Health Econ.* 1993;11:325–339.

11. Homedes N. The disability-adjusted life year (DALY): definition, measurement and potential use. Human Capital Development and Operations Policy Working Paper, World Bank. Available at: www.worldbank.org/html/extdr/hnp/hddflash/workp// wp_00068.html. Accessed October 2, 2003.

12. Anand S, Hanson K. Disability-adjusted life years: a critical review. *J Health Econ.* 1997;16:685–702.

13. Mathers CD, Murray CJ, Salomon JA, et al. Healthy life expectancy: comparison of OECD countries in 2001. *Aust N Z J Public Health.* 2003;27:5–11.

14. Sadana R, Tandon A, Mathers CD, et al. Comparable measures of population health with a focus on OCED countries. In: Martin JP, ed. *A Disease-Based Comparison of Health Systems.* Paris, France: Organisation for Economic Co-operation and Development; 2003:261–274.

15. Shibuya K, Mathers CD, Boschi-Pinto C, Lopez AD, Murray CJ. Global and regional estimates of cancer mortality and incidence by site, II: results for the global burden of disease 2000. *Bio Med Central Cancer.* 2002;2:37. Available at: http://www.biomedcentral.com/1471-2407/2/37.

16. Mathers CD, Sadana R, Salomon JA, Murray CJL, Lopez AD. Healthy life expectancy in 191 countries. *Lancet.* 1999;357:1685–1691.

12

Discounting Made Simple

Discounting is the process used to account for the time value of money or some other entity of value. In regard to money, a thousand dollars in hand at the present time is more valuable than a thousand dollars in hand in the future.[1] That thousand dollars received five years from now or ten years from now has less value than money now, and therefore it must be reduced (discounted) by an appropriate degree.[1]

There are two realities in healthcare: benefits are derived and costs are expended. To truly understand the value of an intervention, the principle of discounting needs to be applied to both benefits and costs associated with the intervention. The costs expended and the benefits immediately received from an intervention need not be discounted, but the principle becomes increasingly important as additional costs are expended and additional value is conferred in the form of quality-adjusted life-years (QALYs) gained after an intervention.

NET PRESENT VALUE ANALYSIS
OF HEALTHCARE INTERVENTIONS

The discounting of *future benefits (QALYs gained,* in the situation of health benefits), *costs* to their respective benefits, and costs today can be thought of as a net *present value analysis,* uniquely applied to healthcare. When utilized with healthcare interventions, the net present value analysis takes into account the present value of both healthcare expenditures and health benefits derived. Again, the rationale is that money and good health in hand now are worth more than money and good health in the future.

The rationale for discounting[2] includes the intuitive reasoning that:

1. Money and good health in hand now are worth more than money and good health in the future since individuals prefer current consumption to future consumption. Viewed in another perspective, money and good health in hand now can be invested to earn more money or something else of value with time.

2. When there is monetary inflation, the value of currency decreases over time.

3. Any risk associated with cash flow in the future reduces the value of the future cash flow.

B enefits gained = QALYs gained = outcome

A net *present value analysis* reduces future costs incurred and benefits gained (QALYs) to their present costs and benefits, respectively.

DISCOUNTING COSTS

Discounting costs is the process of moving cash flows expected in the future back to present dollars.[2] It is the reverse of *compounding*, which is the process by which cash flows are converted from present dollar values to future dollar values.

D *iscounting* is the process that accounts for the time value of money or some other entity of benefit (QALYs, in the case of health benefits).

Discounting is a straightforward calculation and can be described best through an example. If $1,000 is spent n years from now, and we assume a fixed rate of interest of 10%, then that $1,000 is worth $1,000/(1.10)^n$, today. This follows from the idea that this value [$1,000/(1.10)^n$], invested at a 10% annual return for n years, will yield $1,000 at the end of the n years. Therefore, if something of value is gained in the future, it does not have as much value as if it were gained today.

A dollar now is worth more than a dollar in the future because:
■ the dollar now has the opportunity to grow with time if invested,
■ monetary inflation decreases the value of money over time, and
■ any risk associated with future cash flow reduces the value of that cash flow.

DISCOUNTING OUTCOMES (VALUE GAINED)

Economists have recommended that health benefits (QALYs gained) be discounted in addition to costs.[3,4] The rationale? Weinstein and Stason[4] argue that QALYs are discounted not because a year of life in the future is not worth as much as a current year of life, but because the "steady-state relationship between dollars and health benefits mandates the discounting of health benefits (QALYs) in addition to dollar health costs." They walk readers through a simple scenario to demonstrate the fundamental break in logic that occurs if benefits are not discounted at the same rate as costs in an economic evaluation. We are not so certain about this rationale, but we believe it can also be argued that individuals prefer good health now and good health now is more valuable than good health in the future because good health now can be productively put to use for endeavors that will produce additional income or other entities of value over time. Whichever the underlying rationale, it is generally agreed that both costs and outcomes should be discounted at the same annual rate in healthcare economic analyses.[5-7]

We and most others do not confer greater value to years in one period of life over another in performing cost-utility analysis, although the disability-adjusted life-year (DALY) does so.[8] The fact that the DALY gives more value to the middle years of life leads to bias against the very young and older patients. That alone negates its use in cost-utility analyses from the political point of view.

THE PREFERRED ANNUAL DISCOUNT RATE

The Panel for Cost-Effectiveness in Health and Medicine,[5-7] a group initially organized by the US Public Health Service to set cost-effectiveness standards, recommended that healthcare costs and outcomes (QALYs gained) both be discounted at a rate of 3% per year. There is economic rationale for a 3% annual rate; over the past decade, this is what could have been earned over and above in a safe, or riskless, investment such as a short-term US Treasury bill.[8] We encourage interested readers to pursue this topic in further detail.[9]

> The Panel for Cost-Effectiveness in Health and Medicine[6,7] recommends that both costs and outcomes (value gained in QALYs) for an intervention be discounted at 3% per year.

THE IMPORTANCE OF COMPARABLE DISCOUNT RATES

The discount rate used for cost-utility analyses must be the same for studies to be comparable. Minor changes in the discount rate can lead to substantial changes in benefits (QALY) and cost results, particularly over long periods of time in analyses that model cost-effectiveness many years in the future. For the comparability of studies, it is therefore reasonable to perform sensitivity analyses using at least 3% and 5% annual discount rates in addition to an undiscounted analysis. This allows for the effects of the discount rate to be distinguished, and facilitates comparability with studies that may use a different discount rate.

HOW DISCOUNTING AFFECTS THE OUTCOME

If the costs are predominantly incurred at the start of an intervention, its cost-effectiveness will be less than if the costs are incurred at a later date. For example, $1,000 expended now for 0.1 QALY received now results in a $/QALY (cost-utility) of $1,000/0.1 = $10,000, while $1,000 spent in five years (3% annual discount rate) for 0.1 QALY received now results in a $/QALY of $[\$1,000/(1.03)^4]/(0.1) = \$8,600$.

If the health benefits are received early after the intervention, rather than years later, the intervention will be more cost-effective. Using the same example, if $1,000 is spent for 0.1 QALY received now, the $/QALY is $1,000/0.1 = $10,000, while $1,000 spent for 0.1 QALY in five years yields a $/QALY of $1,000/[0.1/(1.03)^4] = $11,628 when QALYs are discounted at a 3% annual rate.

As with many other opportunities in life, receiving a benefit now and paying for it later is more attractive, and in this case more cost-effective, than paying now and receiving the benefits at a later date.

HOW COSTS ARE DISCOUNTED

Discounting is typically not undertaken for costs or benefits (QALYs gained) during the first year after treatment. Health benefits incurred at the beginning of the second year after treatment are, however, discounted at 3%. The costs expended and value gained for *each* year, starting at the beginning of the second year forward, must be discounted at a different rate. The resultant values for each year are then added to arrived at the total discounted costs and the total discounted value (QALYs).

The discounting of benefits (QALYs) is shown in Table 12.1. Costs are discounted in exactly the same way. Discounting is accomplished by dividing the outcome and the costs, respectively, at the beginning of each year, starting one year after an intervention. Accordingly, outcomes and costs remain unchanged for the first year. For example, if there is a 3% annual discount rate and 0.5 QALY is gained each year, the discounted outcome for Year 1 (the first year) is $0.5/1.03^0$, the discounted outcome for Year 2 (the second year) is $0.5/1.03^1$, the discounted outcome for the Year 3 (the third year) is $0.5/1.03^2$, that for Year 4 (the fourth year) is $0.5/1.03^3$, and so on. This can become tedious when performed manually for periods of 70 or 80 years, although programs such as Microsoft Excel can readily undertake such calculations.

> We prefer to start discounting QALYs and costs beginning at the start of the second year after an initial intervention. Accordingly, the QALYs gained and costs incurred are not discounted during the first year.

Must Costs and Outcomes Be Discounted Starting at the Beginning of the Second Year After Treatment?

Not necessarily. Discounting could be started at three months after an intervention or six months after an intervention, especially if large costs are incurred at that time. If $1,000 is discounted at a 3% annual rate and we decide to discount earlier than at the start of the year after the initial intervention, the discount rate is intermediate between 1.00 and 1.03. With an annual discount rate of 3%,

TABLE 12.1

Discounting of Benefits Gained at Various Annual Discount Rates*

Annual Discount Rate	Discounted QALY Value				Total Discounted QALYs
	Year 1	Year 2	Year 3	Year 4	
0%	0.5	+ 0.5	+ 0.5	+ 0.5	= 2.0
3%	0.5	+ 0.5/1.03	+ 0.5/(1.03)^2	+ 0.5/(1.03)^3	= 1.91
5%	0.5	+ 0.5/1.05	+ 0.5/(1.05)^2	+ 0.5/(1.05)^3	= 1.86
10%	0.5	+ 0.5/1.10	+ 0.5/(1.10)^2	0.5/(1.10)^3	= 1.74

QALY indicates quality-adjusted life-year.

* Assuming a 0.5-QALY gain per year for five years and application of the rate at the beginning of a yearly period, starting at Year 2. QALYs gained in the future are converted to their present value using various discount rates. The higher the discount rate, the lower the present value of QALYs.

discounting costs spent three months after the initial intervention is accomplished by dividing the costs by 1.0075. If the discount rate is 3% per year and the costs are discounted starting at six months after the intervention, the discount rate for costs and outcomes incurred from six months to 12 months is 1.5%. While discounting starting at three months or six months is slightly more accurate than beginning at the end of one year, the variation is relatively minor and discounting tables and calculators often do not calculate in less than single digits. Thus, we generally prefer to start discounting at the end of one year.

The costs expended at the time of an initial intervention are not discounted, no matter what the discount rate. If $1,000 is discounted at a 3% annual rate

TABLE 12.2

Discounting of Costs at Other Than Yearly Intervals After the Initial Intervention

Cost	Time After Intervention	Discount Rate/Year	Cost/ Divisor	Discounted Cost
$1,000	0	3%	$1,000/1.00	$1,000
$1,000	3 months	3%	$1,000/1.0075	$992
$1,000	6 months	3%	$1,000/1.015	$985
$1,000	1 year	3%	$1,000/1.030	$971
$1,000	1.5 years	3%	$1,000/1.045	$957
$1,000	10 years	3%	$1,000/1.03^{10}	$744
$1,000	70 years	3%	$1,000/1.03^{70}	$126
			Total:	**$5,775**

and we decide to discount starting six months after the intervention, the discount rate is 1.5% and the discounted value of funds spent at this time is $1,000/1.015. Assuming an annual discount rate of 3%, costs occurring at other than yearly intervals after the initial intervention are discounted by dividing them as shown in Table 12.2.

Is There Another Way to Discount?

Costs and benefits (QALYs gained) can also be discounted at the rates shown, and for the years shown, by multiplying by the appropriate multiplier (Tables 12.3, 12.4, 12.5) starting at the beginning of the second year after the intervention. This is just a variation on the theme of multiplying by a number less than 1.0, rather then dividing by a number greater than 1.0. For example, discounting 0.5 QALY at the beginning of the second year after the intervention can be accomplished by multiplying $(1/1.03) \times 0.5$ or dividing 0.5 by 1.03. Again, costs are typically discounted on a yearly basis, but they can be discounted more frequently, particularly if there are large expenditures during the first year or two after treatment. Whether the discounting takes place at yearly intervals or more often, however, the costs and outcomes (QALYs) must be discounted in the same fashion.

CORE CONCEPTS

- *Discounting* is the economic tool used to account for the time value of money (costs) and outcomes (QALYs or value gained). It is the reverse of *compounding*. A net *present value analysis* of healthcare interventions discounts future costs and value gained (QALYs) to their present value.

TABLE 12.3

Using Multipliers to Discount Health Benefits (QALYs)

		Outcomes		
QALY Gained	**Time After Intervention**	**Annual Discount Rate**	**Multiplier**	**Discounted QALYs (Multiplier × 0.5 QALY)**
0.5	0	3%	1.0	0.5
0.5	3 months	3%	0.992	0.496
0.5	6 months	3%	0.985	0.4925
0.5	1 year	3%	0.971	0.4855
0.5	1.5 years	3%	0.957	0.4785
0.5	10 years	3%	0.744	0.372
0.5	70 years	3%	0.126	0.063

TABLE 12.4

Using Multipliers to Discount Costs*

Cost	Time After Intervention	Annual Discount Rate	Multiplier	Discounted Cost (Multiplier × 0.5 QALY)
$1,000	0	3%	1.0	$1,000
$1,000	3 months	3%	0.992	$992
$1,000	6 months	3%	0.985	$985
$1,000	1 year	3%	0.971	$971
$1,000	1.5 years	3%	0.957	$957
$1,000	10 years	3%	0.744	$744
$1,000	70 years	3%	0.126	$126
			Total:	$5,775

* Note that the discounted costs are the same as those shown in Table 12.2.

TABLE 12.5

Discounting Multiplier Table for Outcomes and Costs*

Year	Annual Discount Rate				
	0%	1%	3%	5%	10%
0	1	1	1	1	1
0.25 (3 months)	1	0.9975	0.9925	0.9876	0.9756
0.50 (6 months)	1	0.9950	0.9852	0.9756	0.9524
0.75 (9 months)	1	0.9925	0.9780	0.9638	0.9302
1	1	0.9901	0.9709	0.9524	0.9090
1.5	1	0.9852	0.9569	0.9302	0.8696
2	1	0.9803	0.9426	0.9070	0.8264
3	1	0.9706	0.9151	0.8638	0.7513
4	1	0.9609	0.8885	0.8227	0.6830
5	1	0.9514	0.8626	0.7835	0.6209
6	1	0.9420	0.8375	0.7462	0.5645
7	1	0.9327	0.8131	0.7107	0.5132
8	1	0.9234	0.7894	0.6768	0.4665
9	1	0.9143	0.7664	0.6446	0.4241
10	1	0.9053	0.7441	0.6139	0.3855
11	1	0.8963	0.7224	0.5847	0.3505
12	1	0.8874	0.7014	0.5568	0.3186
13	1	0.8786	0.6810	0.5303	0.2897

continued

TABLE   12.5 continued

Discounting Multiplier Table for Outcomes and Costs*

	Annual Discount Rate				
Year	0%	1%	3%	5%	10%
14	1	0.8699	0.6611	0.5051	0.2633
15	1	0.8613	0.6419	0.4810	0.2394
16	1	0.8528	0.6232	0.4581	0.2176
17	1	0.8443	0.6050	0.4363	0.1978
18	1	0.8360	0.5874	0.4155	0.1799
19	1	0.8277	0.5703	0.3957	0.1635
20	1	0.8195	0.5537	0.3769	0.1486
21	1	0.8114	0.5375	0.3589	0.1351
22	1	0.8034	0.5219	0.3418	0.1228
23	1	0.7954	0.5067	0.3256	0.1117
24	1	0.7875	0.4919	0.3101	0.1015
25	1	0.7797	0.4776	0.2953	0.0923
26	1	0.7720	0.4637	0.2812	0.0839
27	1	0.7644	0.4502	0.2678	0.0763
28	1	0.7568	0.4371	0.2551	0.0693
29	1	0.7493	0.4243	0.2429	0.0630
30	1	0.7419	0.4120	0.2314	0.0573
31	1	0.7346	0.4000	0.2204	0.0521
32	1	0.7273	0.3883	0.2099	0.0474
33	1	0.7201	0.3770	0.1999	0.0431
34	1	0.7129	0.3660	0.1904	0.0391
35	1	0.7059	0.3554	0.1813	0.0356
36	1	0.6989	0.3450	0.1727	0.0323
37	1	0.6920	0.3350	0.1644	0.0294
38	1	0.6851	0.3252	0.1566	0.0267
39	1	0.6783	0.3158	0.1491	0.0243
40	1	0.6716	0.3066	0.1420	0.0221
41	1	0.6650	0.2976	0.1353	0.0201
42	1	0.6584	0.2890	0.1288	0.0183
43	1	0.6519	0.2805	0.1227	0.0166
44	1	0.6454	0.2724	0.1169	0.0151
45	1	0.6390	0.2644	0.1113	0.0137
46	1	0.6327	0.2567	0.1060	0.0125
47	1	0.6264	0.2493	0.1009	0.0113
48	1	0.6202	0.2420	0.0961	0.0103
49	1	0.6141	0.2350	0.0916	0.0094

TABLE 12.5 continued

Discounting Multiplier Table for Outcomes and Costs*

	Annual Discount Rate				
Year	0%	1%	3%	5%	10%
50	1	0.6080	0.2281	0.0872	0.0085
51	1	0.6020	0.2215	0.0831	0.0077
52	1	0.5960	0.2150	0.0791	0.0070
53	1	0.5901	0.2088	0.0753	0.0064
54	1	0.5843	0.2027	0.0717	0.0058
55	1	0.5785	0.1968	0.0683	0.0053
56	1	0.5728	0.1910	0.0651	0.0048
57	1	0.5671	0.1855	0.0620	0.0044
58	1	0.5615	0.1801	0.0590	0.0040
59	1	0.5559	0.1748	0.0562	0.0036
60	1	0.5504	0.1697	0.0535	0.0033
61	1	0.5450	0.1648	0.0510	0.0030
62	1	0.5396	0.1600	0.0486	0.0027
63	1	0.5342	0.1553	0.0462	0.0025
64	1	0.5290	0.1508	0.0440	0.0022
65	1	0.5237	0.1464	0.0419	0.0020
66	1	0.5185	0.1421	0.0399	0.0019
67	1	0.5134	0.1380	0.0380	0.0017
68	1	0.5083	0.1340	0.0362	0.0015
69	1	0.5033	0.1301	0.0345	0.0014
70	1	0.4983	0.1263	0.0329	0.0013
71	1	0.4934	0.1226	0.0313	0.0012
72	1	0.4885	0.1190	0.0298	0.0010
73	1	0.4836	0.1156	0.0284	0.0010
74	1	0.4789	0.1122	0.0270	0.0009
75	1	0.4741	0.1089	0.0258	0.0008
76	1	0.4648	0.1027	0.0234	0.0006
77	1	0.4602	0.0997	0.0222	0.0006
78	1	0.4556	0.0968	0.0212	0.0005
79	1	0.4511	0.0940	0.0202	0.0005
80	1	0.4466	0.0912	0.0192	0.0004
81	1	0.4422	0.0886	0.0183	0.0004
82	1	0.4378	0.0860	0.0174	0.0004
83	1	0.4335	0.0835	0.0166	0.0003
84	1	0.4292	0.0811	0.0158	0.0003
85	1	0.4250	0.0787	0.0151	0.0003

continued

TABLE 12.5 continued

Discounting Multiplier Table for Outcomes and Costs*

Year	Annual Discount Rate				
	0%	1%	3%	5%	10%
86	1	0.4208	0.0764	0.0143	0.0003
87	1	0.4166	0.0742	0.0137	0.0002
88	1	0.4125	0.0720	0.0130	0.0002
89	1	0.4084	0.0699	0.0124	0.0002
90	1	0.4043	0.0679	0.0118	0.0002
91	1	0.4003	0.0659	0.0112	0.0002
92	1	0.3964	0.0640	0.0107	0.0001
93	1	0.3924	0.0621	0.0102	0.0001
94	1	0.3886	0.0603	0.0097	0.0001
95	1	0.3847	0.0586	0.0092	0.0001
96	1	0.3809	0.0569	0.0088	0.0001
97	1	0.3771	0.0552	0.0084	0.0001
98	1	0.3734	0.0536	0.0080	0.0001
99	1	0.3697	0.0520	0.0076	0.0001
100	1	0.3660	0.0505	0.0072	0.0001

* The costs incurred and/or outcomes conferred after the time shown post intervention are multiplied by a number to the right, depending upon the annual discount rate employed. Discounting is usually started at the beginning of year 2 (or the very end of year 1).

- The rationale for discounting includes the intuitive reasoning that:
  — Money and good health in hand now are worth more than money and good health in the future since individuals prefer current consumption to future consumption. Viewed in another perspective, money and good health in hand now can be invested to earn more money or something else of value with time.
  — When there is monetary inflation, the value of currency decreases over time.
  — Any risk associated with cash flow in the future reduces the value of the future cash flow.
- Both costs and outcomes should be discounted at the same rate.
- While there is some controversy in this regard, the discounting of QALYs is undertaken since good health now can produce future goods of value.

- The Panel for Cost-Effectiveness in Health and Medicine recommends a 3% annual discount rate for healthcare costs and outcomes (QALYs gained).
- Sensitivity analysis varying the base case discount rate of 3% to between zero and 5% should be undertaken to ascertain the effect of discounting and to allow better comparability with other papers in the literature that might not have used discounting or discounted at a rate other than the recommended 3%.

REFERENCES

1. Case KE, Fair RC. *Principles of Economics.* 4th ed. Upper Saddle River, NJ: Prentice Hall; 1996:1–133.

2. Damodaran A. *Corporate Finance, Theory and Practice.* New York, NY: John Wiley & Sons, Inc; 1997:37–65.

3 Drummond ME, O'Brien B, Stoddart GL, Torrance GW. *Methods for the Economic Evaluation of Health Care Programmes.* 2nd ed. New York, NY: Oxford University Press; 1999.

4. Weinstein MC, Stason WB. Foundations of cost-effectiveness analysis for health and medical practices. *N Engl J Med.* 1977;296:716–721.

5. Gold MR, Patrick DL, Torrance GW, et al. Identifying and valuing outcomes. In: Gold MR, Siegel JE, Russell LB, Weinstein MC, eds. *Cost-Effectiveness in Health and Medicine.* New York, NY: Oxford University Press; 1996:82–134.

6. Siegel JE, Weinstein MC, Russell LB, Gold MR. Recommendations for reporting cost-effectiveness analyses: Panel on Cost-Effectiveness in Health and Medicine. *JAMA.* 1996;276:1339–1341.

7. Weinstein MC, Siegel JE, Gold MR, Kamlet MS, Russell LB. Recommendations of the Panel on Cost-Effectiveness in Health and Medicine. *JAMA.* 1996;276:1253–1258.

8. Brown GC, Brown MM, Sharma S. Cost-effectiveness of therapy for threshold retinopathy of prematurity. *Pediatrics.* 1999;104:e47.

9. Luce BB, Manning WG, Siegel JE, Lipscomb J. Estimating costs in cost-effectiveness analysis. In: Gold MR, Siegel JE, Russell LB, Weinstein MC, eds. *Cost-Effectiveness in Health and Medicine.* New York, NY: Oxford University Press; 1996:176–213.

13

Decision Analysis

A healthcare economic analysis involves two separate processes. First, one must determine the preferred course of action when uncertainty exists. This can be done through the use of decision analysis. A well-conducted decision analysis should integrate all potential outcomes associated with vying treatment alternatives. Potential outcomes included in the analysis should incorporate the benefits as well as the outcomes that may be adverse in nature. In addition, these outcomes need to be valued in terms of their desirability from the patient perspective. Through the use of decision analysis, one treatment alternative is typically demonstrated to be superior—or more desirable—than another.

For example, let us assume that two nonsteroidal anti-inflammatory drugs have the same clinical benefit in alleviating pain. In addition, on the surface it appears as though both drugs have similar adverse effect profiles. At first glance, the drugs may therefore be considered equivalent by clinicians, patients, and drug formulary committees. However, upon further scrutiny it is noted that the incidence and severity of potential adverse effects differ between the two. By weighing all aspects of the clinical benefits and the side effects, one treatment will almost certainly be proven to be superior to the other.

Decision analysis incorporates elements of evidence-based medicine, but values them in terms that are germane to patients—the *desirability* of different outcomes. Through its use, different treatment alternatives can be compared to one another in global terms. Decision analysis is especially valuable as well for another reason: the fact that it can demonstrate that one intervention is preferable to another when clinical judgment and primary evidence-based outcomes cannot effectively differentiate between the value conferred by two seemingly similar interventions. Decision analysis is an important first step in creating an economic healthcare analysis, and a necessary precursor for determining the value of an intervention.

> Decision analysis, by incorporating all benefits and adverse effects associated with an intervention, can demonstrate that one intervention is preferable to another when clinical judgment and primary evidence-based outcomes cannot effectively differentiate between the value conferred by two seemingly similar interventions.

MODELING THE PROBLEM

Unless a fully prospective economic evaluation is being performed, relevant cost and effectiveness data must be combined through analytic modeling to determine a cost-utility ratio. Clearly, an economic evaluation can be very complex and incorporate a large number of variables. Consequently, the purpose of modeling the problem is to simplify reality to a level where it is of practical use.

The first task in modeling a problem is to decide on a time horizon. Ideally, long-term data will be available for the health program of interest, but in many cases only a specified period of effectiveness data will be available. Understanding the health program that is being modeled will also play a role in determining the time horizon that should be considered. For example, if an economic evaluation is designed to study the cost-effectiveness of a smoking cessation program, the main health outcome of interest may be survival at the end of a lifetime (ie, 25 to 50 years in the future), and a long-term time horizon will be necessary.

It is often advisable to perform a short-term analysis where primary data are available. If the primary data are not available, a longer-term analysis can be modeled into the future. For example, data from the North American Symptomatic Carotid Endarterectomy Trial (NASCET) and the European Carotid Surgery Trial (ECST) show that endarterectomy results in a five-year, 21% absolute risk reduction compared to aspirin therapy in patients with a symptomatic carotid artery stenosis of 70% to 99%.[1-3] The benefits have been demonstrated to be maintained at ten years.[3] In this instance, the study can be modeled directly from data for the first ten years. Assuming that the average patient lives for 20 years following endarterectomy, the data can either be carried forward from the ten-year point to the 20-year point or modeled according to whether other evidence-based data show that the benefit increases or decreases over the next ten years. If in doubt as to which time frame is best, both the ten-year and 20-year time frames can be modeled.

> The time frame for a healthcare economic analysis can vary, depending upon the availability of the data and the information required from the health program modeled.

> When long-term data are not available, many researchers *carry forward* or model the most recent data.

BASIC DECISION ANALYSIS

Basic decision analysis, also called *straightforward* or *simple* decision analysis, is a methodology that allows for the calculation of the most probable outcome of an intervention or a strategy. It is used to determine the preferred treatment option when there is a scenario of uncertainty. The models employed in this chapter (Figures 13.1, 13.2, 13.3. 13.4, and 13.5) were developed with TreeAge Data 4.0 decision analysis software from TreeAge Software (www.treeage.com).[4]

> Decision analysis demonstrates the preferred strategy under a situation of uncertainty, by valuing all possible outcomes of an intervention.

There is a large body of literature on medical decision analysis, and we recommend the reader consult other texts[5,6] for a detailed description of modeling methods and points of consideration. Decision analysis has its roots in economics and game theory and has been used for decades.

In essence, decision tree models are a sequence of decisions and chance events over time where every chance event is assigned a probability.[7-9] Each path through the decision tree consists of a combination of decision and chance nodes and is associated with a final pathway designated by a terminal node (Figure 13.1).[10,11] Each decision alternative is evaluated with weighted utility values calculated from data entered at the terminal nodes of the decision analysis tree and the proportions of weighting entered below the branches. The preferred decision is defined as the alternative with the largest expected utility.

> Decision analysis allows for decisions to be made using information that is relevant to patients—their *desirability* of different potential outcomes.

While the outcomes associated with terminal nodes (triangles) are often in the form of utility values, other values (dollars, $/QALY, life-years, visual acuity, decibel level, and so on) can be used depending upon what is being studied. In this book we use only QALYs as outcomes for both straightforward and Markov decision analysis trees. If a problem is straightforward and does not have to be modeled for recurrent risk, a basic decision tree will often be adequate (Figures 13.1, 13.2).

The nodes in Figure 13.1 are represented as follows:

1. The rectangle is a *decision node*. The decision here is whether to treat or not to treat with antibiotics.

2. Each oval is a *chance node*. With each decision there is a chance of living and a chance of dying. The chance of each outcome is indicated under the respective branch in decimal form (decimal x 100 = %). For example, with antibiotic treatment there is a 90% chance of living and a 10% chance of dying. With no antibiotic treatment, there is a 10% chance of living and a 90% chance of dying.

3. Each triangle is a *terminal node* representing an outcome. The utility values to the right of the terminal nodes are those associated with specific outcomes (1.0 corresponds to full recovery and normal health, while a value of 0.0 corresponds to death).

The utility values associated with each outcome are weighted according to the chance of occurrence to give the most probable utility value outcome (located in the rectangular boxes just to the right of the oval decision nodes) for each major

FIGURE   13.1

Straightforward Decision Tree for Bacterial Pneumonia. The tree, as is the case for all decision analysis trees, progresses from left to right, with increasing numbers of branches as it advances.

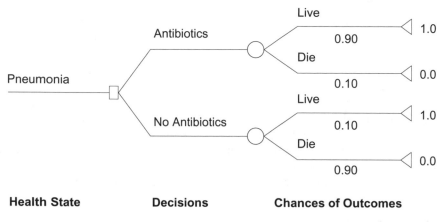

Health State   Decisions   Chances of Outcomes

FIGURE   13.2

Solved Basic Decision Tree for Pneumonia Corresponding to Figure 13.1

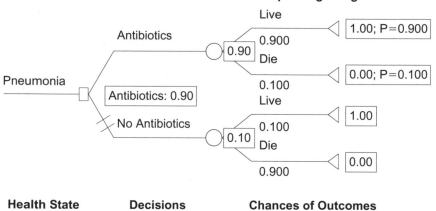

Health State   Decisions   Chances of Outcomes

branch emanating from the decision node (Figure 13.2). The preferred strategy here is treatment with antibiotics, and the utility value for the *reference case* (average case) treated with antibiotics is 0.90. For no treatment with antibiotics, the utility value outcome is 0.10. Thus, there is a 0.90 − 0.10 = 0.80 utility value gain for the average patient with bacterial pneumonia treated with antibiotics vs the average patient with bacterial pneumonia not treated with antibiotics. If the treatment benefit lasts for the 20-year life expectancy of the average patient, the undiscounted gain in value from the treatment for the reference case is 0.80 (in utility value improvement) × 20 (years) = 16.0 QALYs.

> **D**ecision analysis determines expected gains in quality of life associated with an intervention and compares them with those expected from other interventions and/or no treatment.

What Program Should We Use?

There are multiple decision analysis programs available. A review of the more common programs commercially available can be viewed at a Web site sponsored by the Decision Analysis Society.[12] We currently use TreeAge Software's TreeAge Data 4.0 decision analysis software with the Healthcare User's Manual.

Many variables can be incorporated into a decision analysis tree (Figure 13.3). At times the number of variables can run into the hundreds. Here is an example of a somewhat more complicated tree in which multiple adverse effects of treatment are valued.

FIGURE 13.3

Decision Analysis for Osteoarthritis Comparing No Treatment With NSAID Treatment Over a 12-Month Period

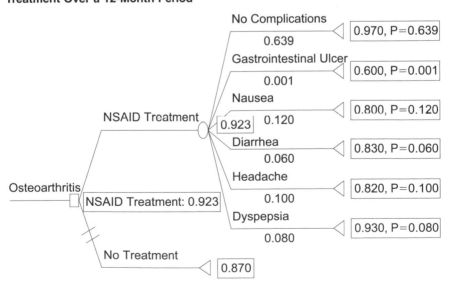

NSAID indicates nonsteroidal anti-inflammatory drug; P, probability.

The utility value associated with no treatment in Figure 13.3 is 0.870. The utility value associated with nonsteroidal anti-inflammatory drug (NSAID) treatment without complications is 0.970, while the utility values corresponding to each of the adverse effects located on the branches of the NSAID treatment arm are shown to the right of each triangular node (gastrointestinal ulcer = 0.600, nausea = 0.800, and so on). The incidence of each terminal node outcome in the NSAID treatment arm is shown beneath its corresponding arm in decimal form (% = decimal form × 100). The utility values associated with the multiple variables in the treatment arm are weighted to achieve the final treatment utility value outcome. The final utility value outcome for the reference case with NSAID treatment is 0.923. Because the 0.923 utility value outcome with treatment is higher than the 0.870 utility value outcome associated with no treatment, the preferred strategy is treatment with the NSAID.

MARKOV MODELING

Modeling becomes more difficult when recurrent events over time (especially recurrent risks) are considered in the analysis. For example, consider a situation where a hypothetical patient has a surgery that may or may not be successful. Suppose that if the surgery is successful, the patient lives normally for his or her remaining life, but if the surgery is not successful, another surgery will be performed. This process can be highly iterative when a number of unsuccessful surgeries are modeled. To analyze this problem, a transition-state model is required, and is commonly performed using a Markov-cycle decision tree.

In a Markov model, a hypothetical participant must always be in one of a finite number of Markov states (or distinctive health states) that are defined by the analyst. The hypothetical participant may change health states at the end of each time period, or cycle, according to predefined transition probabilities. The hypothetical patient is then given appropriate credit, also called a reward, in the form of a utility multiplied by time, or QALY, for each cycle he or she spends in a given Markov state. The QALYs gained during each cycle are added to arrive at the total number of QALYs rewarded during a set period of time. The number of QALYs rewarded with one treatment can be compared to those rewarded with another treatment or those rewarded with no treatment.

For example, if a cohort of patients has a 5% chance of dying per year, 95% of that cohort will pass through the year and 5% will die. In this instance, the patient can be in two health states: alive or dead. The utility value associated with death is 0.0. If the patients who live have a utility value of 1.0, 0.95 QALY is rewarded to the average person (reference case) in the cohort during the first year. At the end of a second year, 5% of the 95% (4.75%) of remaining patients die and 90.25% of the original cohort lives. At a utility value of 1.0, the average person is rewarded 0.9025 QALY during the second year. This cycle continues until an end time is specified (for example, 20 years) or until virtually all patients in the cohort have died. If a treatment reduces the yearly incidence of death to 3%, the difference between the QALYs gained in the untreated group (5% of the remaining cohort dies per year) and the treated group (3% of the remaining cohort dies per year) over a set period of time can be compared similarly.

Markov models can have transition probabilities that are constant or that can vary.[4,13,14] Models with transition probabilities that remain constant are known as *Markov chains,* while models with transition probabilities that change over time are known as *Markov processes.* An *absorbing state,* or health state from which there is no transition, is another important concept in Markov modeling. For example, in the above scenario, death is an absorbing state since no transition from this state is possible.

> **M**arkov modeling measures the recurrent risk of an event (such as the yearly chance of dying from a myocardial infarction in a patient who has already had one myocardial infarction).

The cycles typically are one year in length, but theoretically could be one month, one week, or even one day. The expected number of QALYs for each decision alternative is calculated mathematically. Readers who want more information regarding the use of Markov models in decision analysis should refer to articles by Sonnenberg and Beck[13] and Naimark et al.[15]

An example of Markov modeling for data presented in the Sixth Report of the Joint National Committee on Prevention, Detection, Evaluation, and Treatment of High Blood Pressure[16] is shown in Figure 13.4.

According to the Sixth Report of the Joint National Committee on Prevention, Detection, Evaluation, and Treatment of High Blood Pressure,[16] treatment of hypertension yields an absolute risk reduction of 0.7% per year for cardiac death. Without treatment, there is approximately a 5.7% chance of dying per year, while treatment reduces the risk to 5.0%. At the beginning of the initiation of the intervention to treat hypertension, all theoretical patients in the treatment and nontreatment groups are alive. While Markov modeling results are *reference case* results, meaning that the outcome is for the average person in a decision arm, it is easier to think of each arm as a model for a cohort of patients going through the cycles.

In the example shown in Figure 13.4, 1.0 QALY is gained by going through each yearly cycle the average patient lives. Because 95% of the treated cohort lives, the treated group gains 0.95 QALY during the first year of the cycle. In the untreated group, 94.3% of the cohort lives through the first cycle, so 0.943 QALY is awarded. No QALYs are awarded for patients who have died.

In this example the square node is a *decision node,* the oval node with an M in it is a *Markov node,* the empty oval node is a *chance node,* and the triangular nodes are *terminal nodes.* The two health states modeled are live and cardiac death. The model attributes 1.0 QALY for each year lived (at a utility value of 1.0) and 0.0 for death. The model encompasses 15 cycles (15 years), or the average life expectancy of the 70-year-old reference case.

The numbers under the large Markov Information boxes are probabilities at the beginning of the cycle (100% alive and 0% dead), and the numbers under

FIGURE 13.4

Markov Decision Analysis Tree Modeling the QALYs Gained by the Average 70-Year-Old Person (Reference Case) From Treatment of Hypertension to Reduce Cardiac Death

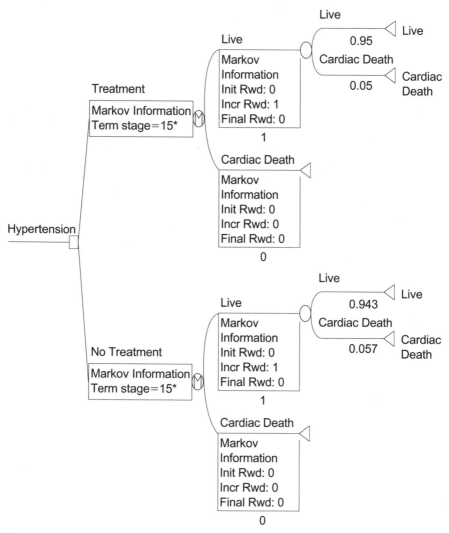

Final Rwd indicates final reward (or reward in QALYs given upon leaving the cycle); Incr Rwd indicates incremental reward (or the reward gained from having gone through a cycle); Init Rwd, initial reward (or the reward in QALYs given upon entering a health state at the beginning of a Markov yearly cycle).

* Term stage = 15 in the two smaller Markov Information boxes farthest to the left indicates that the health states are modeled over a period of 15 years for both the treated group and the untreated group.

the four far right triangular terminal nodes are the probability of each event for the cohort by the end of each yearly cycle. In the treated group, 95% of patients are alive and 5% have died a cardiac death by the end of the first year (first cycle). In the untreated group, 94.3% of patients are alive and 5.7% of patients have died a cardiac death by the end of the first cycle. With each cycle, more patients move from the live state to the dead state, but not vice versa, as death is an *absorbing state,* or a state from which transition is not possible. The solved Markov model from Figure 13.4 is shown in Figure 13.5.

As shown in Figure 13.5, at the beginning of the first yearly cycle, all subjects are alive (P = 1.000). The average person gains 9.73 QALYs with treatment for hypertension over the 15-year life expectancy, while 9.27 QALYs are gained by the average person without treatment. Thus, 9.73 − 9.27 = 0.46 QALYs are gained over the 15-year period with treatment vs no treatment.

The final probability of an outcome at the end of the 15-year cycle is indicated by FP in the figure. In the treated hypertensive group, 46.3% of patients are alive at the end of the 15-year cycle and 53.7% of patients have died, while in the untreated hypertensive group 41.5% of patients are alive at the end of the 15-year cycle and 58.5% of patients have died.

The annual discount rate can also be integrated in a decision analysis with Markov modeling, as shown in Figure 13.6.

In Figure 13.6, despite the 3% annual discounting for the treated and untreated groups, the percentages of patients living and dying in each group remain unchanged compared to Figure 13.5. As expected, however, the value gained from treatment is less in the discounted model (8.05 − 7.69 = 0.36 QALY) than in the undiscounted model (9.73 − 9.27 = 0.46 QALY).

MONTE CARLO SIMULATION

A cost-effective model can also be defined as either *deterministic* or *stochastic.*[10,13] A deterministic model generally employs expected value decision making where the expected outcome of a decision tree is calculated mathematically. The preceding hypertension example is deterministic. A stochastic model, on the other hand, is a simulation that is performed a large number of times; alternatively, it can be thought of as a sampling of the variance of the model.

The most common procedure for a stochastic model is to use a Monte Carlo simulation. In a stochastic model, in contrast to a deterministic model, the outcome will change each time the model is simulated; however, the mean will approximate the mean value of the deterministic model after a large number of trials have been performed.

The advantage of using a stochastic model is that a distribution of the outcome, value range, mean, median, and 95% confidence interval can be calculated and visualized. By integrating probabilistic distributions, the potential outcomes are elucidated to let a patient know the percentage chance that he or she will fall within a particular health state. For example, the deterministic model may show that treatment A is superior to treatment B, while the stochastic

FIGURE 13.5

Solved Markov Model from Figure 13.4

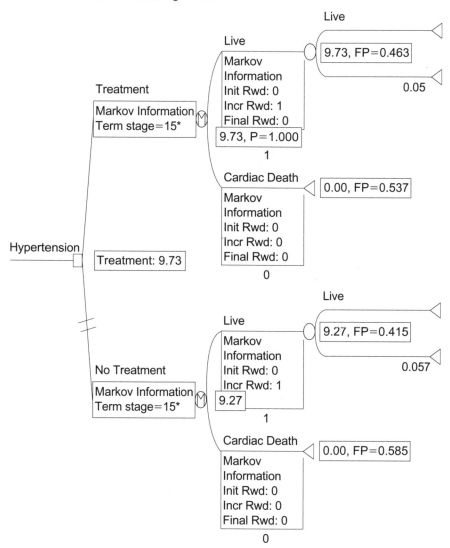

Final Rwd indicates the final reward (or that awarded as a patient leaves the cycle, which is 0 for the treatment and no treatment arms in this case); FP final probability; Init Rwd, the initial reward (or that awarded upon entering a cycle, which is 0 for treatment and no treatment arms in this case); Incr Rwd, the incremental reward (which is 1.0 for the proportion of the cohort that is alive at the end of the yearly cycle); P, probability.

* Term stage = 15 in the two smaller Markov Information boxes farthest to the left means that the health states are modeled over a period of 15 years for both the treated cohort and the untreated cohort.

FIGURE 13.6

Solved Markov Model From Figure 13.3 but With 3% Annual Discounting of the QALYs Gained During the Incremental Reward Phase in Both the Treatment and No Treatment Arms. Utilizing a 3% annual discount rate for the incremental awards, the average person gains 8.05 QALYs with treatment for hypertension over the 15-year life expectancy, while an average of 7.69 QALYs are gained by the average person without treatment. In this instance, 8.05 − 7.69 = 0.36 QALY is gained over the 15-year period with treatment vs no treatment.

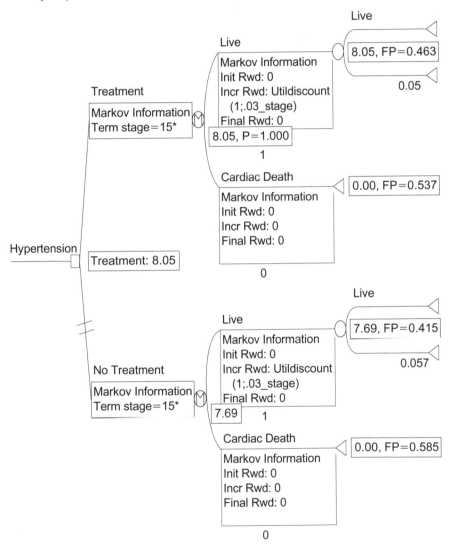

Final Rwd indicates final reward; FP, final probability of an outcome (Live or Cardiac Death) at the end of the 15-year cycle; Incr Rwd, incremental reward; Init Rwd, initial reward; M, Markov node.

* Term stage = 15 in the two smaller Markov Information boxes farthest to the left indicates that the health states are modeled over a period of 15 years for both the treated group and the untreated group.

model with Monte Carlo simulation will show in what percentage of instances, albeit small, treatment A is inferior to treatment B.

> Monte Carlo simulation is a *stochastic* model in which a simulation is performed many times. The outcome changes with each simulation, but the mean approximates that of a *deterministic* model calculated using a decision analysis tree.

Most decision analysis software programs have a Monte Carlo simulation procedure that allows the analyst to actually perform a hypothetical trial of the cost-effective model. In a primary *(first-order)* Monte Carlo simulation, the model is performed using the reference-case point estimates and a hypothetical cohort is put through the individual trials using random number generators. The outcome is an "observed" cost-utility analysis. This cost-utility ratio will be similar to the expected value cost-utility ratio, and the average "observed" cost-utility ratio will closely approximate the expected cost-utility ratio, if the simulation is performed a large number of times. Through using this method, a measure of uncertainty in the model can be determined, and statistical tests can be employed. A primary Monte Carlo simulation does not, however, consider the inherent variability of the variables in the model.

In a secondary *(second-order)* Monte Carlo simulation, during each trial, some (or all) of the variables are sampled from their respective distributions and then random number generators are used to determine an expected cost-utility ratio. For instance, if the life expectancy of a patient with HIV infection is ten years with a standard deviation of three years, then each time the trial is run, a life expectancy will be derived through a random number generator that will pick a number from a normal (mean ten, standard deviation three) distribution. Each time the process is performed, that hypothetical patient will live for a different amount of time (with the long-term average being ten years). In a complicated analysis with good effectiveness and outcome data, it is possible for a large number of variables to be defined statistically as distributions and sampled in this manner. When a secondary Monte Carlo simulation is performed, a distribution of the cost-utility ratio can be graphically displayed, thereby giving an idea of the variability inherent in the model.

THE IDEAL MODEL

When modeling the cost-effectiveness of a program, it is important that the model be sufficiently complex that it is able to incorporate relevant data. However, if it is too complex, it can go farther than the data appropriately allow, or can be too difficult for readers to understand. An analyst should use the simplest modeling technique possible that incorporates all relevant data and adequately represents the problem. A deterministic approach will generally be sufficient; however, in some situations a more complicated stochastic model may be necessary.

One major criticism of modeling in cost-effective or decision analysis is that it is difficult to reproduce. A basic caveat of the scientific method, first described by Galileo, is that data used in formulating hypotheses are able to be reproduced. Consequently, if the situation allows, the analyst should use a common decision analysis program and provide enough information that a reader or reviewer could reproduce the results. If the analysis is complex, the analyst should provide an overview in the actual report or publication and an appendix that makes available more detailed methods of the analysis. While models for health state interventions will likely never be perfect, this should not discourage researchers from creating reproducible good models that are more valuable to the patient than current anecdotal management.

Sensitivity analysis, which is discussed in more detail later in this book, confers more confidence that a model is of functional value. For example, let us assume a model yields a $/QALY (cost-utility, or dollars spent per QALY gained) for an intervention of $10,000. If the utility values employed are then varied, for example, to reflect the upper and lower boundaries of their 95% confidence intervals, as are the costs and other input parameters, and the $/QALY gained ranges from $5,000 to $15,000, we can be confident that the analysis is robust and the intervention is indeed cost-effective (assuming that interventions that are less than $50,000/QALY gained are considered cost-effective).[17–19]

Hussein Hollands, MSc, contributed to this chapter.

CORE CONCEPTS

- The response to a healthcare intervention can be modeled into the future. If long-term data are not available, a short-term or intermediate-term analysis can be performed, or the most recent data can be carried forward.

- Decision analysis demonstrates the most probable outcome of an intervention.

- Decision analysis demonstrates the preferred treatment option when faced with uncertainty.

- Decision analysis can compare the outcome of an intervention with the outcome of another intervention or with no treatment.

- Markov modeling measures the recurrent risk of an event (such as the yearly risk of having a recurrent myocardial infarction following an initial myocardial infarction).

- A *deterministic* model generally employs expected value decision making where the expected outcome of a decision tree is calculated mathematically.

- A *stochastic* model is a simulation that is performed a large number of times; alternatively, it can be thought of as a sampling of the variance of the model.

- *Monte Carlo simulation* is a stochastic model that uses reference-case point estimates to perform a hypothetical trial of a cost-utility model. In doing so it can calculate the range, mean, median, and 95% confidence interval for a model.

■ A cost-utility model should be sufficiently complex to incorporate relevant data, yet not so complex that it cannot be understood and reproduced by others.

REFERENCES

1. North American Symptomatic Carotid Endarterectomy Trial Collaborators. Beneficial effect of carotid endarterectomy in symptomatic patients with high-grade carotid stenosis. North American Symptomatic Carotid Endarterectomy Trial Collaborators. *N Engl J Med.* 1991;325:445–453.

2. Paciaroni M, Eliasziw M, Sharpe BL, et al. Long-term clinical and angiographic outcomes in symptomatic patients with 70% to 99% carotid artery stenosis. *Stroke.* 2000;31:2037–2042.

3. Rothwell PM, Gutnikov SA, Warlow CP. European Carotid Surgery Trialists Collaboration: reanalysis of the final results of the European Carotid Surgery Trial. *Stroke.* 2003;34:514–523.

4. TreeAge Software, Inc. *DATA 4.0 Healthcare User's Manual.* Williamstown, Mass: TreeAge Software, Inc; 2003:293–378.

5. Sox HC, Blatt MA, Higgins MC, Marton KI. *Medical Decision Making.* Toronto, Canada: Butterworths; 1988:406.

6. Weinstein MC, Fineberg HC. *Clinical Decision Analysis.* Philadelphia, Pa: WB Saunders; 1980.

7. Detsky AS, Naglie G, Krahn MD, Naimark D, Redelmeier DA. Primer on medical decision analysis: part 1—getting started. *Med Decis Making.* 1997;17:123–125

8. Detsky AS, Naglie G, Krahn MD, Redelmeier DA, Naimark D. Primer on medical decision analysis: part 2—building a tree. *Med Decis Making.* 1997;17:126–135.

9. Pauker SG, Kassirer JP. Decision analysis. *N Engl J Med.* 1987;316:250–258.

10. Krahn MD, Naglie G, Naimark D, Redelmeier DA, Detsky AS. Primer on medical decision analysis: part 4—analyzing the model and interpreting the results. *Med Decis Making.* 1997;17:142–151.

11. Naglie G, Krahn MD, Naimark D, Redelmeier DA, Detsky AS. Primer on medical decision analysis: part 3—estimating probabilities and utilities. *Med Decis Making.* 1997;17:136–141.

12. Decision Analysis Society. Decision Tree and Influence Diagram Software. Available at: http://faculty.fuqua.duke.edu/daweb/dasw6.htm. Accessed August 29, 2004.

13. Sonnenberg FA, Beck JR. Markov models in medical decision making: a practical guide. *Med Decis Making.* 1993;13:322–338.

14. Petitti DB. *Meta-Analysis, Decision Analysis and Cost-Effectiveness Analysis.* 2nd ed. New York, NY: Oxford University Press; 2000:140–158.

15. Naimark ND, Krahn MD, Naglie D, Redelmeier DA, Detsky AS. Primer on medical decision analysis: part 5—working with Markov processes. *Med Decis Making.* 1997;17:152–159.

16. Joint National Committee on Prevention, Detection, Evaluation and Treatment of High Blood Pressure. Figure 7: Combined results of five randomized trials of anti-hypertensive treatment in the elderly. In: *The Sixth Report of the Joint National Committee on Prevention, Detection, Evaluation and Treatment of High Blood Pressure.* Bethesda, Md: National Institutes of Health; November 1997. N/H publication 90-4080.

17. Heudebert GR, Centor RM, Klapow JC, et al. What is heartburn worth? A cost-utility analysis of management strategies. *J Gen Intern Med.* 2000;15:175–182.

18. Kallmes DF, Kallmes MH. Cost-effectiveness of angiography performed during surgery for ruptured intracranial aneuryms. *AJNR Am J Neuroradiol.* 1997;18:1453–1462.

19. Smith KG, Roberts MS. Antiviral therapies for herpes zoster infections: are they economically justifiable? *Pharmacoeconomics.* 2000;18:95–104.

14

Costs

While the subject of costs may initially appear straightforward, it is not. But it is comprehensible. Lack of standardization for parameters to calculate the value conferred by an intervention, as well as lack of standardization for costs, has prevented establishment of a value-based medicine (VBM) database. In this chapter we discuss the various types of healthcare costs and recommend which costs to use in a cost-utility analysis to create a VBM database.

TYPES OF COSTS

The costs associated with an intervention should be valued as the difference in resource use between an intervention and the alternative intervention (or no treatment). Consequently, costs should refer to the *incremental* resources consumed or saved.[1] Costs should be measured in dollars of a specific year and specific currency if other than the US dollar. Some suggest that costs or outcomes (quality-adjusted life-years [QALYs]) that are insignificant in the context of analysis be excluded.[2] Nonetheless, the definition of insignificant is unclear.

> *Incremental costs* are those consumed or saved secondary to a healthcare intervention. Without the intervention, they would not have occurred.

When measuring costs in an economic evaluation, the costs are generally divided into *direct* costs and *indirect* costs[3,4] (Table 14.1).

Direct Costs

Direct healthcare costs.   Direct healthcare costs are defined as the value of goods, services, and other resources consumed in the provision of an intervention or in dealing with the side effects or other current and future consequences linked to the intervention.[1] Direct healthcare costs include the costs of:

1. providers,
2. acute hospitalization,

3. ambulatory surgery centers,
4. skilled nursing facilities,
5. rehabilitation,
6. nursing home care,
7. home health care,
8. pharmaceuticals,
9. laboratory tests,
10. diagnostic studies (radiologic, pathologic, and others),
11. durable goods, and
12. other medical treatments relating to the procedure, as well as any potential costs in the future that result from the health program or intervention.

Direct healthcare costs are the costs we recommend for use in cost-utility analyses.

We advocate the use of direct healthcare costs (provider, hospitalization, pharmaceutical, testing, and other medical costs) for use in cost-utility analysis.

Direct nonhealthcare costs.   Direct nonhealthcare costs encompass the following:

1. childcare costs,
2. caregiver costs (nonfamily),
3. caregiver costs for friends and family,
4. transportation costs for care,
5. housekeeping costs,
6. retraining costs, and
7. social services costs.[4]

The time that unpaid caregivers, such as family members and friends, take in helping a patient at home or elsewhere should be included. This time can be considered as lost time from work and can be converted to dollar form by using the average wage in the community.

While time lost from work for family and friend caregivers, as well as childcare and transportations costs, and the remainder are considered direct costs, we believe including these *nonhealthcare costs* in cost-utility analysis adds a considerable degree of complexity and uncertainty. We therefore do not recommend including direct nonhealthcare costs in a typical cost-utility analysis at this time, especially since there is no body that standardizes these costs. Including direct nonhealthcare costs in cost-utility analysis will produce an even greater disparity among cost-utility analyses. Once again, the key is to create good cost-utility analyses. Waiting additional years until these costs are standardized to yield perfect cost-utility analyses and the perfect VBM database only means the tasks will never be accomplished, and we will continue to rely upon anecdotal evidence.

It is imperative to create a good cost-utility database. Inability to create the perfect database has prevented it from happening to date.

Indirect Costs

Indirect costs, also referred to as *productivity costs*,[3] are those associated with the loss (or gain) in productivity due to a health program or intervention. This includes loss of time or productivity due to morbidity or mortality and the gain of time and productivity due to decreased morbidity and the prevention of mortality. This lost productivity can be quantified by measuring lost patient time and wages, lost family caregiver wages, lost tax revenue, decreased productivity due to death, and disability payments. Lost tax revenue, however, should not be counted twice. Thus, if lost patient wages are counted, lost tax revenue should not be counted as well. Lost patient time has a value, depending upon whether the patient is working or not. For nonworking time lost, the conversion to monetary form can be undertaken using the minimum wage, the wage of those necessary to help maintain a household, or other variants.

Indirect costs are included in the societal perspective for cost-utility analysis, but they are not used in the third-party insurer perspective. The types of healthcare economic costs are listed in Table 14.1.

Future Costs

When determining what healthcare costs to include in a cost analysis, consider any healthcare costs in the future that are associated with the intervention. Examples of costs to include are those associated with the treatment of rejection and the treatment of opportunistic infections in patients who have undergone solid organ transplantation and those associated with bowel obstruction due to strictures occurring at years after intra-abdominal surgery. However, there is controversy as to whether healthcare costs unrelated to the intervention should be included if they occur in years that are added to life expectancy because of the intervention.

Future healthcare costs directly related to a healthcare intervention should be included in a cost-utility analysis. An example is the cost of the treatment of rejection in patients who have undergone solid organ transplantation.

There are valid arguments to both sides of this discussion whether to include unrelated costs. Some suggest these costs can be included or excluded at the discretion of the analyst performing a reference case analysis.[3] The clinical situation of smoking cessation provides an example of why seemingly unrelated future costs may be important. The healthcare costs of smokers are estimated to be 40% higher than those of nonsmokers, but in a population in which no one smokes the long-term healthcare costs are estimated to be 7% higher among

TABLE 14.1

Types of Healthcare Economic Analysis Costs

	Perspective		
	Third-Party Insurer	Government	Societal
DIRECT COSTS			
Healthcare Costs*			
Provider†	Yes	Yes	Yes
Hospital, Acute†	Yes	Yes	Yes
Ambulatory Surgical Center (ASC)†	Yes	Yes	Yes
Skilled Nursing Facility†	Yes	Yes	Yes
Rehabilitation†	Yes	Yes	Yes
Nursing Home Care†	Yes	Yes	Yes
Home Health Care†	Yes	Yes	Yes
Pharmaceutical†	Yes	Yes	Yes
Laboratory Tests†	Yes	Yes	Yes
Diagnostic Studies†	Yes	Yes	Yes
Durable Goods†	Yes	Yes	Yes
Nonhealthcare Costs			
Care Provided by Friends and Family	No	No	Yes
Transportation Costs*	No	Yes	Yes
Childcare Costs*	No	Yes	Yes
Housekeeping*	No	Yes	Yes
Retraining*	No	Yes	Yes
INDIRECT COSTS			
Lost Patient Wages‡	No	Yes	Yes
Lost Patient Time (nonwork)	No	No	Yes
Lost Tax Revenue	No	Yes	No
Lost Productivity from Premature Death‡	No	Yes	Yes
Disability Payments	No	Yes	Yes

* These costs contribute to the gross domestic product (GDP), or the costs of all *goods and services* produced in the country annually. All direct healthcare costs contribute to the GDP.

† Costs we recommend using in a cost-utility analysis.

‡ These costs subtract from the GDP.

Provider costs = those of physicians and nonphysicians, Durable goods are larger expensive items, such as a hospital bed, an oxygen-producing machine, a wheelchair, an infusion pump, and so on.

Source: Luce et al[3] and Smith and Brown.[4]

men and 4% higher among women.[5] Thus, if all smokers immediately stopped smoking, healthcare costs would initially be lower, but after 15 years would increase to greater than at present. This occurs because the resultant older population has more chronic diseases. These future healthcare costs would not have occurred without smoking cessation and therefore should likely be included in a long-term economic analysis of smoking cessation programs when a societal perspective is undertaken. The argument could even be made that these costs of chronic disease occur as a direct healthcare result of smoking cessation. With the third-party insurer perspective, however, we believe the exclusion of such future healthcare costs related to increased longevity is the most apropos course, especially since they introduce a variable with an extraordinary number of permutations and thus the ability to further confound any cost-utility analysis.

> With the third-party insurer perspective, we recommend that future costs incurred due to the increased longevity conferred by healthcare interventions not be included in a cost-utility analysis.

Nonhealthcare costs, such as those for food and shelter, that occur in the years of life added due to the intervention under study are not generally included in an economic evaluation. All future costs that are included, however, must be discounted for the time value of money.

PERSPECTIVE: WHOSE COSTS TO USE?

When evaluating a cost-utility analysis, one of the most important questions that must be answered is the cost perspective the methodologist has taken to determine the analysis, and whether this perspective is appropriate for the policymaker or others who review the study. There are several cost perspectives encountered in the healthcare economic literature:

- **the third-party insurer perspective,**
- the self-insured, employer plan perspective,
- **the societal perspective,**
- the governmental perspective, and
- the patient perspective.

Among these perspectives, the third-party insurance and societal perspectives (in bold) are the most commonly used perspectives for healthcare economic analysis.

Third-Party Insurer Perspective Costs

The third-party insurer perspective typically takes into account the incremental treatment costs *incurred by the insurer* (or other third-party payer) and the health outcome in terms of value improvement, or QALYs, gained by the patient. For instance, the decision of whether total hip arthroplasty is cost-effective from the insurers' perspective includes the *direct healthcare costs* of physicians, acute short-stay hospitalization, pharmaceuticals, diagnostic studies, laboratory services, and rehabilitation. We address the most commonly utilized reimbursement cost-basis system for these direct healthcare costs, the Medicare system, later in this chapter.

The third-party insurer perspective takes into account:
1. the incremental costs of treatment incurred by the insurer, and
2. the incremental health outcome in terms of value gained, or QALYs gained, by the patient.

We recommend use of third-party insurer perspective costs with patient-perceived value (QALYs) when performing cost-utility analysis.

Direct nonhealthcare costs, such as the lost time of caregivers, childcare costs, and transportation costs, are ignored in the third-party perspective, as are indirect healthcare costs, such as the disability costs obviated by improved ambulation after surgery or the wages made possible due to benefit from the surgery. (Wages gained and disability costs made unnecessary are considered negative costs, meaning they are subtracted from the other costs in the societal perspective.) Clearly, inclusion of the saving of disability costs and the wages gained, which would occur if one were conducting the analysis from the societal perspective, would have a more favorable impact on the overall cost-utility analysis. The societal perspective often yields a more favorable cost-utility ratio for healthcare interventions than the third-party insurer perspective.

Self-Insured Employer Plan Perspective Costs

Self-insured employer perspective costs are very similar to those of the third-party insurer. The major difference is that loss of patient productivity and sick leave pay are also relevant for the self-insured employer, whereas this is not the case with a public insurer (Medicare, Medicaid), a commercial insurer (under age 65 private insurer), or a managed care plan. The self-insured employer perspective is not often used for cost-utility analysis or other healthcare economic analyses.

Societal Perspective Costs

The broadest view of costs for healthcare economic analyses is the societal perspective. The viewpoint of a policymaker is often the societal perspective, which includes direct healthcare costs, direct nonhealthcare costs, and indirect costs (Table 14.1). Direct healthcare costs actually contribute to gross domestic product (GDP), or the goods and services produced annually within the US, as do direct nonhealthcare costs with the exception of free care provided by nonworking family and friends. Conversely, the indirect costs of lost patient wages due to disability and/or premature death both lower GDP.

> Healthcare interventions are generally more cost-effective when performed using the societal perspective than with the third-party insurer perspective.

Unless a cost-utility analysis is undertaken from a specific viewpoint (for example, from the perspective of a third-party insurer or hospital), some have recommended that the most general perspective, the societal perspective, be used.[2] If the societal perspective is undertaken, it is relatively easy and informative to provide other perspectives in a cost-utility analysis, as virtually all costs are already included within the societal perspective (Table 14.1). Whichever costs are used, they must clearly and unequivocally defined.

> The costs used in a healthcare economic analysis must be clearly and unequivocally defined.

Governmental Perspective Costs

Governmental perspective costs are similar to societal perspective costs in most ways (Table 14.1). In regard to direct nonhealthcare costs, the government is not concerned with care provided by friends and family, and in regard to indirect costs, the government is not interested in loss of patient leisure time. These costs are therefore not included in the governmental perspective. The government is, however, interested in the tax revenue gained from health improvement and consequent gainful employment, as well as the tax revenue lost due to disability, death, and consequent loss of employment.

Patient Perspective Costs

From the patient perspective, virtually all costs can be included since each one can affect a patient in some way. Thus, the patient perspective is most similar to the societal perspective.

Are There Standardized Costs to Use in Cost-Utility Analysis?

The Panel on Cost-Effectiveness in Health and Medicine has recommended that the societal perspective be undertaken for cost-utility analyses.[3] Nonetheless, there is no agreement as to exactly what costs should be utilized in the societal perspective, and this is a major problem. Costs less relevant than the ones we have addressed (training for new medical procedures, nutritionist costs, preparation of medications, prevention costs, and so on[4]) can also be included, but just the use of one or two different costs in cost-utility analyses could make the studies incomparable. Furthermore, there are no recommendations in regard to the cost basis. For example, costs can be based upon the Medicare Fee Schedule, the reimbursement rates of any number of commercial (non-Medicare) insurers, or a combination of public and private insurers. Thus, the costs and cost basis used in one published analysis often differ considerably from those used in another. As such, they contribute to the incomparability of most studies.

The costs and cost basis for the costs used in cost-utility analysis often differ, making most studies incomparable.

What Costs Should Be Used for Cost-Utility Analysis?

At this time, we recommend that third-party insurer costs, also known as direct healthcare costs, be used for cost-utility analyses (Table 14.1). No matter what variant of costs are used, the value outcome remains the same—measured in QALYs.

Recommended costs for cost-utility analysis: direct healthcare costs.

Why Don't We Routinely Use the Societal Perspective?

While the societal perspective is theoretically the ideal because it accounts for all the economic consequences of a healthcare intervention, the third-party perspective is less complex since it includes only direct healthcare costs related to an intervention.

Considering the difficulty of creating a database of VBM quality standards, we believe perspectives other than the third-party insurer perspective add additional parameters and uncertainty to make the task of creating the database extraordinarily difficult, if not impossible. For example, obtaining data to define direct nonhealthcare costs, such as childcare costs, transportation costs, and caregiver costs associated with all interventions, is both labor-intensive and expensive. Additionally, these costs can vary considerably in different areas of the country. The calculation of indirect costs, such as disability costs, lost wages, lost productivity, and social service costs, is also difficult to gather, labor-intensive, expensive, and variable depending upon the locale.

In a perfect world, use of the societal perspective would be highly desirable. Once a VBM database is created, it can be refined when all costs are later standardized, but creating a usable initial VBM database is the key goal at present.

> While use of the *societal perspective* for cost-utility analyses is highly desirable, the current lack of standardization of: 1) which costs to include, 2) the cost basis, and 3) the locale dramatically diminish the ability to compare the studies.

> Because of the lack of consensus on societal costs standards, we believe the simpler *third-party insurer perspective* should currently be used to create a VBM database.

THE COST BASIS

We use direct healthcare costs for cost-utility analysis. But whose costs do we use? There are hundreds of payers in the United States, all with varying reimbursement schedules. Should we use Medicare costs, commercial insurer (under age 65 years) costs, managed care company costs, a weighted mix of the above, or some other variant?

Medicare

Medicare, the US government health insurer for 35 million people 65 years or older and those who are disabled, is the largest healthcare insurer in the country. Medicare uses the Resource-Based Relative Value Scale (RBRVS) to create a Medicare Fee Schedule to reimburse providers for healthcare services rendered.[6] The RBRVS is based upon a system that quantifies physician work value and cost of practice indices.

Medicare requires a disease diagnosis from the *International Classification of Diseases, Ninth Revision, Clinical Modification* (ICD-9-CM)[7] for payment, as well as a corresponding procedure code from the Current Procedural Terminology (CPT®) medical code system, a proprietary intervention classification system owned by the American Medical Association.[8] Any cost-utility information system used to create a database for VBM used in public policy must therefore be compatible with the ICD-9-DM and CPT medical codes.

> Cost-utility analyses should be compatible with ICD-9-DM and CPT medical codes.

We recommend utilizing the costs shown in Table 14.2 as the cost basis because they are the most standardized used by payers. In short, the values are from the Medicare system, with the exception of pharmaceutical costs and nursing home care costs, the latter of which should be based on the average Medicaid reimbursement. Outpatient pharmaceuticals are not covered under the Medicare system as of this time, but they will be covered in 2006 according to the Medicare Prescription Drug, Modernization and Improvement Act.

We also recommend that the third-party insurer perspective costs used be those of the average Medicare payment across the country because most health-care insurers in the US, public and private, base their fee schedules in some fashion on Medicare payment standards. These standards, listed in the following section, can be found on the Centers for Medicare and Medicaid Services Web site at www.cms.hhs.gov.

Specific Medicare patient deductibles and copayments can be found in the Medicare manual, *Medicare and You, 2004*,[9] which can be obtained by calling 800 MEDICARE. A brief review of these costs follows.

In making the recommendation to use Medicare reimbursements (and the average wholesale price [AWP] for drugs) for third-party insurer costs, the deductibles and copayments required for patients should be included in the cost. For example, Medicare requires participants to pay a yearly deductible payment for provider services and for the first hospitalization of the year. In addition, Medicare typically pays 80% of an approved provider reimbursement set for an intervention, while a patient's secondary insurer pays the remaining 20%, or the 20% comes directly from the patient as out-of-pocket expenses. Outpatient mental health services are the exception to the 80:20 rule. The patient or secondary insurance is required to pay 50% of the cost, while Medicare pays the other 50%; there is thus a 50-50 split.

Rather than using solely the amount Medicare pays, however, the *Medicare-approved charge* for an intervention for each of the above services (Table 14.2) should be used in cost-utility analysis. This number includes any copayments or deductibles. Concerning pharmaceuticals, the AWP, the most standardized price, should be used regardless of any copayment or deductible charge. The standard

TABLE 14.2

Cost Basis for Cost-Utility Analysis

Direct Healthcare Cost	Standardized Reference Source*
Provider	Average national Medicare reimbursement
Hospital, Acute	Average national Medicare reimbursement
Ambulatory Surgery Center	Average national Medicare reimbursement
Skilled Nursing Facility	Average national Medicare reimbursement
Rehabilitation	Average national Medicare reimbursement
Nursing Home Care	Average national Medicaid reimbursement
Home Healthcare	Average national Medicare reimbursement
Pharmaceuticals	Average wholesale price (AWP)
Clinical Tests	Average national Medicare reimbursement
Durable Goods	Average national Medicare reimbursement

* Average national Medicare reimbursement refers to the average national Medicare-approved charges.

of AWP could possibly change in the near future due to passage of the Medicare Prescription Drug, Modernization and Improvement Act.

> M*edicare-approved charges,* rather than *Medicare payment* for a service, should be used in cost-utility analysis.

Physicians and Other Providers

The Medicare Fee Schedule, which reimburses physicians according to CPT medical codes published by the American Medical Association, utilizes the RBRVS, a government-mandated relative value scale that incorporates practice expenses and the amount of work required for a healthcare intervention.[10] This Relative Value Scale assigns Relative Value Units (RVUs) to each intervention. These RVUs are multiplied by a conversion factor to yield the fee payment for the intervention. The conversion factor for 2004 is $37.34. Thus, if an intervention is valued at 4 RVUs, the approved reimbursement is 4 × $37.34 = $149.36. Different practice expenses in different areas of the country cause provider reimbursement to vary geographically. Therefore, the national average payment should be used for cost-utility analysis calculations. Physical therapy, occupational therapy, and speech therapy services are covered in a similar manner.

Acute Care Hospitals

Acute care hospitals are paid using a prospective payment system based upon 540 diagnosis related groups (DRGs). Each diagnosis is reimbursed a set amount with the option to bill an additional fraction for very complex cases. Payment also varies depending upon location of the facility, so the national average payment should be used for cost-utility analysis calculations.

While the average approved DRG rate should be used in cost-utility analysis, during each yearly cycle the patient (or secondary insurance) is required to pay $840 toward the first hospitalization for a stay of one to 60 days, $210 per day for days 61 to 90 of a hospital stay, and $420 per day for days 91 to 150 of a hospital stay. The patient or secondary insurance covers all days beyond 150 days. The $840 copayment paid for the first hospitalization of the year is not required for additional hospitalizations during that year. These copayments should be considered relevant direct costs since they occur as a component of Medicare-approved charges.

Ambulatory Surgery Centers

Ambulatory surgery centers (ASCs) are reimbursed according to a preset fee established by Medicare. Only approved interventions can be performed in surgery centers, although the list is extensive and enlarges on a regular basis. For 2004, there are nine ASC payment groups ranging from $340 in Group 1 for something as basic as removal of a skin lesion to $1,366 in Group 9 for repair of an umbilical hernia.

Skilled Nursing Facilities

Medicare has established a prospective payment system for skilled nursing facilities. Per diem (daily) payment rates are based upon a case-mix adjustment and a
geographical adjustment. The first 20 days require no patient copayment, while
up to $105 is required from days 21 to 100, and all costs are borne by the patient
beyond the 100th day.

Rehabilitation Fees, Clinical
Tests, and Durable Goods

The costs associated with rehabilitation fees, clinical tests, and durable goods are
all paid according to a scale for each established by Medicare. Durable goods
include large-item devices such as wheelchairs, oxygen machines, hospital beds,
and so on. As is the case with provider fees, Medicare pays 80% of the amount it
approves for durable goods and outpatient rehabilitation fees, while a secondary
insurance or the patient directly covers the remainder. Clinical laboratory
services require no patient or secondary insurance payment for Medicare-
approved services.

Nursing Homes

Medicare covers some nursing home costs, but it does not generally pay for long-
term nursing home care. Nursing home care, however, is paid for by state
Medicaid programs when the patient lacks funds to pay. The average, daily
national Medicaid payment is a reasonable number to use for nursing home costs.

Home Health Payments

Medicare has developed a specific payment schedule for home healthcare and
requires no copayment.

Pharmaceuticals

In regard to pharmaceuticals, the AWP from the *Red Book* is the most standardized price available for drugs.[11] Nonetheless, the AWP is an arbitrary price set by
each of the pharmaceutical manufacturers for its drugs rather by than any over-
seeing entity or common organization. The Centers for Medicare and Medicaid
Services, the parent organization of Medicare, has not yet set standards for the
cost of most pharmaceuticals. Nonetheless, they will likely be developed at some
point to accompany the Medicare Prescription Drug, Modernization and
Improvement Act, which takes effect in 2006.

Hospice Care

Medicare pays for 95% of an approved amount for hospice care. Again, the
Medicare-approved charges should be used in cost-utility analyses.

Hussein Hollands, MSc, contributed to this chapter.

CORE CONCEPTS

■ *Incremental costs* are those incurred or saved as a result of a healthcare intervention. Without the intervention they would not have occurred.

■ *Direct healthcare costs* are those associated with goods, services, and other resources that are consumed in the provision of an intervention or in dealing with the side effects or other current and future consequences linked to the intervention.

■ Direct healthcare costs include:
  — physician services costs,
  — acute hospital costs,
  — ambulatory surgery center (ASC) costs,
  — skilled nursing facility costs,
  — rehabilitation costs,
  — nursing home costs,
  — home health care costs,
  — pharmaceutical costs,
  — clinical test costs,
  — diagnostic study costs, and
  — durable goods costs.

■ Direct nonhealthcare costs include:
  — care provided by friends and family,
  — transportation costs,
  — childcare costs,
  — housekeeping costs, and
  — retraining costs.

■ Indirect healthcare costs (productivity costs) include:
  — lost patient wages,
  — lost patient nonwork time,
  — lost tax revenue,
  — lost productivity from premature death, and
  — disability payment costs.

■ The third-party insurer perspective is the most appropriate to use for cost-utility analysis and the creation of value-based standards at the current time.

■ National average Medicare-approved charges are the most appropriate to calculate all direct healthcare costs except for pharmaceutical costs and nursing home costs.

■ Pharmaceutical costs are most appropriately calculated using the average wholesale price (AWP).

■ Nursing home costs are most appropriately calculated using national average Medicaid-approved charges.

REFERENCES

1. Weinstein MC, Siegel JE, Gold MR, Kamlet MS, Russell LB. Recommendations of the Panel on Cost-Effectiveness in Health and Medicine. *JAMA*. 1996;276: 1253–1258.

2. Torrance GW, Siegel JE, Luce BR. Framing and designing the cost-effectiveness analysis. In: Gold MR, Siegel JE, Russell LB, Weinstein MC, eds. *Cost-Effectiveness in Health and Medicine*. New York, NY: Oxford University Press; 1996:54–81.

3. Luce BR, Manning WG, Siegel JE, Lipscomb J. Estimating costs in cost-effectiveness analysis. In: Gold MR, Siegel JE, Russell LB, Weinstein MC, eds. *Cost-Effectiveness in Health and Medicine*. New York, NY: Oxford University Press; 1996:176–213.

4. Smith A, Brown GC. Understanding cost-effectiveness: a detailed review. *Br J Ophthalmol*. 2000;54:794–798.

5. Barendregt JJ, Bonneux L, van der Maas PJ. The health care costs of smoking. *N Engl J Med*. 1997;337:1052–1057.

6. Centers for Medicare and Medicaid Services, Relative Value Scale. Available at: www.cms.hhs.gov. Accessed June 8, 2003.

7. Hart AC, Hopkins CA. *International Classification of Diseases, Ninth Revision, Clinical Modification*. Salt Lake City, Utah: Ingenix; 2003.

8. Kirschner CG, Davis SJ, Duffy T, et al. *Physicians' Current Procedural Terminology 2000*. Chicago, Ill: AMA Press; 2000.

9. *Medicare and You, 2004*. Baltimore, Md: Centers for Medicare and Medicaid Services; 2004.

10. Davis JB. *Medical Fees in the United States: Nationwide Charges for Medicine, Surgery, Laboratory, Radiology and Allied Health Services*. Los Angeles, Calif: Practice Management Information Corporation; 2003.

11. Cohen HP, ed. *2003 Drug Topics Red Book*. Montvale, NJ: Thompson Healthcare Inc; 2003.

Value-Based Medicine
The Top Tier of the Value-Based Medicine Pyramid

15

Economic Healthcare Analyses

The economic evaluation of healthcare delivery, be it diagnostic studies, pharmacologic interventions, or surgery, has the potential to influence health policy significantly and ultimately the health of millions of Americans.[1,2] Recently, government agencies, industrial partners, policymakers, and academic researchers have realized the need to collaborate to create policy based on scientific fact. Specifically, policymakers and governing bodies are interested in basing their policy decisions on rigorous scientific evidence, while academics want their research to be more relevant to people who apply it. Economic evaluations of healthcare products and services—if performed using rigorous scientific methods—are, arguably, among the most relevant research studies available to policymakers as aids to healthcare decision making.

When new technologies become available, policymakers in the government, managed care industry, and/or the hospital industry must decide whether investments should be made in these technologies. These decisions are especially difficult given the large capital and operation expenses typically incurred in supporting health technologies. More often than not, decisions made by healthcare managers are based on the minimization of costs. Clearly, this strategy not only ignores much relevant information, but it also leads to loss of productivity and ultimately erodes stakeholder value. In essence, many interventions that cost more deliver considerably more value for the dollar than interventions that are much less expensive. The important issue, however, is not to spend less for healthcare interventions, but rather to gain the most value from these interventions for the resources expended. We believe that the economic evaluation of health technology—in the form of cost-utility analysis—incorporates *all* of the variables that *should be* incorporated in appropriate healthcare decision making.

> Healthcare decisions based solely upon minimization of costs lead to loss of productivity and the erosion of stakeholder value in health care.

The important issue for healthcare spending is not to spend less money, but to derive the greatest value possible for the resources expended.

Managers from many different sectors are used to making investment decisions and frequently rely on analytic tools that compare financial returns to initial investments. These include internal rate of return, economic value added, and net present value (NVP) analysis. Net present value analysis compares future financial returns, which have been corrected for the time value of money, to initial cash outlays. Conceptually, *healthcare economic analyses* can be thought of as being similar to a *net present value analysis*, due to the following reasons:

- They involve cash investments. These investments can take the form of capital expenditures on tangible assets, such as buildings and equipment, or operational costs, such as human resources.

- They quantify benefits accrued. These are measured in dollars in NPV analyses and in dollars and health outcomes in healthcare economic analyses.

- The principles of discounting and sensitivity analyses are incorporated into both methodologies.

- Both involve a comparison of the benefits accrued to the financial investments in terms of an overall summary statistic.

- Both methodologies can allow for multiple projects to be compared to one another.

When referring to a healthcare program in this chapter, we are speaking about any intervention that will cost money and is being considered for implementation for the purpose of improving health. This definition is purposely broad and can include entities such as a new drug delivery system, a genetic screening program, or the decision by a managed care organization to add a new medication to its formulary. Prior to undertaking an economic evaluation of a particular health intervention, however, it should previously have been proven clinically effective using the best evidence-based principles discussed in Chapter 4.

Healthcare economic evaluations can be subdivided into four subgroups[3]:

- cost-minimization analysis,
- cost-benefit analysis,
- cost-effectiveness analysis, and
- cost-utility analysis.

In this chapter we briefly examine each of the subtypes of healthcare economic analysis and the ability of each to evaluate the consequences of healthcare interventions.

COST-MINIMIZATION ANALYSIS

Cost-minimization analysis compares two interventions of equal effectiveness to ascertain which is less costly. In a cost-minimization analysis a critical assumption is made that the effectiveness of the health programs under consideration are equivalent. Consequently, the costs of two or more equally effective programs are compared and the program with the lower cost is the preferred option.

For example, consider a situation in which an equivalence trial shows there is no statistically significant difference between two drugs for treatment of hypercholesterolemia. In this situation a cost-minimization analysis would assume there is no difference in effectiveness between the two options and would investigate the costs associated with both treatment options to determine the preferred choice.

> Cost-minimization analysis compares two interventions of equal effectiveness to ascertain which is less costly.

Cost-minimization analysis is not used as often as other forms of healthcare analyses.[4] The major problem with cost-minimization analysis is that two healthcare interventions are generally not exactly equivalent. For example, with the treatment of hypercholesterolemia, the therapeutic efficacy of each drug in reducing serum cholesterol may be similar, but the side effects, the severity of side effects, and the incidence of side effects associated with each drug are surely different, thereby causing the drugs to confer unequal value.

The intervention of cholecystectomy, or removal of the gallbladder, is also illustrative for cost-minimization analysis. Laparoscopic cholecystectomy and conventional cholecystectomy with a much larger incision may yield the same long-term result, but the disutilities of increased pain and longer recovery time with the conventional variant prevent precise comparability. Comparison of laparoscopic cholecystectomy performed in an ambulatory surgery center vs the same laparoscopic cholecystectomy performed in a hospital setting, however, would be reasonable interventions to consider for comparison with cost-minimization analysis. Cost-minimization analysis comparing surgical facilities that perform only one procedure, vs facilities that perform that same procedure and other various types of procedures, has shown that the more specialized facility is less costly.[5]

COST-BENEFIT ANALYSIS

Cost-benefit analysis compares the costs expended on an intervention with the costs saved as a result of the intervention. Costs can clearly be measured monetarily, but for effectiveness to be measured in this way, it is necessary to convert health outcomes into dollars. Consequently, the analyst must place a monetary value on all health outcomes pertinent to the analysis, including length of life, quality of life, or other health consequences. If the outcome of interest is simply years of life, the analyst can use annual earnings per life-year saved as a monetary measure of effectiveness. However, when other factors such as quality of life and potential complications must be considered, analysts will usually measure effectiveness using a willingness-to-pay method. In this technique, subjects are asked how much money they would be willing to pay to completely avoid a select negative health outcome. A cost-benefit analysis should report results in the form of a net benefit in dollars, or the difference between the monetary value of the health benefits derived minus the cost of the health program.[3]

> Cost-benefit analysis measures the dollars saved by an intervention for the dollars expended.

Assigning a price of a health outcome, however, is a very difficult and controversial task that may be possible in only a limited number of situations. The main disadvantage with this method is that people from different sociodemographic backgrounds may be willing to pay vastly different dollar amounts for the same health outcome.[6,7] Clearly socioeconomic status is highly associated with a person's willingness to pay for a health outcome. In addition, whether a person lives in a country with a universal healthcare system or whether the person has full health insurance will dramatically affect the person's willingness to pay. These differences can drastically bias a study toward or against a certain demographic section of the population.

Cost-benefit analysis in a more limited form—without taking quality of life into account—is more feasible. For example, the cost of cochlear implant surgery for a deaf patient can be compared to the dollars saved by obviating disability payments as result of the surgery, as well as the increased contribution to gross domestic product (GDP) when the patient is able to work more effectively after surgery. The money lost by the average patient during different periods in life due to mild and severe disabilities can be ascertained from the US Census Bureau.[8]

A positive feature of the more limited form of cost-benefit analysis is that the outcome of dollars gained from dollars expended is more readily understood by policymakers than the outcomes in cost-effectiveness analysis and cost-utility analysis. Cost-benefit studies that demonstrate a saving of healthcare dollars on the macroeconomic (national) level are particularly relevant for healthcare policymakers. Such studies are best performed using the *societal perspective* for costs. In select instances, a cost-benefit analysis is complementary to a cost-utility analysis and adds another important dimension.[9]

> Cost-benefit analysis is generally better understood by policymakers than cost-effectiveness analysis or cost-utility analysis.

COST-EFFECTIVENESS ANALYSIS

Cost-effectiveness analysis measures an outcome such as life-years gained, healthy years gained, asthma-free months gained, years of good vision gained, and so on for the costs expended. For the purposes of this book, the quality-adjusted life-year (QALY) will *not* be considered as a cost-effectiveness outcome, but rather as a cost-utility outcome.

A cost-effectiveness analysis, as described by Weinstein and Stason[10] in 1977, requires decision makers to be explicit with respect to the benefits (improvement in length of life and/or quality of life) and values that underlie a resource allocation decision. This type of analysis has since become referred to as cost-utility analysis by Drummond and colleagues.[3] We agree with using the term *cost-utility analysis* for a study that assesses the *value* (improvement in length of life and/or quality of life) measured in QALYs conferred by an intervention for the resources expended, and also agree with reserving the term *cost-effectiveness analysis* for a study that measures the outcome gain in another form (life-years, vision-years, work-years, and so on) for the resources expended.[3]

There is confusion in the literature because the Panel on Cost-Effectiveness in Health and Medicine used the term *cost-effectiveness analysis* interchangeably with *cost-utility analysis*.[11] In doing so, cost-utility analysis was basically considered as a variant of cost-effectiveness analysis, a term that encompasses numerous possible outcomes. Use of the term *cost-utility analysis*, however, is more specific and clearly refers to healthcare economic analyses that measure the dollars expended on an intervention for the value conferred ($/QALY, or dollars expended per quality-adjusted life-year gained).

> Cost-effectiveness analysis measures the dollars expended on an intervention for an outcome (life-years, work-years, vision-years, but not QALYs) gained.

Life-Years Gained

In essence, the outcome for cost-effectiveness analysis is measured in units of effect gained for the resources (dollars) expended. A common unit of effectiveness is time of life, and a cost-effectiveness analysis frequently compares the cost per life-year (year of life) saved between two potential health programs. Although the life-year is perhaps the most common outcome unit used in a cost-effectiveness analysis, there are many cases when this outcome measure will not be useful or appropriate. Life-years saved is not an appropriate outcome measure if the program or intervention is designed to improve *quality* of life (as opposed to the *quantity* of life). In these instances, vision-years (years with good vision) gained, work-years (years in which a person is able to perform a job) gained, disability-free years, or some other variant can be employed. Even then, cost-effectiveness is not as all-encompassing a measure of quality-of-life parameters as is cost-utility analysis.

Life-years saved may be misleading if the improvement in longevity occurs far in the future. For instance, a smoking cessation program for teenagers that increases survival by one year 60 years hence saves one undiscounted life-year, but if the time is discounted at 3% per year, the saving is 1/1.03, or 0.17 life-years. Consequently, it may be more relevant in certain instances to base a cost-effectiveness analysis on an intermediate outcome measure that is assumed to be associated with better health. For instance, the number of pack-a-day smokers who have quit over a six-month period or the asthmatic attacks avoided per year due to a certain drug could be calculated as measured outcomes for the expenditure. Regardless of the outcome unit chosen for the analysis, the purpose of a cost-effectiveness analysis is to compare the cost per health outcome between the health programs under consideration. The superb compilation of 500 life-saving interventions by Tengs et al[12] gives a excellent appreciation of the varied uses of cost-effectiveness analysis in the form of life-years saved. The 500 interventions were divided into three groups:

- medical interventions,
- injury reduction interventions, and
- toxin control interventions.

Medical interventions are self-explanatory, including the treatment of infectious diseases, the use of vaccinations, and the use of mammograms for the detection of breast cancer. *Injury reduction interventions* include the institution of flammability standards for children's clothes, placing monitors on school buses, the performance of random automobile inspections, and setting highway speed limits. *Toxin control interventions* encompass regulations governing the treatment of noxious substances such as benzene emissions, lead levels in water, asbestos use, and radiation control. The inflation-adjusted mean costs in 2004 US dollars instead of the original 1993 dollars used by Tengs et al[12] for each are shown in Table 15.1.

Needless to say, the expenditure of $81 million for each life-year saved by banning asbestos in automatic transmission components seems a questionable use of resources when an influenza immunization costs $175 per life-year saved and many people in the United States are not immunized.[11]

COST-UTILITY ANALYSIS

Cost-utility analysis measures the *value* conferred by an intervention for the costs expended. The *value* conferred incorporates the improvement in *length of life* and *quality of life* and is measured by the QALY (quality-adjusted life-year gained).

A utility is a measure of the strength of preference for a particular health outcome and has a theoretical foundation in economics and decision theory. Essentially, a utility is a measure of the worth a person places on a certain outcome or health state. Using utilities, the quality of life associated with a health state that may have multiple important facets can be measured and reported with one number. Common methods of utility valuation are the time-tradeoff technique, standard-gamble technique, the willingness-to-pay technique, and rating scales. (We examined the details of utility theory in Chapters 8, 9, and 10.)

TABLE 15.1

Mean Cost to Save One Year of Life

Group	Cost in US Dollars (2004)
Medical interventions	$24,298
Injury reduction interventions	$62,329
Toxin control interventions	$3,623,000

Cost-utility analysis is the form of healthcare economic analysis that permits an analyst to combine different health outcomes of a program into one overall measure of *value*, thus allowing for more complete assessment of the effectiveness of a health intervention. The most sophisticated form of healthcare economic analysis, cost-utility analysis allows for health researchers to integrate this value gained from an intervention with the resources expended. Unlike *cost-benefit analysis*, with *cost-utility analysis* the analyst is not forced to perform the difficult task of assigning monetary values to health outcomes.

Cost-utility analysis measures the dollars expended on an intervention for the *value* (improvement in length of life and/or quality of life) gained.

The outcome measure for cost-utility analysis is the resources (dollars) expended per QALY gained. Measuring a health outcome in terms of QALYs allows an analyst to incorporate both morbidity and mortality into a single measure. Thus, a cost-utility analysis can investigate the cost per QALY gained from the implementation of a particular health intervention compared to any alternative intervention or no intervention. Cost-utility analysis allows a comparison of virtually all interventions in health care, no matter how disparate, using this standardized, value-based outcome measure.

Cost-utility analysis uses the outcome of $/QALY (dollars spent per quality-adjusted life-year gained).

A review of the different forms of healthcare economic analysis is shown in Table 15.2.

Throughout the remainder of this text, we concentrate on cost-utility analysis, the instrument that allows us to construct a database of value-based medicine quality standards. While the other forms of healthcare analysis are important, none is as comprehensive in scope as cost-utility analysis. Cost-utility analysis has the potential to incorporate all costs, all benefits, and all adverse effects associated with any healthcare intervention to arrive at a final outcome of *resources expended* for the *value gained* measured in terms of $/QALY.

Cost-utility analysis is the most comprehensive form of healthcare economic analysis.

Hussein Hollands, MSc, contributed to this chapter.

CORE CONCEPTS

■ There are four basic forms of healthcare economic analysis:
— cost-minimization analysis,
— cost-benefit analysis,

TABLE 15.2

Types of Healthcare Economic Analysis

Analysis	Outcome	Shortcomings
Cost-minimization	Dollars expended for equivalent interventions to compare which is less costly	Rarely used; very few interventions are exactly equivalent
Cost-benefit	Dollars expended on an intervention compared to the dollars gained as a result of the intervention	Usually ignores quality of life; difficult to evaluate length of life and quality of life in terms of money
Cost-effectiveness	Dollars expended for a specific outcome gained (life-years, vision-years, work-years, and so on, but not QALYs)	Does not take both length of life and quality of life into account
Cost-utility	Dollars expended per quality-adjusted life-year gained ($/QALY)	Most complex; utility values may not be available

QALY indicates quality-adjusted life-year; $/QALY, dollars expended per quality-adjusted life year gained.

- — cost-effectiveness analysis, and
- — cost-utility analysis.

- Cost-minimization analysis assesses two interventions of identical effectiveness to ascertain which is less costly.

- Cost-benefit analysis compares the costs expended on an intervention with the costs saved as a result of the intervention.

- Cost-effectiveness analysis measures the costs expended for an outcome such as life-years gained, healthy years gained, years of good vision gained, and so on (excluding quality-adjusted life-years).

- Cost-utility analysis measures cost expended for the value (improvement in length of life and quality of life) conferred by an intervention using the outcome measure of $/QALY (dollars expended per quality-adjusted life-year gained).

REFERENCES

1. Alpert B. Tough test: new biotech drugs haven't been subject to cost-effectiveness reviews, but that may change. *Barrons.* August 16, 2004:28–29.

2. Sharma S. New instruments: patient reported health outcomes. *Ret Physician.* 2004;1(suppl):12–14.

3. Drummond MF, O'Brien B, Stoddart GL, Torrance GW. *Methods for the Economic Evaluation of Health Care Programmes.* 2nd ed. Toronto, Canada: Oxford University Press; 2000:96–231.

4. Briggs AH, O'Brien BJ. The death of cost-minimization analysis? *Health Econ.* 2001;10:179–184.

5. Cresswell PA, Allen ED, Tompkinson J, et al. Cost effectiveness of a single functioning treatment center for cataract surgery. *J Cataract Refract Surg.* 1996;22:940–946.

6. Frew E, Wolstenholme JL, Whynes DK. Willingness-to-pay for colorectal cancer screening. *Eur J Cancer.* 2001;37:1746–1751.

7. O'Brien B, Viramontes JL. Willingness-to-pay: a valid and reliable measure of health state preference? *Med Decis Making.* 1994;14:289–297.

8. Disability data. Available at: www.census.gov. Accessed July 10, 2003.

9. Membreno J, Brown MM, Brown GC, Sharma S, Beauchamp GR. A cost-utility analysis of therapy for amblyopia. *Ophthalmology.* 2002;109:2265–2271.

10. Weinstein MC, Stason WB. Foundations of cost-effectiveness analysis for health and medical practices. *N Engl J Med.* 1977;296:716–721.

11. Torrance GW, Siegel JE, Luce BR. Framing and designing the cost-effectiveness analysis. In: Gold MR, Siegel JE, Russell LB, Weinstein MC, eds. *Cost-Effectiveness in Health and Medicine.* New York, NY: Oxford University Press; 1996:54–81.

12. Tengs TO, Adams ME, Pliskin JP, et al. Five-hundred life-saving interventions and their cost-effectiveness. *Risk Anal.* 1995;15:369–390.

16

Cost-Utility Analysis

Cost-utility analysis is the instrument that allows us to create a comparable cost-utility database across all medical specialties that will serve as the foundation for value-based medicine (VBM) quality standards for healthcare interventions. Once a sufficient VBM database is developed, those interventions that are harmful, of no benefit, or of negligible benefit can be examined more closely to ascertain which should be:

- deleted from our therapeutic armamentarium,
- improved, and/or
- allotted less reimbursement.

The converse is true as well: with a sufficient VBM database, procedures that are extremely cost-effective could be considered for increased reimbursement.

Do we call an intervention *cost-utilitarian*? While it is cost-utility analysis that allows us to create a VBM database, the term *cost utility* of an intervention is foreign to all but those interested in quality-of-life measures and healthcare economic analysis. Because the primary goal is to incorporate VBM into everyday practice, we use the term *cost-effective* to refer to an intervention that has a cost utility (dollars spent per quality-adjusted life year [$/QALY]) within the range considered to be cost-effective. We believe that labeling an intervention *cost-effective* will be much better accepted than calling the intervention *cost-utilitarian*. However, when reviewing a study in the literature, the reader should recognize when the term *cost-effectiveness* refers to cost-utility analysis or cost-effectiveness analysis.

In the remainder of the book, the term *cost-effectiveness* will refer to cost-utility analysis. The *incremental cost-effectiveness* or *cost-effectiveness ratio* again will refer to cost-utility analysis using the outcome of $/QALY gained.

Interventions that undergo cost-utility analysis should be referred to as *cost-effective* rather than *cost-utilitarian*, as the latter term may confuse those not intimately familiar with the healthcare economic literature.

WHAT IS COST-EFFECTIVE?

Current Standards

In 1992, Laupacis et al[1] published cost-utility standards in the *Canadian Medical Association Journal* that have since become widely used in the healthcare literature. They classified an intervention with a cost utility of less than $20,000/QALY gained as very cost-effective, while an intervention costing greater than $100,000/QALY gained was not considered cost-effective. Careful analysis of the methodology, however, reveals that the limits were quite arbitrary. Despite the fact that the year was 1992 and the currency was Canadian dollars, most papers on cost-utility analysis still adhere to the figure of $100,000/QALY gained as the upper limit of cost-effectiveness. The currency-adjusted (Canadian to US dollars) and inflation-adjusted (1992 to 2003) upper limit of $100,000 actually equates to $115,000 in 2004 US dollars, a figure that is surprisingly close to the original limit of Laupacis et al.[1] Nonetheless, these comparative figures are not especially valid because cost-utility analyses performed in Canada and the United States utilize an entirely different cost basis.

Other authors in the United States have suggested a cost utility of $50,000 as the upper limit of cost-effectiveness for an intervention.[2,3] Data from the US Food and Drug Administration suggest that society is willing to pay up to $373,000 for 1 QALY, or one year of living at a utility value of 1.0 (perfect health).[4]

Some authors have used $50,000/QALY gained as the upper limit for cost-effectiveness, while others have set the upper limit at $100,000/QALY gained (in US dollars).

Future Standards

Once a database of comparable cost-utility analyses is established, new standards will certainly be developed for the upper limit of cost-effectiveness of an intervention. In part, the upper limit will be decided by how much society is willing to expend on healthcare. The standards will vary from country to country, depending upon the resources each country has and makes available.

Future standards for cost-utility analysis will be developed once there is a large cost-utility database and society decides what it is willing to pay for healthcare.

We anticipate that the cost-utility database of interventions will likely be normally distributed. Thus, standard deviations will be established. A cutoff of one standard deviation above the average would place approximately 17% of interventions above the cost-effective range, while two standard deviations would place 2.5% of interventions above the cost-effective range, and three standard deviations would place 0.5% of interventions above the cost-effective range. The interventions funded will be determined by the resources a given country is willing to assign to healthcare. Other factors, such as the incidence of interventions, the public perceived value, lobbying by interest groups, the introduction of new interventions, and the changing prevalence of disease burden in general will also be factors that play roles in the decision-making process.

From a database we have created to date for cost-utility analyses, and considering the resources spent on healthcare services in the United States, we believe that *cost-utility standards will allow all citizens in the United States to receive virtually all healthcare interventions that provide value.* While the naysayers may protest that some will be denied access to select interventions, we believe that all patients will be far better off and their quality of healthcare improved because interventions that do not work or have a net harmful effect will be targeted.

Few in the public sector realize that a number of our healthcare interventions are of minimal benefit, of no benefit, or harmful. Value-based medicine will enable us to weed out interventions that have essentially no benefit or are harmful so that only beneficial interventions will be provided for everyone. Value-based medicine should be viewed as the *antirationing tool* that improves quality of care and conserves wasted resources that can be used to pay for healthcare services for those who are uninsured and currently experience severe rationing.

AVERAGE VS INCREMENTAL COST-UTILITY ANALYSIS

Cost-utility analysis compares the cost and value conferred by a healthcare intervention with the cost and value conferred by an alternative intervention or with no treatment. For instance, if one is evaluating a new drug for the reduction of blood pressure, the cost-utility analysis should compare the new treatment against the current standard of care. A comparison of the cost and conferred value associated with an intervention with the cost and conferred value associated with the *next-best alternative intervention* is defined as an *incremental cost-utility ratio.*

> The term *cost-utility ratio* is often used synonymously with the term *cost utility.* It is therefore common practice to say that an intervention has either a *cost-utility ratio* of $50,000/QALY or a *cost utility* of $50,000/QALY.

> An *incremental cost-utility ratio* compares the cost and conferred value (QALYs) associated with an intervention with the cost and conferred value associated with the next-best *alternative intervention.*

Some have differentiated between an incremental (or marginal) cost-utility ratio and an average cost-utility ratio.[5] In contrast to the *incremental* cost-utility ratio, for which the differences in cost and effectiveness are calculated when the treatment in question is compared to the next-best alternative, the *average* cost-utility ratio measures the costs and effectiveness independently of any alternative strategy.[5] An average cost-utility ratio therefore compares the incremental costs and incremental value gain associated with an intervention to no treatment. A list of the cost-utility of various healthcare interventions is shown in Table 16.1.

> An *average cost-utility ratio* compares the cost and the conferred value (QALYs) associated with an intervention to no treatment.

Through using a true incremental cost-utility ratio, it is possible to discern the real opportunity cost of a program, or the health outcomes that could have been achieved by forgoing the health program of interest and implementing the next-best available option. By examining health policy in this way, it is possible to compare the cost utility (cost-effectiveness) of various different health interventions in a consistent manner.

Hussein Hollands, MSc, contributed to this chapter.

CORE CONCEPTS

- Cost-utility analysis is the instrument that allows the creation of a cost-utility database across all medical specialties that will serve as the foundation for VBM quality standards for healthcare interventions.
- Healthcare interventions are best referred to as *cost-effective* rather than *cost-utilitarian* since the latter term confuses those not intimately familiar with the healthcare economic literature.
- Current standards for cost-utility analysis results are arbitrary at best.
- Some authors have used $50,000/QALY as the upper limit of cost-effectiveness, while others have set the upper limit at $100,000/QALY.
- Value-based medicine should be viewed as the antirationing tool that improves quality of care and highlights interventions that deliver no value or cause a net value loss.
- There are currently more than sufficient resources in the US healthcare system to pay for interventions that provide value for all citizens.
- Value-based medicine provides a mechanism to conserve wasted resources that can be used to pay for healthcare services for those who are currently uninsured and experience severe rationing.
- An *incremental* cost-utility ratio compares the cost and value gain associated with a healthcare intervention with the cost and value gain associated with the next-best alternative, intervention.
- An *average* cost-utility ratio compares the cost and value gain associated with a healthcare intervention to no treatment.

TABLE 16.1

Cost-Utility of Various Healthcare Interventions*

Intervention	$/QALY	Year of Publication
Eradication of *H. Pylori* With Dyspepsia[6]	$1,198	1997
Cataract Extraction[7]	$2,020	2002
Maintenance of Treatment of Recurrent Depression[8]	$5,000	1995
Cochlear Implant in Children[9]	$9,029	2000
Proton Pump Inhibitor Over Histamine 2-Receptor Antagonist Treatment for Heartburn[2]	$10,400	2000
Normoglycemic Control of Type 2 Diabetes[10]	$16,002	1997
CT For Equivocal Neurological Symptoms[11]	$20,290	1997
Chemoprophylaxis After Occupational Exposure to HIV[12]	$37,000	1997
MRI for Equivocal Neurological Symptoms[11]	$101,670	1997
Endstage Diabetic Renal Disease[13]		
Simultaneous K-P Transplant	$102,422	1998
Living Donor Kidney Transplant	$123,923	1998
Cadaver Kidney Transplant	$156,042	1998
Dialysis	$317,746	1998
Three-Day Chemoprophylaxis of Prosthetic Joint Patients During Dental Treatment[14]	$1,100,000	1991

CT indicates computed tomography; HIV, human immunodeficiency virus; K-P, kidney-pancreas; MRI, magnetic resonance imaging; QALY, quality-adjusted life year.

* Very few of these cost-utility analyses are exactly comparable due to the facts that 1) the utility-value acquisition methodology is not standardized; 2) the utility-value respondents vary; 3) the cost perspective is not standardized; 4) the cost basis is not standardized; 5) the years of the studies differ; 6) the time frames differ; and 7) other variables differ.

REFERENCES

1. Laupacis A, Feeny D, Detsky AS, Tugwell PX. How attractive does a new technology have to be to warrant adoption and utilization: tentative guidelines for using clinical and economic evaluations. *CMAJ.* 1992;146:473–481.
2. Heudebert GR, Centor RM, Klapow JC, et al. What is heartburn worth? A cost-utility analysis of management strategies. *J Gen Intern Med.* 2000;15:175–182.

3. Kallmes DF, Kallmes MH. Cost-effectiveness of angiography performed during surgery for ruptured intracranial aneuryms. *AJNR Am J Neurorad.* 1997;18:1453–1462.

4. Medical devices, patient examinations and surgeons' gloves, test procedures and acceptance criteria. *Federal Register,* 21 CFR, Part 800, Docket No. 03N-0056, Vol 68, No. 61; 2003.

5. Detsky AS, Naglie IG. A clinician's guide to cost-effectiveness analysis. *Ann Intern Med.* 1990;113:147–154.

6. Ebell WH, Warbasse L, Brenner C. Evaluation of the dyspeptic patient: a cost-utility study. *J Fam Pract.* 1997;44:545–555.

7. Busbee B, Brown MM, Brown GC, Sharma S. Incremental cost-effectiveness of initial cataract surgery. *Ophthalmology.* 2002;109:606–612.

8. Kamlet MS, Paul N, Greenhouse J, Kupfer D, Frank E, Wade M. Cost-utility analysis of maintenance for recurrent depression. *Control Clin Trials.* 1995;16:17–40.

9. Cheng AK, Rubin HR, Powe NR, et al. Cost-utility analysis of cochlear implant in children. *JAMA.* 2000;284:850–856.

10. Eastman RC, Javitt JC, Herman WH, et al. Model of complications of NIDDM, II: analysis of the health benefits and cost-effectiveness of treating NIDDM with the goal of normoglycemia. *Diabetes Care.* 1997;20:735–744.

11. Mushlin AI, Mooney C, Holloway RG, Detsky AS, Mattson DH, Phelps CE. The cost-effectiveness of magnetic resonance imaging for patients with equivocal neurological symptoms. *Int J Technol Assess Health Care.* 1997;13:21–34.

12. Pinkerton SD, Holtgrave DR, Pinkerton HJ. Cost-effectiveness of chemoprophylaxis after occupational exposure to HIV. *Arch Int Med.* 1997;157:1972–1980.

13. Douzdijan V, Ferrara D, Silvestri G. Treatment strategies for insulin-dependent diabetics with ESRD: a cost-effectiveness decision analysis model. *Am J Kidney Dis.* 1998;31:794–802.

14. Jacobson JJ, Schweitzer SO, Kowalski CJ. Chemoprophylaxis of prosthetic joint patients during dental treatment: a decision analysis. *Oral Surg Oral Med Oral Pathol.* 1991;72:167–177.

Guide to Performing
a Cost-Utility Analysis

Seven fundamental steps must be undertaken to perform a cost-utility analysis evaluation properly. These steps include the following:

1. Define the question.
2. Define all germane outcome(s) associated with all treatment alternatives, utilizing the best evidence-based data.
3. Assign utility values to the outcomes.
4. Measure the total value conferred by the intervention using decision analysis.
5. Estimate the costs.
6. Calculate the undiscounted cost-utility ratio and then discount the incremental value gained and the incremental costs accrued to their present values, to arrive at a discounted cost-utility ratio.
7. Perform sensitivity analysis to handle uncertainty.

While we focus on the nuts and bolts of performing a cost-utility analysis in this chapter, most of the basic principles outlined here are also applicable to cost-minimization analysis, cost-benefit analysis, and cost-effectiveness analysis.

1. DEFINE THE QUESTION

The first step in performing a cost-utility analysis is to determine the exact problem that needs to be addressed for what group of patients and with what health state. In defining the question, the following seven variables should be addressed:

- the intervention options to be compared (reference case, individual),
- the diseases (health states) to be studied (third-party insurer, societal and so on),
- the target population,
- the study perspective (reference case, individual),
- the cost perspective (third-party insurer, societal, and so on),

- the time frame, and
- the outcomes.

At the same time we choose the question to be answered, we also choose the study perspective, typically that of the *reference case*. By using the reference case perspective, or that of the average person undergoing an intervention, we are best able to appreciate a single incremental cost-utility ratio (ICER) associated with the intervention to allow a direct comparison of ICERs associated with diverse interventions across disparate specialties in medicine. The cost perspective (societal, third-party insurer, patient, governmental, or other) should also be defined at this time.

> Use of the *reference case study perspective* facilitates the comparison of different cost-utility analyses and allows for more direct and relevant comparisons of ICERs derived from different interventions.

When conducting a cost-utility analysis, one must clearly define the question that needs to be answered. Once the question is defined, a review of the literature, discussion with opinion leaders, and a review with patients will identify all possible potential treatment options that will be modeled to answer the question. Once the treatment options are identified, all outcomes associated with all alternatives must also be defined. These outcomes should include both those that are beneficial to patients, such as the alleviation of pain and suffering or the improvement of an outcome such as vision or blood pressure, in addition to adverse outcomes that could be as minor as a rash developing while taking a new medicine to as serious as the risk of immediate death from an anaphylactic reaction. In addition, the target population of the program alternatives should be clear, as the analysis results may not be applied generally to a different population.

To better understand these concepts, let us consider two examples: one from the individual case level, and the other from the societal level. In the first case clinicians may want to decide whether a new anticoagulation medication is the preferred strategy for preventing stroke in an older patient with atrial fibrillation due to cardiomyopathy. In the second example, an insurer may want to determine if a screening program for the human immunodeficiency virus (HIV) should be implemented for pregnant women.* Let us consider both of these decisions through the lens of our aforementioned seven critical questions.

For the question about whether to use a new drug in patients with atrial fibrillation, the seven defining variables of the first fundamental step of *define the question* in performing a cost-utility analysis are as follows.

---

* While we have suggested that cost-utility analyses should generally be performed using the third-party insurer perspective to allow comparability and the feasible creation of a value-based medicine database (Chapter 14), the implementation of a governmental program could well require use of the societal perspective. The researcher should therefore be familiar with the costs included in this perspective (Chapter 14). But again, the third-party cost perspective should be used whenever possible.

1. **The intervention options to be compared:** treatment with a new anticoagulant vs standard anticoagulation.

2. **The health state(s) to be studied:** atrial fibrillation occurring secondary to cardiomyopathy.

3. **The target population:** Medicare beneficiaries.

4. **The study perspective:** reference case (the average person undergoing the intervention for the disease under study in the target population).

5. **The cost perspective:** third-party insurer.

6. **The time frame:** because atrial fibrillation is a chronic condition, the time frame will include the remainder of the average person's life in each cohort.

7. **The outcomes:** stroke and no stroke.

In regard to outcomes, the use of stroke and no stroke is markedly oversimplified. Including the various outcomes of stroke severity and death would make the study much more relevant, as would the inclusion of any potential differences in the side effects of the medicines.

For the question concerning the screening of all pregnant women for HIV, the seven defining variables of the first fundamental step of *define the question* are:

1. **The intervention to be compared:** screening for HIV vs no screening.

2. **The health state to be studied:** pregnancy.

3. **The target population:** all pregnant women.

4. **The study perspective:** reference case.

5. **The cost perspective:** societal.

6. **The time frame:** remaining life expectancy, as the early discovery of HIV likely results in less morbidity and mortality over a long-term period.

7. **The outcomes:** HIV positive and HIV negative.

Again, note that for this study, the outcomes of HIV positive and HIV negative are markedly oversimplified and do not allow the researcher to capture the value accrued in each of these decision arms. To measure the total benefits conferred by using this screening test, the sequelae (death, severe infection, adverse treatment effects, and others) of the health states of being HIV positive and HIV negative must also be considered as outcomes. It is the difference in benefit accrued between these sequelae in the two groups that is critical in deciding the final value conferred by obtaining the HIV test.

After each option in a cost-utility analysis is clearly defined, an analyst will outline all relevant implications of the options with respect to health outcomes and costs. In this stage of the analysis it may be important to consult with experts in the field (physicians, nurses, other health professionals, or program managers) to determine all possible health outcomes. To visualize these possibilities, it may be useful to draw a flow diagram, using a hypothetical cohort of people who begin the program, and follow that cohort through every possible event outcome. The time frame of the study should be considered here as well.

Duration of Treatment Benefit

In identifying what outcome measurement to use, the purpose of the program or intervention must be considered. Mortality data are a basic and very useful outcome measure in a cost-utility analysis and can be used as the sole outcome measure, or incorporated with quality-of-life information, to produce quality-adjusted life-years (QALYs). In either instance, it is critical to know the expected years of life conferred by, or associated with, different treatment options. In some cases, mortality data are reported in terms of statistical survival rates or hazard ratios. For instance, the relative risk or odds ratio of a treatment or intervention's five-year survival may be the only outcome reported in a published paper. Consequently, a conversion between survival data and the mean actual length of life for the *reference case*, or average case, must be employed.

If survival data are not available, or do not fully explain the health outcome conferred by a program, an analyst must use another more appropriate method to measure value. Rather than use total time of benefit for a cost-utility analysis, it is often easier to use an intermediate outcome measure that is assumed to be associated with better health. The major advantages of using an intermediate health outcome in a cost-utility analysis or cost-effectiveness analysis are ease, simplicity, and the fact that a clinical trial may only span a specific interval. For instance, it may be easier and more efficient to use an intermediate health outcome such as asthmatic attacks saved when comparing the cost-effectiveness of two asthma-treating drugs over a one-year period. The major disadvantage of using an intermediate health outcome is that the cost-utility or cost-effectiveness of the program or treatment in question cannot be compared across many interventions without knowing the full long-term benefit conferred by each intervention.

2. DEFINE ALL GERMANE OUTCOME(S) ASSOCIATED WITH ALL TREATMENT ALTERNATIVES, UTILIZING THE BEST EVIDENCE-BASED DATA

Not all costs or possible health outcomes will be relevant to the final cost-utility analysis because some may have a very small effect or be irrelevant to the questions being asked; however, at this point it is useful to include as much information as possible. This will facilitate a more comprehensive understanding of the problem and allow the analyst to choose what is truly relevant at a later time.

Once a decision has been made about which health outcome measures will be used in a cost-utility analysis, the effectiveness of the various treatment alternatives on these outcomes must be determined. A description of the primary evidence-based data (frequently a randomized clinical trial), including the methodology, and pertinent results should be included to highlight the efficacy of a treatment, service, or program.

Specifically, the probability of the different health outcome measures must be estimated. Ideally, to determine the cost-utility of a program, a full prospective study would be employed to measure the quality of life associated with the intervention of interest and the relevant costs associated with the intervention in an experimental fashion. In this way, the study would be designed to meet the exact specifications of the analyst and the data would be easily transferable to the cost-utility model. Repeating thousands of clinical trials already in the peer-reviewed literature to obtain quality-of-life values, however, is an impossibly costly task. Thus, a methodology must be utilized that will take the data from clinical trials and convert them to a value-based format for use in cost-utility analysis.

The Randomized Clinical Trial

In most situations, a prospectively designed, full economic evaluation is not practical and analysts must use previously published secondary data to estimate effectiveness. A randomized controlled trial (RCT) is the gold standard in epidemiology and is considered *level 1* evidence (Chapter 4); consequently, a suitable RCT should be used if it is available. However, there are a number of reasons why an RCT may not be available or appropriate for use in an economic evaluation.

First, a fully powered and properly designed RCT is difficult and expensive to perform, and in many cases can be considered unethical; thus, there may be many instances where an RCT has not been performed in the area of interest. Second, there may be situations in which an RCT exists, but the sample of participants used in the trial is different from the population of interest in the economic evaluation. Depending on the extent of these differences, the results of the trial may not be applied generally to the study population in the cost-utility analysis, in which case the RCT will be of limited value. Finally, most RCTs are designed to determine the efficacy of a treatment as opposed to the effectiveness. The *efficacy* of a treatment refers to how effective it is in an ideal setting (that is, when patients are monitored to stay with the treatment regimen), while *effectiveness* refers to how the treatment works in a real-world setting. If a cost-utility analysis is based on efficacy data, then the trial data may not be a good representation of how the program or treatment will work in a real-world setting, thus biasing the results of the economic evaluation.

> The *efficacy* of a treatment refers to how effective it is in an ideal setting. The *effectiveness* refers to how a treatment works in a real-world setting.

Utilizing the highest level of evidence available is critical for any cost-utility analysis. Because the perfect randomized clinical trial never has been performed, and never will be, the healthcare analyst must decide which clinical data provide the highest level of evidence and clinical relevance. This often requires input from specialists familiar with the intervention under study, as a literature review alone may not reveal the associated and accepted medical practices, especially from the laboratory and diagnostic study viewpoints. For example, in an immunosuppressed solid organ transplant patient with cytomegalovirus viremia, how often should a cytomegalovirus serum antigen level be drawn? Or in a patient with low-grade fever after simultaneous kidney and pancreas transplantation, what workup should be undertaken? In these instances, adequate information may only be available from clinicians who are closely familiar with management and the clinical literature relevant to the intervention(s) of interest. For someone who is not intimately familiar with an intervention, culling information from the literature alone is very difficult and can result in the oversight of importance aspects of therapy.

Other Evidence-Based Data

If a suitable randomized clinical trial is not available, an analyst may choose to use data derived from other study designs such as a prospective cohort study or retrospective case-control study. In the absence of a suitable randomized clinical trial, a prospective cohort study can sometimes be the best option. (See Chapter 4 for more information on alternative study designs.) An analyst may also want to consult with a trained epidemiologist to better evaluate the quality of available literature and to determine possible biases in observational studies that should be considered. In many situations, a tradeoff between level of evidence (or internal validity) and general applicability to the situation and population of interest will exist and must be considered by the analyst.

If a number of clinical trials exist that address the same issue using a similar study design and methodology, then results can be combined in a meta-analysis. A meta-analysis can be particularly useful when a number of different studies provide widely varying or contradictory results. It can also be useful if a number of individual studies have insufficient power to detect a significant difference individually, but a combination of the studies has sufficient power to detect a difference of interest. Meta-analyses on a particular topic can be obtained from the published literature or can be performed by the analyst for the purpose of the cost-utility analysis. For those with additional interest in meta-analysis, we refer the reader to the excellent text of Petitti.[1]

If some effectiveness data are not known, then it may be possible to estimate it after consultation with experts in the field. However, this does not follow the scientific method and should only be used as a last resort. If an expert opinion is used, a sensitivity analysis should be performed on that variable to ensure that it does not affect results drastically.

A cost-utility analysis may use one randomized clinical trial to estimate all probabilities that are needed to describe the health outcomes completely, or a combination of various studies and study designs may be used. This could include a combination of randomized clinical trials, meta-analyses, observational studies, or expert opinions. The appropriate data to use in a cost-utility analysis will depend on the published literature in the area, the resources of the analysts, and the purpose of the study. For instance, a cost-utility analysis performed in-house by a hospital for resource allocation will require different variables than a cost-utility analysis performed by a pharmaceutical company for a new drug to be included on a formulary. The latter cost-utility analysis would likely be based on an approved randomized clinical trial and follow a strict set of guidelines, while the former could be based on the best data readily available to the analyst.

3. ASSIGN UTILITY VALUES TO THE OUTCOMES

Utility values themselves can be gathered from the literature or from surrogate respondents such as providers, administrators, researchers, or a cross section of the general community. As we discussed in Chapter 9, however, time-tradeoff utility values from patients with a disease give the most accurate representation of the quality of life associated with a health state. The final decision as to which utilities to use in a cost-utility analysis will depend on the specific situation, the availability of data, and the preference of the investigators. However, we recommend the use of patient-based utilities; we believe the patients themselves who live with a particular disease are truly in a position to determine how their quality of life is affected by their disease and by interventions for it.

> Correlate the outcomes of the clinical trials with utility values, preferably those obtained from *patients* using *time-tradeoff methodology*.

If one has to rely on an analysis derived from a set of utilities that are not patient-based, then at a minimum, we recommend that the utility methodology include some form of disease state explanation to the participant that captures as completely as possible the disease or health state in question. A written description of a disease state is referred to as a *scenario* and includes a broad-based description that should include all relevant measures or domains of health. Researchers describe these domains differently, but they usually contain aspects of health such as physical/mobility function, emotional/psychological function, sensory function, cognitive function, pain, dexterity, and self-care.

Utility Values and Clinical Trials

When undertaking a cost-utility analysis, there must be a practical way of converting a health outcome into a utility value to use in QALY form. In some circumstances, data will already exist on the effectiveness of the program that incorporates some measure of quality of life. For example, some clinical trials will not only report clinical outcomes, but they will also report changes in quality of life measured with utilities or a multiattribute health classification system. In this case, incorporating the data into a cost-utility analysis should be straightforward. In addition, if the cost-utility of a program is being studied prospectively (that is, a prospective study is being undertaken to determine cost and effectiveness simultaneously using a well-defined epidemiological study design), then quality-of-life measurements can be incorporated as an outcome measure in the prospective study and can be easily incorporated into the modeling.

Most current epidemiological investigations, however, do not include health-related quality-of-life information in their outcomes. Consequently, quality-of-life data must be obtained from previous research in the field. For instance, Duncan and colleagues[2] reported patient-based time-tradeoff utility values associated with stroke categorized according to the Modified Rankin Scale, a function-based instrument used to evaluate stroke changes in clinical trials.[3] When the outcome of a clinical trial for the treatment of stroke is measured using the Modified Rankin Scale, utility values can be substituted directly from the study by Duncan et al.[2]

4. MEASURE THE TOTAL BENEFIT DERIVED BY THE INTERVENTION USING DECISION ANALYSIS

Analyses are modeled using decision analysis software. Currently, we prefer to use TreeAge Software's TreeAge Data 4.0 (www.treeage.com). In many instances, basic (straightforward or simple) decision analysis can be utilized. Markov modeling analysis can be used in cases with recurrent outcomes, including the recurrent chance of death for the reference case analysis, and a combination of both straightforward decision analysis and Markov modeling may be necessary for some cases.

> Perform a decision analysis, usually with utility values at the terminal nodes to establish the difference in utility value between treatment options. This difference can then be multiplied by the duration of treatment benefit to ascertain the value (QALYs) conferred by the intervention.

With straightforward decision analysis, the utility value outcomes for the interventions undergoing comparison are contrasted and the lower value is subtracted from the higher value to ascertain the incremental utility gained. This incremental utility value difference between two alternatives is generally multiplied by the time of benefit of the intervention to ascertain the total value (in QALYs gained), while with Markov modeling, the computer program output is already in QALYs because time is factored in. With the Markov method, the QALYs accrued by the alternative intervention (or no intervention) over the time period are subtracted from those accrued by the primary intervention of interest to give the total value gained by the intervention.

As noted, a *reference-case analysis* cost-utility analysis, or the case of the average person with a disease, should be undertaken. While using an age-specific model for every patient might yield more accurate data, we believe the ramifications of basing the value of a healthcare intervention on age are politically unacceptable. In addition, reference-case analyses are necessary to compare different interventions across diverse specialties.

5. ESTIMATE THE COSTS

As we discussed in Chapter 12, the third-party insurer cost perspective uses direct healthcare costs (provider costs, hospital and other facility costs, pharmaceutical costs, laboratory and diagnostic costs) in cost-utility analysis. We also recommend using the most standardized cost basis, which in the United States is the Medicare reimbursement schedule (found at www.cms.hhs.gov). Most insurers in the United States base their reimbursement in some fashion upon the Medicare schedule.

> Use the third-party cost perspective and direct costs with the national average Medicare reimbursement schedule as the cost basis. For outpatient drugs, use the *average wholesale price* (AWP).

An exception to the use of Medicare data is the expenditure for skilled nursing facilities. Because the Medicaid program covers expenditures for nursing home care to a much greater degree than Medicare, the average Medicaid reimbursement schedule is therefore preferable to the Medicare reimbursement schedule to use for this service.

A second exception to the use of Medicare data is the expenditure for prescription drugs. As of the writing of this text, the most standardized current system for pharmaceutical costs is the average wholesale price (AWP) available from the *Red Book*.[4] Once the Medicare Prescription Drug, Modernization and Improvement Act is fully instituted in 2006, it is likely that a different, standardized cost basis affiliated with Medicare will be utilized.

6. CALCULATE THE UNDISCOUNTED COST-UTILITY RATIO AND THEN DISCOUNT THE INCREMENTAL VALUE GAINED AND THE INCREMENTAL COSTS ACCRUED TO THEIR PRESENT VALUES TO ARRIVE AT A DISCOUNTED COST-UTILITY RATIO

As discussed in Chapter 12, both costs and outcomes (QALYs gained) are discounted in cost-utility analysis. The Panel on Cost-Effectiveness in Health and Medicine recommended using a 3% annual discount rate,[5] which we believe is still reasonable in today's markets.

> Discount both the value gained (in QALYs) and direct healthcare costs at a 3% annual rate using a net present value analysis.

Most cost-utility analyses utilize a 3% and/or a 5% annual discount rate, but while 3% and 5% rates might seem similar at first glance, the cost-utility of the same intervention using each of theses rates can differ considerably, particularly over long time periods. By utilizing 0%, 3%, and 5% discount rates, the researcher will have a reasonable idea how much varying the discount rate will vary the final result of the cost-utility analysis. The researcher can then more readily compare the study with other studies in the literature that use varying discount rates. In theory, only studies that employ the same discount rate can be directly compared.

7. PERFORM A SENSITIVITY ANALYSIS TO HANDLE THE UNCERTAINTY

When modeling a health intervention vs an alternative, there are many potential uncertainties to consider. The most important in a cost-utility analysis are the *parameter* uncertainties, which refers to the inherent variability associated with point estimates used in the model. These can include health outcomes (such as length of life and/or quality of life), costs, probabilities, and/or discount rates.

To increase the robustness of a model, one-, two-, three-, or *n*-way sensitivity analyses can be performed by varying one or more parameters in the model. One-way sensitivity analysis is performed by changing one variable at a time, two-way sensitivity analysis changes two variables simultaneously (such as utility values and discount rate), three-way sensitivity analysis changes three variables simultaneously (utility values, discount rate, and survival), and so on.

> Perform sensitivity analysis by altering the variables in which there is the least confidence.

Sensitivity analyses should be performed in all economic evaluations to determine the robustness of the analysis. In cases in which 95% confidence intervals are available for parameters such as the clinical efficacy of an intervention, utility values, or costs, it is reasonable to calculate a cost utility using the upper and lower limits of the 95% confidence intervals. If the values fall within the accepted range of cost-effectiveness across all the sensitivity analyses, the overall analysis is considered to be *robust*.

> *Sensitivity analysis* takes into account (or corrects for) the uncertainty associated with healthcare economic analyses.

Performing sensitivity analysis is straightforward in a simple model, but it can become intricate when there are many parameters and the model is complex. In a complex model there can be a very large number of one-way sensitivity analyses to perform and exponentially more two-, three- and *n*-way sensitivity analyses possible. In this situation the analyst must use discretion in deciding what parameters to vary. It is important that sensitivity analyses be performed on the parameters that are the most uncertain (for instance, if a utility was derived from an expert panel, or if a probability was derived from a study that was not randomly designed). It is also important that sensitivity analysis be performed on variables that have a large impact on the overall outcome of the study.

Sensitivity analysis should be performed on the parameters that:
1. are the most uncertain, and
2. have the greatest impact on the analysis.

When performing a cost-utility analysis, we recommend that one-way sensitivity analyses be performed by the analyst on as many variables as possible. An analyst should also perform two- and three-way analyses on parameters that have a large degree of uncertainty or are highly influential in the model. The analyst should report a sufficient amount of information without overburdening the reader. An appendix of additional sensitivity analyses can be included for those who want more information.

SUMMARY OF RECOMMENDED COST-UTILITY VARIABLE STANDARDS

A summary of the cost-utility variable standards that we believe will greatly facilitate the performance of comparable cost-utility analyses to create value-based medicine standards is listed as follows. As we have built upon the work of others, we are certain that others will utilize these parameters and improve upon them with time. But the use of these parameters to create value-based medicine standards, even though imperfect in some ways, will be far superior to the system of incomparable thousands of interventions most commonly utilized in healthcare today.

Cost-Utility Variable Standards

- **Study perspective:** reference case
- **Cost perspective:** third-party insurer (using direct healthcare costs)

Direct Healthcare Cost	Standardized Reference Source
Provider	Average National Medicare Reimbursement
Hospital, Acute	Average National Medicare Reimbursement
Ambulatory Surgery Center	Average National Medicare Reimbursement
Skilled Nursing Facility	Average National Medicare Reimbursement
Rehabilitation	Average National Medicare Reimbursement
Home Healthcare	Average National Medicare Reimbursement
Clinical Tests	Average National Medicare Reimbursement
Durable Goods	Average National Medicare Reimbursement
Nursing Home Care	Average National Medicaid Reimbursement
Pharmaceuticals	Average Wholesale Price (AWP)

■ **Utility values:** utility values as listed here:

Methodology: time-tradeoff
Source: patients
Comorbidities: should not be used to discriminate against those who are disabled

■ **Costs:** direct healthcare costs as listed here
■ **Annual discount rate:** 3% for QALYs and costs
■ **Sensitivity analysis:** should perform at least one-way and often two-way; those input variables in which we have the least confidence should be analyzed.

Hussein Hollands, MSc, contributed to this chapter.

CORE CONCEPTS

■ The seven steps necessary to perform a cost-utility analysis include the following:
— Define the question.
— Define all germane outcomes utilizing the best evidence-based data.
— Assign utility values to the outcomes.
— Estimate the costs.
— Measure the total benefit derived by the intervention using decision analysis.
— Calculate the undiscounted cost-utility ratio and then discount the incremental value (QALYs) gained and the incremental costs accrued to their present value to arrive at a discounted cost-utility ratio.
— Perform sensitivity analysis to handle uncertainty.

■ The seven defining variables encompassed by the first fundamental step of *define the question* in a cost-utility analysis include:
— the intervention options to be compared,
— the diseases (health states) to be studied,
— the target population,
— the study perspective,
— the cost perspective,
— the time frame of the study, and
— the outcomes.

■ The *efficacy* of a treatment refers to how effective it is in an ideal setting (ie, when patients are monitored to stay with the treatment regimen), while *effectiveness* refers to how the treatment works in a real-world setting.

- A reference case study perspective (case of the average person) should be performed for the population under study in a cost-utility analysis, as this form of analysis allows the greatest comparability of cost-utility analyses.

- The third-party insurer cost perspective is suggested for the performance of a cost-utility analysis. Direct healthcare costs are recommended for use in the third-party insurer perspective, but not direct nonhealthcare costs or indirect healthcare costs.

- The recommended preferences for use as utility values in cost-utility analysis include:

  — time-tradeoff utility analysis values

  — utility values obtained from patients who have experienced the health state under study, and

  — values in which comorbidities are not used in a fashion that discriminates against the disabled.

- Both costs and value gained (QALYs) from an intervention should be discounted at a 3% annual rate.

- Sensitivity analysis should be performed on those variables in which we have the least confidence.

REFERENCES

1. Petitti DB. *Meta-Analysis, Decision Analysis and Cost-Effectiveness Analysis.* New York, NY: Oxford University Press; 2000:68–139.

2. Duncan PW, Lai SM, Keighley J. Defining post-stroke recovery: implications for design and interpretation of drug trials. *Neuropharmacology.* 2000;39:835–841.

3. Siironen J, Juvela S, Varis J, et al. No effect of enoxaparin on outcome of aneurysmal subarachnoid hemorrhage: a randomized, double-blind, placebo-controlled clinical trial. *J Neurosurg.* 2003;99:953–959.

4. Stein HP, ed. *2003 Drug Topics Red Book.* Montvale, NJ: Medical Economics Company; 2003.

5. Weinstein MC, Siegel JE, Gold MR, Kamlet MS, Russell LB. Recommendations of the Panel on Cost-Effectiveness in Health and Medicine. *JAMA.* 1996;276:1253–1258.

18

Cost-Utility Analysis Reference-Case Study With Standardized Parameters

The greatest hindrance to a good cost-utility analysis database for use in the practice of value-based medicine (VBM) is the expectation of creating the perfect database with perfect methodology. While some criticize a system that they consider less than perfect, we prefer the option of going with this system rather than utilizing the current haphazard medical practice system that does not quantify the patient value of interventions, much less compare the value and integrate the resources spent for them.

> The greatest hindrance to the creation of a good cost-utility database for use in the practice of VBM is lack of action while waiting for the *perfect* database.

In this chapter we present a relatively uncomplicated cost-utility analysis for the *reference case* of a person with bacterial pneumonia using a third-party insurer perspective. (The recommendations we made in Chapter 17 are utilized herein.) We are dogmatic in performing the analysis because we believe the lack of a set, comprehensible format has greatly contributed to the general lack of acceptance and use of cost-utility analysis for public policy to date.

CASE HISTORY

National Medicare data show that pneumonia is the second leading discharge diagnosis for the Medicare population in acute care hospitals.[1] For a large community hospital in central Pennsylvania, for example, it is the leading discharge diagnosis. The regional Medicare insurance carrier believes that reimbursement for the treatment of bacterial pneumonia may be too high and asks the hospital to substantiate the reimbursement it receives. The hospital then comes to physicians on the staff in the Pulmonary Medicine Department and requests assistance in justifying the reimbursement. The physicians, having read this book, decide that a cost-utility analysis for the treatment of bacterial pneumonia will suit their purpose of demonstrating the value conferred by the treatment for the costs expended. An analysis of the cases of bacterial pneumonia treated at the hospital reveals that 70% of patients have either hypertension, diabetes, coronary artery disease, or arthritis.

As described in Chapter 17, the seven fundamental steps undertaken in performing a cost-utility analysis are as follows:

1. Define the question. The seven *defining variables* inherent in this first fundamental step include defining:
   — the intervention options to be compared,
   — the diseases (health states) to be studied,
   — the target population,
   — the study perspective,
   — the cost perspective,
   — the time frame, and
   — the outcomes.
2. Define all germane outcomes utilizing the best evidence-based data.
3. Assign utility values to the outcomes.
4. Measure the total value conferred by the intervention using decision analysis.
5. Estimate the costs.
6. Calculate the undiscounted cost-utility ratio and then discount the incremental value gained and the incremental costs accrued to their present values to arrive at a discounted cost-utility ratio.
7. Perform sensitivity analysis to handle the uncertainty.

1. Define the Question

The question in this instance is whether the treatment of bacterial pneumonia is cost-effective. The seven defining variables inherent in "defining the question" are as follows:

- **Treatment options:** the options to be compared are treatment vs no treatment.
- **Disease(s) to be studied:** bacterial pneumonia
- **Target population:** Medicare patients
- **Study perspective:** reference case
- **Cost perspective:** third-party insurer
- **Time frame:** life expectancy of the reference case
- **Outcomes:** normal health and death

The study will be performed for the *reference case*, or the average case, which happens to be that of a 70-year-old person.[2] The age of a patient other than that of the reference case (70-year-old person) is not specifically incorporated since the use of age biases cost utility against older patients and reference case cost utility can better be compared with the cost utilities of other interventions.

The comorbidities of hypertension, diabetes, coronary artery disease, and arthritis are also not included in the analysis because these entities:

- discriminate against the value of pneumonia treatment in such an individual compared to a person in otherwise good health, and

- complicate the analysis factorially by increasing the number of cost-utility analyses needed to incorporate various combinations of these comorbidities.

2. Define All Germane Outcomes Utilizing the Best Evidence-Based Data

We go to the literature and choose the highest level of evidence to decide the outcome probabilities. Let us assume in this instance that with antibiotic treatment there is a 90% chance of having a full recovery and a 10% chance of dying, while without treatment there is a 10% chance of making a full recovery and a 90% chance of dying from the pneumonia. Thus, the possible outcomes are *full recovery* and *death*.

3. Assign Utility Values to the Outcomes

In this step, we first convert the outcomes from clinical trials into utility value form, then we apply them in decision analysis. Decision analysis tells us the most probable outcome with antibiotic treatment and with no treatment. *In this instance, we assume that making a full recovery is associated with a utility value of 1.00, while death is associated with a utility value of 0.00.*

4. Measure the Total Value Conferred by the Intervention Using Decision Analysis

The evidence-based literature tells us that there is a 90% chance of living with antibiotic treatment, while there is a 10% chance of dying with antibiotic treatment. Without antibiotic treatment, there is a 10% chance of living and a 90% chance of dying. These percentages are incorporated into the decision analysis tree as shown in Figure 18.1.

The decision analysis tree in Figure 18.1 shows that the average resultant utility value outcome with treatment is 0.90 and without treatment is 0.10, yielding a gain of 0.80 utility points with treatment over no treatment for the reference case. Consequently, for each year of life after treatment, the average quality-adjusted life-year (QALY) gain for a cohort of pneumonia patients treated with antibiotics is 0.90, while the average QALY gain for a cohort of untreated pneumonia patients is 0.10. Antibiotic treatment, compared to no treatment, leads to an annual QALY gain of $0.90 - 0.10 = 0.80$. To calculate the total value gained from treatment, the utility value gain per year is multiplied by the duration of

FIGURE 18.1

Decision Analysis Tree Comparing Treatment With Antibiotics vs No Treatment for Bacterial Pneumonia*

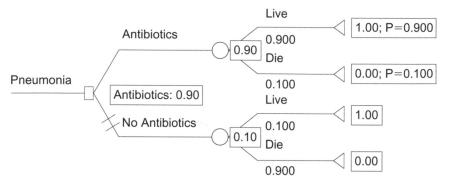

P indicates probability.

* The rectangular node is a *decision node* where the decision to treat with antibiotics or not to treat is made. The round nodes are chance nodes at which the reference case will be assigned to live or die. The numbers beneath the arms of the tree on the right are the percentages for each outcome in decimal form, and the utility values associated with each outcome are located just to the right of their triangular terminal nodes.

treatment benefit (we are assuming it is years of remaining life). The life expectancy for the 70-year-old reference case is 15 years,[3] and therefore the total value gained from treatment is 0.80 (utility gain) × 15 (years) = 12.0 QALYs.

5. Estimate the Costs

For the third-party insurer perspective, the costs are the incremental, direct healthcare costs associated with treatment over no treatment (Table 18.1). The incremental Medicare Fee Schedule costs of treatment (available at www.cms.hhs.gov) and timing of the costs are listed. The average wholesale price (AWP) is used for the outpatient antibiotics.[4]

6. Calculate the Cost-Utility Ratio and Then Discount the Incremental Value Gained and the Incremental Costs to Their Present Values to Arrive at a Discounted Cost-Utility Ratio

Both the costs associated with an intervention and the value gained (QALYs) from the intervention must be discounted, preferably at a 3% annual rate over the 15-year life expectancy of the reference case, a 70-year-old person. Table 18.2 outlines the costs and outcomes associated with the treatment of bacterial pneumonia discounted at a 3% annual rate.

TABLE 18.1

Incremental Healthcare Costs Associated With Antibiotic Treatment for Bacterial Pneumonia

Expenditure	Amount	Time of Cost
Hospitalization x 1 Week	$5,000	1st week
Physician Cost	$600	1st week
Antibiotics (Outpatient)	$200	1st week
Computed Tomographic Scan of Lung	$800	1 year
Computed Tomographic Scan of Lung	$800	2 years

TABLE 18.2

The Costs and the Outcomes Associated With Treatment of Bacterial Pneumonia Discounted at a 3% Annual Rate

Time (Years)	Incremental Costs	Discounted Costs	QALYs Gained	Discounted QALYs Gained
0–1	$5,800	$5,800	0.8	$0.8/(1.03)^0 = 0.800$
1–2	$800	$800/(1.03)^1 = 776	0.8	$0.8/(1.03)^1 = 0.776$
2–3	$800	$800/(1.03)^2 = 754	0.8	$0.8/(1.03)^2 = 0.754$
3–4	0	0	0.8	$0.8/(1.03)^3 = 0.732$
4–5	0	0	0.8	$0.8/(1.03)^4 = 0.711$
5–6	0	0	0.8	$0.8/(1.03)^5 = 0.690$
6–7	0	0	0.8	$0.8/(1.03)^6 = 0.670$
7–8	0	0	0.8	$0.8/(1.03)^7 = 0.650$
8–9	0	0	0.8	$0.8/(1.03)^8 = 0.631$
9–10	0	0	0.8	$0.8/(1.03)^9 = 0.613$
10–11	0	0	0.8	$0.8/(1.03)^{10} = 0.600$
11–12	0	0	0.8	$0.8/(1.03)^{11} = 0.578$
12–13	0	0	0.8	$0.8/(1.03)^{12} = 0.561$
13–14	0	0	0.8	$0.8/(1.03)^{13} = 0.545$
14–15	0	0	0.8	$0.8/(1.03)^{14} = 0.529$
Totals	$7,400	$7,330	12.0	9.837

QALY indicates quality-adjusted life-year.

For this case, the incremental costs (those attributable to the intervention) occur during the first two years after the onset of pneumonia. The value gained from the intervention, however, remains unchanged because the reference case maintains the 0.8 QALY gain per year until death. Because the costs occur early and the value gained occurs later, it is expected that the cost utility will be higher, or less cost-effective, than if the costs and value gained are not discounted, vs discounted at a 3% yearly rate.

The difference in utility value between antibiotic treatment and no treatment is 0.80 utility points, yielding a 0.8 QALY gain per year with treatment. To calculate the cost utility, or $/QALY gained, from the intervention, the cumulative costs are divided by the QALYs gained over the total period of benefit (lifetime of the reference case, or 15 years). The undiscounted $/QALY, or cost-utility of the intervention, is $7,400/12.0 = $617. The discounted (3%/year) $/QALY, or cost utility of the intervention, is $7,330/9.837 = $745.

We will still use the term *cost-effective* when speaking to the public about an intervention that has a favorable cost-utility. The treatment of pneumonia at $745/QALY is therefore highly cost-effective using the conventional standard of $100,000 as the upper limit for cost-effectiveness.[5]

As expected, the discounted cost-utility ratio—when both costs and outcomes are discounted—is higher (less cost-effective) than the undiscounted cost-utility ratio because the costs are expended early on during the disease, while the benefits (QALYs gained) accrue over the remaining lifetime of the reference case.

7. Perform a Sensitivity Analysis to Handle the Uncertainty

We can alter any of the input variables (cost, utilities, discount rate, incidences of outcomes, and so on) with particular emphasis on those about which we are less certain. In Figure 18.2 we alter each of the outcome incidences by 20% toward the median (live with treatment goes from 90% to 70% and death goes from 10% to 30%; live without treatment goes from 10% to 30% and death goes from 90% to 70%).

FIGURE   18.2

Sensitivity Analysis for the Treatment of Bacterial Pneumonia Altering the Percentages of Patients Who Live and Die in the Antibiotic Treatment and No Treatment Groups

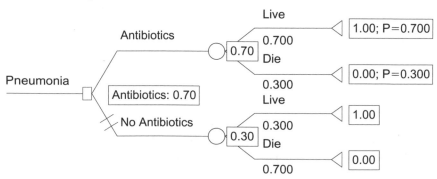

With altered incidences of life and death, the outcomes changes (QALYs gained) from 0.8 per year to 0.4 (0.70 to 0.30) per year. While the discounted costs remain the same, the new number of QALYs gained must be discounted.

The cost-utility ratio with *one-way sensitivity analysis* (varying only one class of variables) is doubled by varying each of the outcome incidences by 20%, as illustrated in Table 18.3. The cost-utility ratio is still higher when costs and outcomes are discounted, as compared to not discounted, because the costs are expended early on during the disease, while the benefits (QALYs gained) accrue over the remaining lifetime.

If we change a second variable concomitantly with changing the incidence of outcomes, we have a *two-way sensitivity analysis.* A common method employed in sensitivity analysis is to calculate the $/QALY for the upper and lower limits of the 95% confidence interval.[6] For example, the mean discounted cost in this case is $7,330. If the 95% confidence intervals are $7,330 ± $2,070, the lower limit of the interval is $5,260 ($7,330 − $2,070) and the upper limit is $9,400 ($7,330 + $2,070). The $/QALY using the limits of the 95% confidence intervals

TABLE 18.3

One-Way Sensitivity Analysis*

Time (Years)	Incremental Costs	Discounted Costs	QALYs Gained	Discounted QALYs Gained
0–1	$5,800	$5,800	0.4	$0.4/(1.03)^0 = 0.400$
1–2	$800	$800/(1.03)^1 = 776	0.4	$0.4/(1.03)^1 = 0.388$
2–3	$800	$800/(1.03)^2 = 754	0.4	$0.4/(1.03)^2 = 0.377$
3–4	0	0	0.4	$0.4/(1.03)^3 = 0.366$
4–5	0	0	0.4	$0.4/(1.03)^4 = 0.355$
5–6	0	0	0.4	$0.4/(1.03)^5 = 0.345$
6–7	0	0	0.4	$0.4/(1.03)^6 = 0.335$
7–8	0	0	0.4	$0.4/(1.03)^7 = 0.325$
8–9	0	0	0.4	$0.4/(1.03)^8 = 0.316$
9–10	0	0	0.4	$0.4/(1.03)^9 = 0.307$
10–11	0	0	0.4	$0.4/(1.03)^{10} = 0.298$
11–12	0	0	0.4	$0.4/(1.03)^{11} = 0.289$
12–13	0	0	0.4	$0.4/(1.03)^{12} = 0.289$
13–14	0	0	0.4	$0.4/(1.03)^{13} = 0.289$
14–15	0	0	0.4	$0.4/(1.03)^{14} = 0.289$
Totals	**$7,400**	**$7,330**	**6.0**	**4.918**

* The number of QALYs gained and discounted QALYs gained change (Table 18.2) when the percentages of patients who live and die with and without antibiotic treatment are altered. The undiscounted $/QALY gained is $7,400/6.0 = $1,233 and the discounted $/QALY gained (3%/year) is $7,330/4.918 = $1,490. QALY indicates quality-adjusted life-year.

for cost and a total discounted QALY gain of 4.918 (Table 18.3) in the overall analysis is therefore $5,260/4.918 = $1,070 for the lower limit and $9,499/4.918 = $1,931 for the upper limit. Both values are still extraordinarily cost-effective using conventional standards.

FINAL ANALYSIS

The treatment of bacterial pneumonia by antibiotics is highly cost-effective at $745/QALY (quality-adjusted life-year gained) using a 3% annual discount rate and the conventional standard that an intervention with a cost utility of less than $100,000/QALY is cost-effective. Sensitivity analysis confirms that substantially varying the variable of least certainty—the proportion of a cohort dying and living with and without antibiotic treatment—still results in a highly cost-effective therapy. The hospital can now argue with confidence that, if anything, the reimbursement received for the treatment of bacterial pneumonia is very low compared to other interventions.

CORE CONCEPTS

- The seven fundamental steps in performing a cost-utility analysis include the following:
  — Define the question.
  — Define all germane outcomes utilizing the best evidence-based data.
  — Assign utility values to the outcomes.
  — Measure the total value conferred by the intervention using decision analysis.
  — Estimate the costs.
  — Calculate the undiscounted cost-utility ratio and then discount the incremental value gained and the incremental costs accrued to their present values to arrive at a discounted cost-utility ratio.
  — Perform sensitivity analysis to handle the uncertainty.
- The seven defining variables inherent in the first fundamental step (define the question) include:
  — the intervention options to be compared,
  — the diseases (health states) to be studied,
  — the target population,
  — the study perspective,
  — the cost perspective,
  — the time frame, and
  — the outcomes.
- The greatest hindrance to the creation of a *good* cost-utility database is lack of action while waiting for the *perfect* database.

■ Using the upper and lower bounds of the 95% confidence interval surrounding a cost-utility analysis input variable allows for the performance of a more *robust* analysis.

REFERENCES

1. Centers for Medicare and Medicaid Services. Medicare short-stay hospital DRGs ranked by discharges: fiscal year 2000. Available at: http://cms.hhs.gov. Accessed February 20, 2004.

2. Delgado Morales J, Alonso Del Busto R, Pascual Calleja I, et al. Observational study of in-patients in an Internal Medicine Department. *An Med Interna.* 2004;21:3–6.

3. Arias E. United States life tables, 2000. *Natl Vital Stat Rep.* 2002;51:8.

4. Stein HP, ed. *2003 Drug Topics Red Book.* Montvale, NJ: Medical Economics Company; 2003.

5. Laupacis A, Feeny D, Detsky AS, Tugwell PX. How attractive does a new technology have to be to warrant adoption and utilization: tentative guidelines for using clinical and economic evaluations. *CMAJ.* 1992;146:473–481.

6. Sharma S, Brown GC, Brown MM, Hollands H, Shah GK. The cost-effectiveness of photodynamic therapy for fellow eyes with subfoveal choroidal neovascularization secondary to age-related macular degeneration. *Ophthalmology.* 2001;108:2051–2059.

19

Value-Based Nursing

Up until this point in this book, we have primarily described value-based medicine (VBM). The is no reason, however, why VBM ideals cannot be applied to other disciplines in healthcare such as nursing, dentistry, physical therapy, and so on. One field in which quality-of-life issues have been in the forefront for decades is nursing. To the authors, it only seems to be a natural progression that integration of quality-of-life principles with other VBM principles will transpire in nursing practice.

A NATURAL ENDEAVOR: NURSING AND QUALITY OF LIFE

The nursing profession has long been concerned with quality-of-life aspects associated with single diseases and different health states. From the beginning of nursing school onward, emphasis is placed on patient quality-of-life issues both in the classroom and in the clinical setting. Thus, it is not surprising that a recurrent theme in the nursing peer-reviewed literature concerns the quality of life associated with a disease or health state.[1,2] Other nonphysician healthcare professions, such as physical therapy and occupational therapy, also place great emphasis upon quality-of-life issues associated with the healing process.

> The study of quality-of-life issues is a natural fit with the mission of nursing.

The arena of value-based healthcare encompasses all specialties in medicine, nursing, physical therapy, occupational therapy, dentistry, optometry, and other health-related professions. Just as all healthcare providers work together to maximize the quality of patient care in this era of evidence-based medicine (EBM) and evidence-based nursing,[3] the same will happen with VBM and value-based nursing, only at a higher level of quality. Once an information system is provided that more accurately measures the value conferred by an intervention than evidence-based data alone, all healthcare providers will adopt it. Why? Because it will allow for the highest quality of care by better defining which interventions deliver substantial patient-perceived value, which deliver negligible value, which deliver no value, and those that may actually be harmful.

Value-Based Healthcare

One might ask why we did not call this book *Value-Based Healthcare*. The thought certainly entered our minds, but we thought the theoretical leap from EBM to VBM would be less than the leap from EBM to value-based healthcare. We also believe the branding of evidence-based medicine will facilitate the most rapid acceptance of value-based medicine, value-based nursing, value-based pharmacy, and so on.

AN OPPORTUNITY TO ADVANCE VALUE-BASED PRINCIPLES

In nursing, as in medicine, there are interventions that deliver specified amounts of value to patients. In some instances, the value delivered is the same as that delivered by physicians,[4,5] especially with increasing numbers of nurse practitioners. In many instances, however, the value delivered by nursing interventions is complementary to that delivered by medical interventions—and equally as valuable as medical services.

To date, there has been limited attention in nursing directed toward healthcare economic analyses.[6,7] Douglas and colleagues[6] undertook a review of the economic studies of clinical nurse specialists and found 17 studies that reported primary outcome data, cost data, and specifically included a clinical nurse specialist. Specific nursing outcomes were reported in only a minority of studies, and none of the studies reported cost-effectiveness ratios (the value gained for the resources expended). Nonetheless, some studies revealed that interventions undertaken by a clinical nurse specialist were less costly and more effective than alternative forms.

Douglas and colleagues[6] recommend that economic evaluations of the clinical nurse specialist need to be undertaken and "should involve nursing researchers and practitioners so that evaluations reflect the complex and multidimensional nature of [clinical nurse specialist] care and meet the required standard of evidence to influence practice." We agree enthusiastically. Quality-of-life research falls well within the realm of nursing, while the economic background needed to perform cost-utility analysis is as accessible to nursing as it is to those in medicine or other professional healthcare fields.

At this time, the field of value-based nursing is wide open and the application of cost-utility analysis is virtually unlimited.[8] A few nursing interventions that could be studied include rehabilitation to improve dementia,[9] nursing care to improve outcomes with congestive heart failure,[10] nursing interventions to help homebound diabetics,[11] the community psychiatric nurse in primary care,[12] and the improvement in quality of life for patients undergoing cardiac catheterization.[13] The list of possible interventions to study is infinite and limited only by the imagination of the researcher.

NURSING INTERVENTION: A COST-UTILITY ANALYSIS

Studies have shown that the quality of life in patients with congestive heart failure can improve considerably from home nursing.[10,14] Let us assume that a health insurer, however, notices that home nursing care costs more than hospital care for a congestive heart failure cohort. The insurer questions the rationale of home nursing and wants to study the issue before deciding to continue to cover the service. The question of interest is therefore, is it cost-effective for a health insurer to have nurses deliver home care to homebound patients with congestive heart failure?

The data available on two cohorts of patients followed for a two-year period are shown in Tables 19.1 and 19.2. The only treatment difference between the cohorts is that cohort 1 patients had home nursing visits, while cohort 2 patients did not.

Again, we undertake the same steps in performing this cost-utility analysis as with a pharmaceutical, surgical, or other cost-utility analysis (Chapters 17 and 18). The seven fundamental steps in performing a cost-utility analysis include the following:

1. Define the question.
2. Define all germane outcomes utilizing the best evidence-based data.
3. Assign utility values to the outcomes.
4. Measure the total value conferred by the intervention using decision analysis.
5. Estimate the costs.
6. Calculate the undiscounted cost-utility ratio and then discount the incremental value gained and the incremental costs accrued to their present values to arrive at a discounted cost-utility ratio.
7. Perform sensitivity analysis to handle the uncertainty.

TABLE 19.1

Home Nursing Care vs No Home Nursing Care: Outcomes*

	Cohort 1 (Home Nursing Care)	Cohort 2 (No Home Nursing Care)
AHA Functional Capacity Classification Class	II	II
Hospitalizations (Weeks/Year)	1	2
Mortality (Mean Time of 1 Year)	10%	20%

AHA indicates American Heart Association; class II includes patients with cardiac disease resulting in slight limitation of physical activity; ordinary physical activity results in fatigue, palpitation, dyspnea, or anginal pain.[15]

* Two-year results in a cohort of 100 patients with congestive heart failure and home nursing care vs 100 patients with congestive heart failure and no home nursing care.

Home Nursing Care vs No Home Nursing Care: Costs*

Year	Cost
Incremental Nursing Costs: Home Care	
Year 1	$10,500
Year 2	$11,000
Incremental Hospital Costs: No Home Care	
Year 1	$8,000
Year 2	$9,000

* Two-year results in a cohort of 100 patients with congestive heart failure and home nursing care vs 100 patients with congestive heart failure and no home nursing care.

1. Define the Question

The seven defining variables inherent in this first fundamental step are:

- **The intervention options to be compared:** home nursing care
- **The diseases (health states) to be studied:** congestive heart failure
- **The target population:** homebound patients
- **The study perspective:** reference case
- **The cost perspective:** third-party insurer
- **The time frame:** two years
- **The outcomes:** cardiac function, death, and hospitalizations

2. Define All Germane Outcomes Utilizing the Best Evidence-Based Data

In this case, the outcomes are the American Heart Association (AHA) Functional Capacity Classification for congestive heart failure,[15] which is the same in both cohorts. Other outcomes include hospitalization and death.

3. Assign Utility Values to the Outcomes

The utility values needed are those associated with the outcomes of heart failure, hospitalization, and death and are listed in Table 19.3. The 0.85 utility value associated with AHA Functional Capacity Classification Class II[15] comes from the Center for Value-Based Medicine utility value database, and the utility value for acute hospitalization is a point estimate obtained from patients who are acutely ill and hospitalized.[16]

TABLE 19.3

Utility Values Associated With Outcomes

	Group 1 (Home Nursing Care)	Group 2 (No Home Nursing Care)	Utility Value
AHA Functional Capacity Classification Class	II	II	0.85
Hospitalizations (Weeks/Year)	1	2	0.09
Mortality (Mean Time of 1 Year)	10%	20%	0.00

4. Measure the Total Value Conferred by the Intervention Using Decision Analysis

Value is gained in this case over a two-year period. Because a percentage of each cohort dies at a mean time of one year, the mean value gained during the first year will differ from the value gained during the second year. The value gained for each year will therefore have to be calculated separately. The value conferred by home nursing care over the first year of the two-year model is shown in Figure 19.1,

FIGURE 19.1

Decision Analysis Modeling, Year 1. The home nursing care group undergoes one week of acute hospitalization (at a utility value of 0.09) per year, while the no home nursing care group undergoes two weeks of acute hospitalization (at a utility value of 0.09) per year. The difference in utility value between the two cohorts is 0.8348 − 0.8196 = 0.0152. Thus, during the first year 0.0152 incremental QALYs are gained by the home nursing care group. The overall utility value in the no home nursing care group is less because this group is hospitalized for a mean time of weeks (0.040 years) at an inpatient hospital utility value of 0.09, while the home nursing group is hospitalized for only one week.

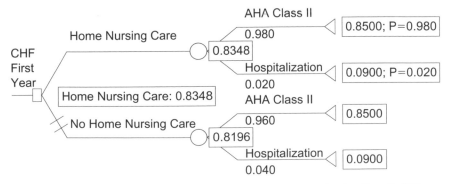

AHA indicates American Heart Association Functional Capacity Classification Class II; CHF, congestive heart failure; P, probability.

while the value conferred by home nursing care during the second year is shown in Figure 19.2.

The value gained in the home nursing care cohort in Figure 19.2 is therefore 0.0152 QALYs gained during year 1 and 0.1002 QALYs gained during year 2, for a total value gained of 0.1154 QALYs over the two-year period.

5. Estimate the Costs

The costs and the timing of the costs are also shown in Tables 19.1 and 19.2. There is the *incremental cost of home nursing care* ($21,500) in the home nursing care cohort and the *incremental cost of 2.0 weeks hospitalization* ($17,000) in the no home nursing care cohort. Overall, the expenses for the average person in the home nursing care cohort exceed those of the average patient in the no home nursing care cohort by $4,500 ($21,500 − $17,000). The net incremental cost in

FIGURE   19.2

Decision Analysis Modeling, Year 2. The difference in utility value between the two cohorts is 0.7498 − 0.6496 = 0.1002. There is a larger utility value difference between the two groups than in the first year because 20% of the no home nursing care cohort has died vs 10% of the home nursing care cohort. During this second year, 0.1002 incremental QALYs are also gained by the home nursing care cohort due to fewer deaths and because this group again experiences one week less of hospitalization in addition to fewer deaths. (Remember that it is sometimes easier to think of the reference case as a cohort of patients when planning the study.)

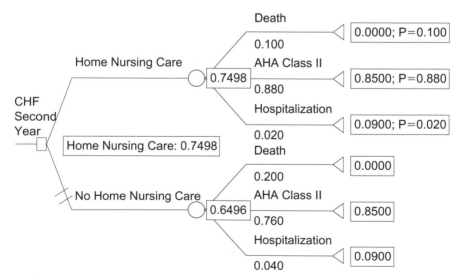

AHA indicates American Heart Association Functional Capacity Classification; CHF, congestive heart failure; P, probability.

the home nursing group is $2,500 ($10,500 − $8,000) in the first year and $2,000 ($11,000 − $9,000) in the second year.

6. Calculate the Undiscounted Cost-Utility Ratio and Then Discount the Incremental Value Gained and the Incremental Costs Accrued to Their Present Values to Arrive at a Discounted Cost-Utility Ratio

The rate of discounting is 3% annually for both value gained and costs expended, as shown in Table 19.4. The undiscounted cost-utility ratio is $4,500/0.1154 = $38,995.

The total discounted incremental cost is $4,442, and the total discounted incremental value gained is 0.1125 QALY. Thus, the discounted cost-utility of home nursing care for patients with congestive heart failure is $4,442/0.1125 QALY = $39,484/QALY. Using the upper limit of cost-effectiveness of $100,000/QALY,[17] the intervention of home nursing care for patients with congestive heart failure is cost-effective.

7. Perform Sensitivity Analysis to Handle Uncertainty

In this analysis, let us assume the variable we have the least assurance about is the utility value associated with acute hospitalization. The utility value for acute hospitalization is 0.09 and the 95% confidence intervals are 0.02 to 0.16. Substitution of the lower and upper confidence values into the first-year and second-year decision analysis trees results in a final analysis as shown in Table 19.5. Both the total value gain and the cost are discounted at a 3% annual rate.

The one-way (changing one variable) sensitivity analysis reveals a narrow range of cost-utility results, all of which are well within the conventional upper limit of $100,000/QALY. The results of this cost-utility analysis suggest the intervention of nurses providing home care to patients with congestive heart failure

TABLE 19.4

Discounting of the Value Gained and the Costs Expended at an Annual Rate of 3%

	Value Gained (QALY)	Discounted Value (QALY)	Costs (2004 US Dollars)	Discounted Costs (2004 US Dollars)
Year 1	0.0152	0.0152	$2,500	$2,500
Year 2	0.1002	0.0973	$2,000	$1,942
Totals	**0.1154**	**0.1125**	**$4,500**	**$4,442**

TABLE   19.5

One-Way Sensitivity Analysis Altering the Utility Value Associated With Acute
Hospitalization (at a 3% Discount Rate for Value Gained and Costs)

Acute Hospitalization Utility Value	Total Value Gain	Cost	Cost Utility
0.02	0.1148 QALY	$4,442	$38,693/QALY
0.09	0.1125 QALY	$4,442	$39,484/QALY
0.16	0.1103 QALY	$4,442	$40,273/QALY

delivers significant patient-perceived value for a reasonable cost. The service of
home health care for patients with congestive heart failure is one that an insurer
should reasonably cover.

THE FUTURE

The nursing profession is beginning to enter into the arena of healthcare economic analysis.[7,18] Because the health-related quality-of-life arena is closely
aligned with nursing theory, principles, and culture in general, going from evidence-based data to value-based data seems a natural step. The additional step
of adding costs to arrive at a cost-utility analysis is eminently feasible.

> The health-related quality-of-life arena is closely aligned with nurs-
> ing theory, principles, and culture.

There is a large void in the cost-utility analysis arena, especially for nursing
interventions. The opportunity is great, and the return on investment for
improving quality of care and maximizing the efficient use of healthcare
resources is extraordinary.

CORE CONCEPTS

- The study of quality-of-life issues is a natural fit with the mission of nursing.
- The health-related quality-of-life arena is closely aligned with nursing principles, theory, and culture.
- There is an extraordinary opportunity for nursing research in the realm of
  value-based nursing.

REFERENCES

1.   Gwede CK. Overview of radiation- and chemoradiation-induced diarrhea. *Semin
     Oncol Nurs.* 2003;19(suppl 3):6–10.

2. Luk WS. The HRQoL of renal transplant patients. *J Clin Nurs.* 2004;13:201–209.

3. Pape TM. Evidence-based nursing practice: to infinity and beyond. *J Contin Educ Nurs.* 2003;34:154–161.

4. Aigner MJ, Drew S, Phipps J. A comparative study of nursing home resident outcomes between care provided by nurse practitioners/physicians versus physicians only. *J Am Med Dir Assoc.* 2004;5:16–23.

5. Kamps AW, Brand PL, Kimpen JL, et al. Outpatient management of childhood asthma by paediatrician or asthma nurse: randomised controlled study with one year follow up. *Thorax.* 2003;58:968–973.

6. Douglas HR, Halliday D, Normand C, et al. Economic evaluation of specialist cancer and palliative nursing: a literature review. *Int J Palliat Nurs.* 2003;9:424–428.

7. Stone PW, Curran CR, Bakken S. Economic evidence for evidence-based practice. *J Nurs Scholarsh.* 2002;34:277–282.

8. Brosnan CA, Swint JM. Cost analysis: concepts and application. *Public Health Nurs.* 2001;18:13–18.

9. Dewing J. Rehabilitation for older people with dementia. *Nurs Stand.* 2003;18:42–48.

10. Konick-McMahan J, Bixby B, McKenna C. Heart failure in older adults: providing nursing care to improve outcomes. *J Gerontol Nurs.* 2003;29:35–41.

11. Huang CL, Wu SC, Jeng CY, Lin LC. The efficacy of a home-based nursing program in diabetic control of elderly people with diabetes mellitus living alone. *Public Health Nurs.* 2004;21:49–56.

12. Gournay K, Brooking J. Community psychiatric nurse in primary care: an economic analysis. *J Adv Nurs.* 1995;22:769–778.

13. Harkness K, Morrow L, Smith K, Kiczula M, Arthur HM. The effect of early education on patient anxiety while waiting for elective cardiac catheterization. *Eur J Cardiovasc Nurs.* 2003:113–121.

14. Vavouranakis I, Lambrogiannakis E, Markakis G, et al. Effect of home-based intervention on hospital readmission and quality of life in middle-aged patients with severe congestive heart failure: a 12-month follow up study. *Eur J Cardiovasc Nurs.* 2003;2:105–111.

15. American College of Cardiology/American Heart Association. Chronic heart failure evaluation and management guidelines: relevance to the geriatric practice. *J Am Geriatr Soc.* 2003;51:123–126.

16. Jansen SJT, Stiggelbout AM, Wakker PP, et al. Patients' utilities for cancer treatments: a study of the chained procedure for the standard gamble and time tradeoff. *Med Decis Making.* 1998;18:391–399.

17. Laupacis A, Feeny D, Detsky AS, Tugwell PX. How attractive does a new technology have to be to warrant adoption and utilization: tentative guidelines for using clinical and economic evaluations. *CMAJ.* 1992;146:473–481.

18. Stone PW. Dollars and sense: a primer for the novice in economic analyses (part II). *Appl Nurs Res.* 2001;14:110–112.

20

Pharmacoeconomics

Pharmaceutical agents are, in large part, responsible for the length-of-life and quality-of-life gains made over the last century. It is likely that this trend will accelerate as new drugs enter the marketplace. Nonetheless, the cost of drugs is a problem for many segments of the population. A brief discourse on pharmacoeconomics—the economics of pharmaceuticals—is helpful in demonstrating the beneficial role of value-based medicine (VBM) in this arena.

OVERVIEW OF PHARMACOECONOMICS

Pharmacoeconomics is a relatively new discipline that applies the VBM principles we have discussed to the use of pharmaceuticals employed in healthcare interventions. Pharmacoeconomics draws from multiple disciplines, such as medicine, pharmacy, economics, business administration principles, nursing, epidemiology, and others. As is the case for VBM in general, there is a great need for standardization of healthcare economic analyses performed in the area of pharmacoeconomics.[1,2] Rascati and colleagues[2] believe there is a global need for training in pharmacoeconomics. We agree unreservedly.

While 95% of policymakers with managed care organizations are aware of at least one instance in which a pharmacoeconomic model played a role in optimizing the formulary positioning of a product, there is no agreement upon which model(s) to use.[3] Most agree, however, that user-friendly, standardized, scientifically sound models are required to advance the science—thus the need for this book and for the same models for pharmaceuticals that we advocated earlier.[3,4] Value-based medicine principles are exceptionally applicable to the science of pharmacoeconomics.

Current Drug Formulary Standards

A large number of drug formulary members from Sweden[5] were polled on what source(s) of information they used in making their decisions. Respondents stated that government guidelines and articles from peer-reviewed journals were important sources of information, but that cost-effectiveness was the most important modality. Nonetheless, they noted three major drawbacks with using cost-utility (cost-effectiveness) studies:

■ There was a lack of pharmacoeconomic competence among formulary members.

■ An adequate supply of relevant studies was lacking.

■ There was difficulty translating the results of the studies into clinical guidelines.

To this we also add:

■ There is a lack of cost-utility analysis standards. There is considerable agreement about this fact in the peer-reviewed literature.[3,4,6]

Suh and colleagues[7] found relatively similar factors that impede the use of pharmacoeconomic studies. They include:

■ a lack of knowledge on how to evaluate such studies,

■ limited reliability of available studies, and

■ the problem of departmental budgetary restraints in regard to creating the studies.

Others also noted a general lack of familiarity with cost-utility analysis that precludes its use.[8,9] There is resistance as well when the population used for a cost-utility analysis is believed to differ from a patient population undergoing treatment.[10] But again we see the recurrent themes of:

■ a lack of cost-utility expertise,

■ a lack of relevant studies, and

■ a lack of translation of study results into clinical guidelines.

Another contributing factor to the lack of use of pharmacoeconomic standards in the United States is that managed care organizations generally use a formulary system that evaluates drugs exclusively on clinical efficacy, safety, and daily acquisition cost, with little attention given to cost-effectiveness.[7] A major reason that value-based standards are not used by managed care organizations is the fact the such standards have not yet been developed.

The lack of comparability of studies is a major problem that contributes to all of the other problems mentioned above. Without comparability of cost-utility studies, the use of a management information system database for pharmaceutical interventions is next to worthless. Those unfamiliar with healthcare economic analyses might not perceive the incomparability of pharmaceutical cost-utility studies due to the current chaotic state of which preferences to use and what other variable standards to incorporate, but they certainly will after reading this text.

> The lack of comparability among pharmaceutical cost-utility analyses is a major impediment to the formation of value-based pharmaceutical standards.

The First Step

The standardization of cost-utility input variables allows a database to be created. As was said in the baseball movie *Field of Dreams*, "If you build it, they will come." Once a value-based pharmaceutical database is available, demand will definitely increase as stakeholders realize it will improve quality of care and maximize the efficacy of the use of resources devoted to pharmaceutical interventions.

The major objective of this book is the clarification cost-utility analysis principles to allow the adoption of VBM. The exact same principles used in surgical and medical cost-utility analyses can be used in the pharmacoeconomic arena. We hope the clarification brings more converts into the VBM arena and allows good comparable studies on the cost-utility of pharmaceutical agents to be published in the peer-reviewed literature. We address clinical guidelines and relevance later in this chapter.

Is Spending More on Pharmaceuticals Bad?

No, not necessarily, if done correctly and drugs are made available to all citizens. Increased spending on pharmaceuticals will likely be very good for patients and the country. There is no other industry group that confers the extraordinary value (improvement in quality of life and length of life) of pharmaceuticals to individuals and society as a whole. In addition to improving quality of life and length of life, pharmaceuticals also reduce the burden of disease and increase worker productivity, thus adding to gross domestic product (GDP). Pharmaceuticals allow us to live more comfortably and will also greatly increase life expectancy in the near future. For example, the drug atorvastatin has shown to halt the progression of coronary atherosclerosis, the major cause of death in the United States in half of the population.[11] In essence, drugs greatly contribute to the overall well-being of patients and to the country as a whole.

> Pharmaceuticals contribute greatly to the overall well-being of patients and the country as a whole.

Problems Associated With Pharmaceutical Spending

As with other healthcare interventions, however, the inefficient use of pharmaceutical agents is bad. Furthermore, not all citizens can access the drugs that benefit them, and that should not be tolerated.

Value-based medicine can ameliorate the inefficient use of drugs and conserve resources that can then be directed to those who currently lack access to beneficial pharmaceuticals. That said, while VBM eliminates harmful interventions and interventions of no value, a specific mechanism must be in place to allow necessary drugs to be distributed to all in need. This mechanism will be developed within the political realm. Value-based medicine improves quality of life and saves money, but society must decide how the money is used to pay for healthcare services and drugs that work for all.

We believe that improving both efficiency of drug use and the equity of drug distribution will create larger markets for pharmaceutical products rather than cost the pharmaceutical companies money that could be devoted to research. And in return, solving the efficiency and equity issues will create an overall healthier society with greater longevity, improved quality of life, greater productivity, and a lessened burden of disease.

> Spending considerable amounts of money on pharmaceutical agents that work well yields great value and a considerable return on investment. Spending it inefficiently does not.

THE ECONOMICS OF PHARMACOECONOMICS

How Much Is Spent?

As outlined in Table 20.1, the prescription pharmaceutical bill in the United States in 1980 was $12 billion, or 4.9% of the $245.8 billion annual healthcare budget. By 2003, the amount spent on prescription pharmaceuticals was $181.5 billion, or 11% of the healthcare budget. Overall, pharmaceutical company sales in the United States in 2003 were $216.4 billion.[12]

In 2004, the estimated prescription pharmaceutical expenditure is estimated to be $203.4 billion, comprising 11.5% of healthcare expenditures, while by 2010 it is estimated to be $376 billion, or 14.2% of the $2.639 trillion overall health expenditure.[13]

Are Drugs a Good Deal?

They can be, even if they are expensive. For example, a drug such as imatinib mesylate (Gleevec), a targeted therapy that saves the lives of patients with previously hopeless cases of chronic leukemia,[14] is cost-effective at almost any price using an upper limit of $100,000/quality-adjusted life-year (QALY).[15–17] On the other hand, an inexpensive drug may not be cost-effective if it provides negligible value. A good example of the latter phenomenon is the use of oral cephalex-

T A B L E   20.1

Prescription Drug Costs as a Percentage of Healthcare Costs

Year	Prescription Drug Costs	Percent of Healthcare Costs
1980	$12 billion	4.9
2004	$203.4 billion	11.5
2010	$376 billion	14.2

in for three days prior to dental treatment to prevent infection in patients with prosthetic joints. The $/QALY for preventing late prosthetic joint infections was shown to be $1.1 million in 1991.[18]

The best way to tell with certainty whether reasonable value is conferred by a pharmaceutical agent is to perform a cost-utility analysis on use of the drug for a specific intervention. While the proportion of healthcare dollars spent on pharmaceutical agents is increasing considerably, the proportion cannot be viewed as simply a number that is rising too high. Why? Because the benefits conferred by drugs in quality of life, length of life, surgical interventions made unnecessary, and the decrease in the burden of disease are all factors that merit incorporation into the therapeutic equation.

> Cost-utility analysis incorporates all benefits conferred by a drug, as well as all the adverse effects associated with that drug.

As is the case with most healthcare interventions, the societal perspective yields the most favorable cost utility for pharmaceutical agents in that it includes the direct nonhealthcare costs made unnecessary, as well as the indirect healthcare costs. As standardized models for direct nonhealthcare costs and indirect healthcare costs become available, the societal perspective will become more reproducible and reliable. But until that time, unless there is a special circumstance, we recommend the third-party insurer perspective to allow enough comparable analyses to be performed to create a value-based pharmaceutical database.

How Is the Money Spent?

A relatively small number of prescription drugs account for a relatively large proportion of prescription drug expenditures. In 2002, the top ten prescription drugs by retail sales accounted for 17% of all prescription drug costs, the top 25 accounted for 30.6% of costs, the top 50 accounted for 43.9% of costs, and the top 100 accounted for 56.8% of costs (Table 20.2).[19]

The average retail cost of a prescription drug in 2002 was $54.57, a 9% increase over the cost in 2001.[20] But even among those who have healthcare

TABLE 20.2

Top Prescription Drugs and Their Market Share in 2002

Prescription Drugs	Percentage of Prescription Drug Costs (Market Share)
Top 10	17%
Top 25	30.6%
Top 50	43.9%
Top 100	56.8%

insurance that covers pharmaceuticals, the recent trend is to increase copayments for each prescription, especially for the more expensive brand-name drugs.

Generic Drugs

Drugs can be sold in *generic form*, meaning that the chemical compound is what is marketed and sold, or they can be sold in the more familiar *brand form* generally developed and marketed by a specific company. A good example of a well-known generic drug is *acetaminophen*, which is more commonly recognized by the specific brand name *Tylenol*.

Overall, generic drugs accounted for 42.1% of total prescription drug sales in 2001 and 45.2% of total prescription drug sales in 2002.[20] The increasing tendency toward the prescription of generic drugs occurred due to patient preference for the lesser cost of generic drugs and the fact that some brand drugs lost their patents, allowing generic substitutes to come onto the market.

Marketing and Research

Approximately $13 billion was spent on the promotion of drugs in 2002. This cost includes 90,000 high-quality jobs directly related to the promotion of pharmaceutical agents.[20]

Pharmaceutical companies spent approximately $32 billion per year on research for new drugs in 2002.[21] In contrast, the 2002 budget of the National Institutes of Health (NIH) was $23.3 billion, of which 92%, or $21.4 billion, was spent directly on research (Table 20.3).[22–24] When clinical research on humans is examined, pharmaceutical companies spent $21.7 billion in 2002, three times the NIH expenditure of $7 billion.[22–24]

Approximately 79% of research and development (R&D) by the major pharmaceutical companies is performed in the United States.[23] Overall, all R&D expenses compose 16.3% of global pharmaceutical sales, but domestic pharmaceutical R&D in the United States composes 18.2% of domestic sales. In regard to overall sales, approximately 73% of the revenue from pharmaceutical sales comes from the United States.

Preclinical (animal and other nonhuman) basic science studies account for 32.5% of the research dollars spent by pharmaceutical companies and patient

TABLE 20.3

Research Expenditures by the National Institutes of Health and the Pharmaceutical Industry in 2002

Research Expenditures	Overall	Clinical Research
National Institutes of Health	$21.4 billion	$7 billion
Pharmaceutical companies	$32 billion	$21.7 billion

clinical studies account for 67.5%.[23] At the National Institutes of Health, approximately 32% of funds are spent on clinical research and the remainder of the research funds are spent for basic science research that may eventually lead to new discoveries.[24] In short, the current pharmaceutical company clinical trials are likely more relevant to patients over the next decade, while much research at the NIH will likely be more relevant over the next generation. Both forms of research are critically important.

Drug approvals run in cycles.[21] The all-time high was 120 drugs approved by the Food and Drug Administration (FDA) per year in each of 1996 and 1997. In 2001 only 24 new drugs were approved, while in 2002 only 17 received clearance. Many drugs coming onto the market are facsimiles of ones that are already on the market. Thus, a comparison of drugs in the same class can reveal that one drug provides more value than the other, especially for the dollars expended. This is an area where pharmaceutical cost-utility analysis can be especially valuable.

Overall, it costs approximately $800 million to bring the average drug to market, from the creation of the drug through its approval by the FDA.[25] Unfortunately, many drugs under development fail to pass the rigorous safety and efficacy criteria for public sale set by the FDA. Obviously, hundreds of millions of dollars can be lost on a single such endeavor.

Cost-utility analysis can be of great help to pharmaceutical companies in evaluating the economic feasibility of potential new drugs, as well as in the area of pricing. Saving money on drugs that have no market or that have questionable value conferred can allow companies to devote their research interests to drugs shown by VBM to have greater worth and potential for helping patients. Spending more dollars on development of drugs that confer the greatest value to the most patients is an endeavor that considerably benefits patients and pharmaceutical manufacturers as well.

Cost-utility analysis can greatly help pharmaceutical companies to evaluate the potential economic feasibility of new drugs under consideration for development or in the pipeline for FDA approval.

Value-based medical data can readily demonstrate the worth of pharmaceuticals to all stakeholders in healthcare, including patients, policymakers, providers, and others. To date, pharmaceutical manufacturers have had difficulty demonstrating this value for select drugs. Value-based medicine can ameliorate this problem, especially when a comparison is made between the amount society spends on healthcare interventions vs injury reduction interventions and toxin control interventions (see Chapter 15).

Value-based medicine allows pharmaceutical manufacturers to readily demonstrate the value of their drugs to all stakeholders in healthcare.

TRANSLATING RESULTS INTO
CLINICAL GUIDELINES FOR PATIENTS

As noted at the beginning of this chapter, those who have intimate familiarity with drug formularies relate difficulties with translating the results of healthcare economic analyses into clinical guidelines. Considering that it is difficult for formulary committee members to evaluate cost-utility studies, it is critical that researchers who perform economic analyses in the area of pharmacoeconomics do so with the thought of clinical usefulness in mind. In essence, these studies should be user-friendly. Authors of value-based analyses have a tendency to make their analyses so comprehensive that the average clinician has difficulty understanding the major message, much less the methodology or quality of the methodology. A crucial factor is to make an analysis comprehensible to the point that it can be applied clinically for the benefit of patients. If no one understands a study but the author(s), it does very little good sitting on the shelf in the *Journal of Incomprehensible Methods.*

VALUE-BASED MEDICINE,
PHARMACEUTICALS, AND COMPARATOR DRUGS

Average cost-utility analysis can compare a pharmaceutical intervention with no treatment, but these analyses generally find such an intervention is within a cost-effective range. More useful, however, are incremental cost-utility analyses that compare treatment with one pharmaceutical agent with that of another agent (comparator drug) used to treat the same health condition. This type of analysis can be particularly useful, especially since many newer pharmaceutical agents are in the same class as drugs previously approved by the FDA.

   Identifying a drug that provides the same value for less cost, greater value for the same cost, or greater value for less cost compared to a comparator is a very reasonable use for a pharmaceutical cost-utility analysis.

A PHARMACEUTICAL COST-UTILITY ANALYSIS

In this section we demonstrate the use of a cost-utility model for the evaluation of pharmaceutical agents. Let us assume that a large clinical trial shows a new

T A B L E   20.4

Adverse Effects Associated With Drugs A and B During a One-Year Period of Use

Adverse Effects	Drug A	Drug B
Headache	10%	12%
Heartburn	8%	7%
Diarrhea	7%	5%
Nausea	11%	9%

nonsteroidal anti-inflammatory drug (Drug B) to have the same therapeutic equivalency of a comparator drug already on the market (Drug A) for the treatment of rheumatoid arthritis. Drug B is marketed as causing less gastrointestinal adverse effects than Drug A. A review of the clinical trial data shows that each drug has the adverse effects listed in Table 20.4 during the one-year period of the study.

The average wholesale price (AWP) for a one-year supply of Drug A is $1,000 and for Drug B is $2,000. A healthcare insurer asks which drug confers more patient value and which drug is more cost-effective for its pharmaceutical formulary.

The seven fundamental steps undertaken in performing a cost-utility analysis for a pharmaceutical intervention are the same as those in medical, surgical, and nursing cost-utility studies:

1. Define the question.
2. Define all germane outcome(s) utilizing the best evidence-based data.
3. Assign utility values to the outcomes.
4. Measure the total value conferred by the intervention using decision analysis.
5. Estimate the costs.
6. Calculate the cost-utility ratio and then discount the value gained and the costs accrued to their present values to arrive at a discounted cost-utility ratio.
7. Perform sensitivity analysis to handle uncertainty.

1. Define the Question

There are two questions in this analysis:

- Which drug confers more value?
- Which drug is more cost-effective?

As with the cost-utility analysis examples outlined in Chapters 17, 18, and 19, we must first answer the seven defining variables inherent in this first fundamental step:

- **The intervention options to be compared:** use of two nonsteroidal anti-inflammatory drugs
- **The diseases (health states) to be studied:** rheumatoid arthritis
- **The target population:** patients with rheumatoid arthritis
- **The study perspective:** reference case
- **The cost perspective:** third-party insurer
- **The time frame:** one year
- **The outcomes:** function with arthritis, the adverse drug effects of headache, heartburn, diarrhea, and nausea

2. Define All Germane Outcomes Utilizing the Best Evidence-Based Data

The value derived from both Drug A and Drug B is equivalent. Each drug improves the patient with rheumatoid arthritis from the American College of Rheumatology Classification of Global Functional Status in Rheumatoid Arthritis Class II (able to perform usual self-care and vocational activities, but limited in avocational activities) to Class I (completely able to perform usual activities of daily living, including self-care, vocational, and avocational activities).[26] The incidence of the adverse effects associated with each drug was shown earlier in Table 20.4.

3. Assign Utility Values to the Outcomes

From the evaluation of patients with rheumatoid arthritis at the Center for Value-Based Medicine, we have found that the utility value associated with Class II rheumatoid arthritis is 0.91 and that associated with Class I rheumatoid arthritis is 0.98. The patient-based time-tradeoff utility values associated with moderate to severe adverse effects are shown in Table 20.5.

4. Measure the Total Value Conferred by an Intervention Using Decision Analysis

To calculate the value conferred by each drug, the benefit and the adverse effects must be integrated into a decision analysis tree to ascertain the mean utility value associated with the use of Drug A and the use of Drug B (Figure 20.1). The utility value for no treatment (0.91) is that associated with the American College of Rheumatology Classification of Global Functional Status Class II (able to perform usual self-care and vocational activities, but limited in avocational activities).[26] The utility value for treatment with no adverse effects (0.98) is that associated with the American College of Rheumatology Classification of Global Functional Status Class I (able to perform usual self-care, vocational activities, and avocational activities).[26] The utility values for adverse effects are derived from Table 20.5.

TABLE 20.5

Patient Time-Tradeoff Utility Values Associated With Adverse Effects

Adverse Effect (Moderate to Severe)	Associated Utility Value
Headache	0.80
Heartburn	0.93
Diarrhea	0.85
Nausea	0.82

FIGURE 20.1

Decision Analysis Tree Comparing Drug A, Drug B, and No Treatment. The tree shows the mean utility value (0.91) of the average person with untreated arthritis, the mean utility value (0.9313) of the average person with arthritis treated with Drug A, and the mean utility value (0.9340) of the average person with arthritis treated with Drug B. The preferred strategy is the use of Drug B since it yields the highest utility value. The number beneath each arm of the tree on the right is the incidence of the outcome listed on the line above it, and the numbers within the rectangular boxes are utility values associated with each outcome.

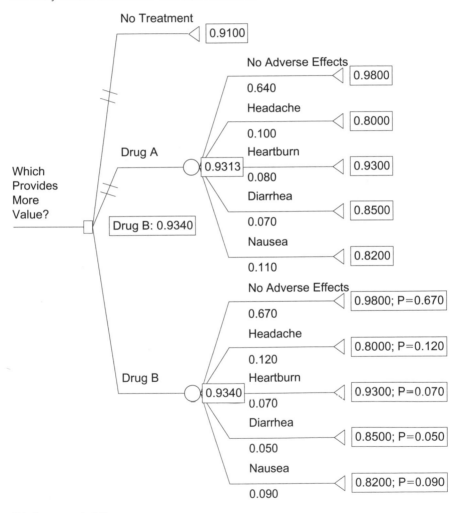

P indicates probability.

The QALY accrual during one year of untreated arthritis is thus 0.91 (0.91 × 1), while that of treatment with Drug A is 0.9340 (0.9340 × 1), and that for treatment with Drug B is 0.9313 (0.9313 × 1) (Table 20.6). The total value gained over no treatment for Drug A is 0.0213 QALY, while for Drug B it is 0.0240 QALY. The total value conferred by Drug B over Drug A is 0.0240 − 0.02313 = 0.0027 QALY.

5. Estimate the Costs

The AWP of Drug A over a one-year period is $1,000, while that associated with Drug B is $2,000.[27] There are no hospital costs, and the costs of seeing a provider are estimated to be the same whether the reference case is treated with Drug A or Drug B or receives no treatment. For simplicity we are supposing that the adverse effects of each drug are not treated with additional pharmaceuticals. The associated costs of each strategy were shown earlier in Table 20.5.

6. Calculate the Cost-Utility Ratio(s) and Discount the Value Gained and the Costs Accrued to Their Present Values to Arrive at a Discounted Cost-Utility Ratio

The average (vs no treatment) cost utility of drug A is $46,948/QALY, while the average cost utility of Drug B is $83,333/QALY. The use of either Drug A or Drug B is considered cost-effective using $100,000/QALY as the upper limit of cost-effectiveness.[17] While Drug B confers more value than Drug A, it is also more expensive than Drug A. Thus, should one use Drug A or Drug B, the latter of which confers greater value?

The incremental cost-effectiveness of Drug B referent to Drug A can also be calculated. In this instance, the incremental yearly QALY (value) gain from the use of Drug B over Drug A is 0.9340 − 0.9313 = 0.0027. The incremental yearly cost associated with using Drug B instead of Drug A is $2,000 − $1,000 = $1,000. Thus the cost utility of using Drug B instead of Drug A is $1,000/0.0027 = $185,185/QALY.

TABLE   20.6

Yearly Value Gain (QALYs) and Costs

	Utility Value	Total Value (QALY) Gain Over No Treatment	Costs	$/QALY, Undiscounted
	0.91	0	NA	NA
Drug A	0.9313	0.0213	$1,000	$46,948*
Drug B	0.9340	0.0240	$2,000	$83,333*

NA indicates not applicable; QALY, quality-adjusted life-year.

* Average cost-effectiveness (compared to no treatment).

Using an upper limit of $100,000/QALY, the use of Drug B instead of Drug A is not considered to be cost-effective. From the clinical point of view, the difference between the drugs is nominal with such a high cost-utility ratio. The data suggest that generally using Drug A as a first-line drug in the insurer's preferred drug list is reasonable unless there are contraindications such as allergy or other idiosyncratic effects.

Because costs and outcomes (QALYs) are generally not discounted during the first year, it is not necessary in this instance. Since the yearly cost and the yearly outcomes remain constant in this case, discounting each at 3% will not alter the $/QALY. Since discounting will not change the final result, it is unnecessary in this particular analysis.

7. Perform a Sensitivity Analysis to Handle Uncertainty

The costs, the utility values, and/or the incidences of adverse effects can all be varied in the sensitivity analysis. It is most critical to examine those variables in which we have the least confidence. The use of 95% confidence intervals is helpful in this regard. The confidence intervals surrounding clinical outcomes, utility values, costs, and other variables about which we have the least certainty should be investigated.

The variable that often has the most influence upon a cost-utility analysis is the degree of clinical benefit, or value, gained. In the above scenario, Drug A and Drug B had an identical clinical benefit (utility value = 0.98) but differing adverse effects. Let us assume that the 95% confidence interval for the utility values associated with treatment with Drug B ranges from 0.96 to 1.00, a seemingly small amount. The resultant decision analysis using the upper limit for the 95% confidence interval (1.00) is shown in Figure 20.2.

The new total value outcomes associated with no treatment, Drug A, and Drug B are shown in Table 20.7. Drug B now delivers sufficient value that it, despite its 100% greater cost than Drug A, is close in cost utility to Drug A.

TABLE 20.7

Yearly Value Gain (QALYs) and Costs

	QALY Gain (Yearly)	QALY Gain Over No Treatment	Costs	$/QALY
	0.91	0	NA	NA
Drug A	0.9313	0.0213	$1,000	$46,948*
Drug B	0.9474	0.0374	$2,000	$53,475*

NA indicates not applicable; QALY, quality-adjusted life-year.

* Average cost-effectiveness (compared to no treatment).

F I G U R E   20.2

Decision Tree Analysis Shown in Figure 20.1 With the Utility Value Outcome Associated With Treatment Using Drug B Changed From 0.98 to 1.00. Drug B is associated with a higher utility value and is still the theoretical preferred treatment strategy according to the decision analysis.

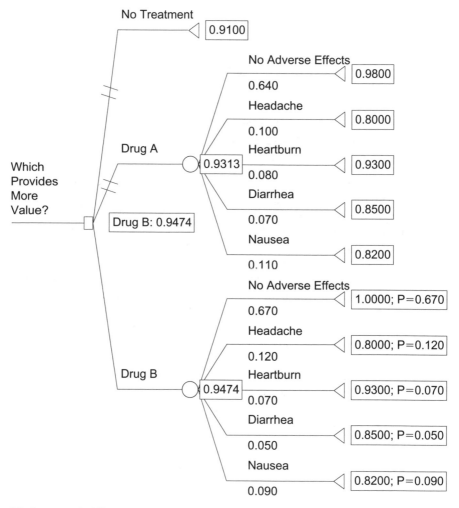

P indicates probability.

The incremental cost-effectiveness of Drug B referent to Drug A is again calculated. In this instance, the incremental yearly QALY (value) gain from the use of Drug B over Drug A is $0.9474 - 0.9313 = 0.0161$. The incremental yearly cost associated with using Drug B instead of Drug A is still $2,000 - 1,000 = 1,000$.

Thus, the cost utility of using Drug B instead of Drug A is now $1,000/0.0161 = $62,112. Using an upper limit of $100,000/QALY, the use of Drug B instead of Drug A is considered cost-effective.

Thus, a seemingly small change in the utility value associated with an outcome (0.98 to 1.00 for Drug B) has resulted in a markedly different cost utility for the drug and a different clinical recommendation. Despite the higher cost of Drug B, it delivers sufficient value to be listed as the first-line drug over Drug A in the health insurer's preferred drug list.

CORE CONCEPTS

- Value-based medicine principles are highly applicable to the science of pharmacoeconomics.
- Value-based medicine has played a minor role to date in regard to the utilization of pharmaceutical interventions because:
  - There is a lack of healthcare economic competence among formulary members.
  - An adequate supply of relevant, value-based studies is lacking.
  - There is difficulty in translating the results of cost-utility studies into clinical guidelines.
  - There is a lack of cost-utility analysis standards.
- Spending money on pharmaceutical agents that work well returns great value to patients and to the country. Spending it inefficiently does not.
- Approximately 73% of the revenue from pharmaceutical sales comes from the United States.
- Approximately 79% of pharmaceutical research and development is performed in the United States.
- Cost-utility analysis can help pharmaceutical manufacturers evaluate new drugs for development as well as those in the pipeline for FDA approval.
- Value-based medicine allows pharmaceutical manufacturers to readily demonstrate the value of their drugs to stakeholders in healthcare.
- Value-based medicine identifies drugs of the same or greater value for less cost.
- Value-based medicine will:
  - allow pharmaceutical dollars to be spent in the most efficient fashion, and
  - facilitate the provision of pharmaceuticals to all patients in need.

REFERENCES

1. Berger ML. The once and future application of cost-effectiveness analysis. *Jt Comm J Qual Improv.* 1999;25:455–461.

2. Rascati KL, Drummond MF, Annemans L, Davey PG. Education in pharmacoeconomics: an international multidisciplinary view. *Pharmacoeconomics.* 2004;22:139–147.

3. Olson BM, Armstrong EP, Grizzle AJ, Nichter MA. Industry's perception of presenting pharmacoeconomic models to managed care organizations. *J Manag Care Pharm.* 2003;9:159–167.

4. Wang Z, Salmon JW, Walton SM. Cost-effectiveness analysis and the formulary decision-making process. *J Manag Care Pharm.* 2004;10:48–59.

5. Anell A, Svarvar P. Pharmacoeconomics and clinical practice guidelines: a survey of attitudes in Swedish formulary committees. *Pharmacoeconomics.* 2000;17:175–185.

6. Sanchez LA. Applied pharmacoeconomics: evaluation and use of pharmacoeconomic data from the literature. *Am J Health Syst Pharm.* 1999;56:1630–1638.

7. Suh DC, Okpara IR, Agnese WB, Toscani M. Application of pharmacoeconomics to formulary decision making in managed care organizations. *Am J Manag Care.* 2002;8:161–169.

8. Anis AH, Gagnon Y. Using economic evaluations to make formulary coverage decisions: so much for guidelines. *Pharmacoeconomics.* 2000;18:55–62.

9. Prosser LA, Koplan JP, Neumann PJ, Weinstein MC. Barriers to using cost-effectiveness analysis in managed care decision making. *Am J Manag Care.* 2000;6:173–179.

10. Grabowski H, Mullins CD. Pharmacy benefit management, cost-effectiveness analysis and drug formulary decisions. *Soc Sci Med.* 1997;45:535–544.

11. Nissen SE, Tuzcu EM, Schoenhagen P, et al, for the REVERSAL Investigators. Effect of intensive compared with moderate lipid-lowering therapy on progression of coronary atherosclerosis: a randomized controlled trial. *JAMA.* 2004;291:1071–1080.

12. Ukens C. How mail order pharmacy gained in market share in 2003. *Drug Topics.* 2004;148.

13. Centers for Medicare and Medicaid Services. Statistics and data. Available at: www.cms.hhs.gov. Accessed March 6, 2004.

14. John AM, Thomas NS, Mufti GJ, Padua RA. Targeted therapies in myeloid leukemia. *Semin Cancer Biol.* 2004;14:41–62.

15. Heudebert GR, Centor RM, Klapow JC, et al. What is heartburn worth? A cost-utility analysis of management strategies. *J Gen Intern Med.* 2000;15:175–182.

16. Kallmes DF, Kallmes MH. Cost-effectiveness of angiography performed during surgery for ruptured intracranial aneuryms. *AJNR Am J Neuroradiol.* 1997;18:1453–1462.

17. Laupacis A, Feeny D, Detsky AS, Tugwell PX. How attractive does a new technology have to be to warrant adoption and utilization: tentative guidelines for using clinical and economic evaluations. *CMAJ.* 1992;146:473–481.

18. Jacobson JJ, Schweitzer SO, Kowalski CJ. Chemoprophylaxis of prosthetic joint patients during dental treatment: a decision utility analysis. *Oral Surg Oral Med Oral Pathol.* 1991;72:167–177.

19. Drug Topics Archive. Top 200 brand and generic drugs by retail dollars in 2002. *Drug Topics.* 2003;7:53, 57.

20. Gebhart F. 2002 Rx market: a look in the rearview mirror. *Drug Topics.* 2003;6:37.

21. PhRMA. Pharmaceutical companies receive FDA approval for 26 NME and biologics, 63 other new medicines, and 172 new uses for medicines in 2002. Press release, January 30, 2003. Available at: www.phrma.org/mediaroom/press/releases/30.01.2003.682.cfm. Accessed March 23, 2004.

22. Office of the Budget, National Institutes of Health. Distribution of NIH Budget, FY 2002. Available at: http://grants.nih.gov/grants/award/trends/distbud02.htm. Accessed September 6, 2004.

23. Pharmaceutical Researchers and Manufacturers of America (PhRMA). *Pharmaceutical Industry Profile 2003.* Washington, DC: PhRMA; 2003.

24. US General Accounting Office. Clinical Research: NIH has implemented key provisions of the Clinical Research Enhancement Act. Report to Congressional Committees, 2002. Available at: www.gao.gov/new.items/d02965.pdf. Accessed September 6, 2004.

25. Tufts Center for the Study of Drug Development. Backgrounder: a methodology for counting costs for pharmaceutical R&D. Available at: http://csdd.tufts.edu/NewsEvents/RecentNews.asp?newsid=5. Accessed March 23, 2004.

26. Hochberg MC, Chang RW, Dwosh I, Lindsey S, Pincus T, Wolfe F. The American College of Rheumatology revised criteria for the classification of global functional status in rheumatoid arthritis. *Arthritis Rheum.* 1992;35:498–502.

27. Stein HP, ed. *2003 Drug Topics Red Book.* Montvale, NJ: Medical Economics Company; 2003.

21

The Paradigm Will Prevail

Many have solutions for the "healthcare crisis" in the United States. With rapidly rising healthcare costs and over 40 million lacking health insurance, hardly a day passes that any major city newspaper does not have an article on healthcare.

Despite the rhetoric, we have yet to see a plan that offers the rewards of value-based medicine (VBM). We are unaware of another information system, methodology, or program that can improve quality of healthcare at the same time it saves the vast resources that VBM can save.

CURRENT USE OF HEALTHCARE ECONOMIC ANALYSIS

Healthcare economic analyses have been used increasingly to evaluate health interventions over the past decade. To demonstrate, the results of a MEDLINE search we performed using the key words *cost-effectiveness* and *cost-utility* came up with 724 hits for the year 2000 as opposed to 191 hits for 1990. This increase can be attributed to a number of sources, including advancement of the scientific methods used in evaluating cost-effectiveness, increasing numbers of healthcare providers who have formal experience in healthcare and business principles, and interest from pharmaceutical companies in demonstrating the value of their products.

Most formulary committees for hospitals, managed care organizations, and public payers (Medicare and Medicaid) in the United States do not require data on the cost utility of a pharmaceutical before funding it through an insurance plan. This will change.

We predict a cost-utility analysis will be a well-accepted standard in select healthcare arenas within a decade. While no one can say where the first major effect will occur, it is likely that pharmaceuticals will be among the first interventions to be affected. In Ontario, the Ministry of Health and Long Term Care requires any pharmaceutical company that submits a request for drug funding through the provincial formulary (which covers drug costs for seniors and those on social assistance) to submit a cost-effectiveness analysis that meets certain criteria. However, formulary committees generally use these submissions subjectively in making final decisions. Australia also requires healthcare economic analyses for inclusion of a pharmaceutical in a drug formulary,[1] while in the United Kingdom the National Institute for Clinical Excellence (NICE) dissemi-nates guidance to the National Health Service.[2]

Existing and potential requirements for funding new pharmaceuticals have pressured drug companies into performing cost-utility analyses both in-house or through academic centers and/or private consulting firms. In addition, other funding agencies, such as federal and state or provincial governments, nonprofit research organizations, and universities, are increasingly interested in the cost-utility of current and novel medical treatments and are funding this research more heavily.

In recent years, the scientific interest in cost-utility analysis has also increased, thus allowing more scientifically rigorous studies to be performed and published.[3] The financial support of those agencies with an inherent interest in the potential results of economic evaluations—including insurers, pharmaceutical companies, and government—has facilitated this academic interest. In addition, the relative abundance of randomized clinical trials being published has allowed for full eco-nomic evaluations to be performed more easily. The recent increase in computing power allows more sophisticated computer programs to be designed and more iterations and complex analyses to be performed more quickly.

THE CHANGING ENVIRONMENT

Although there has been an increasing interest in the economic evaluation of healthcare interventions, the actual applications of scientifically rigorous studies have not been well documented. The most common application of rigorous full economic evaluations for formulary or device committees is as aids to decide whether to fund a new drug or medical device. Even in this case, the cost-utility analysis is used subjectively in the decision-making process. Cost-utility analysis can also be used by private or government insurers, but it is difficult to know how often this is done or how important the cost-utility analysis is in the deci-sions being made.

As the scientific methods of cost-utility analysis develop and become more systematic, and the public begins to understand the importance of basing fund-ing decisions on the *value* of a medical treatment, there will be more potential applications of cost-utility analysis in health policy. At this time, the cost utility of a treatment or medical practice is not currently considered when agencies determine best practice guidelines for medical or public health. In the future, these guidelines will likely consider not only the effectiveness of medical treat-ments, but also their value when compared to comparable alternatives. In addi-tion, as the cost-utility literature becomes more systematic and readily compara-ble, it will be possible to create valid league tables, or lists of health interventions along with their respective cost-utility ratios. If the cost utility of the various programs in a league table have been measured rigorously using similar meth-ods, then the cost utility of a wide variety of health interventions can potentially be compared. Such comparisons can aid in difficult resource allocation decisions so that quality of care can be improved in the most cost-effective manner.

BENEFITS OF VALUE-BASED MEDICINE

For the Patient

Patients lack a standardized source of information that recounts the value of an intervention. Value-based medicine will provide a more sophisticated form of *Consumer Report* for patients to evaluate treatment options using the opinions of other patients who have lived in, and been treated for, the same health state. This VBM database could be used for all interventions: medical, surgical, and pharmaceutical. No such database exists at the present time. Despite the considerable difficulties encountered in creating a VBM database, the eventual results can be clarified to whatever level necessary to allow the information to benefit even those with a nominal understanding of healthcare services.

If an intervention costs $10,000/QALY gained, the patient can be confident that the intervention works well. Even expensive interventions that work well will have a reasonable cost-utility ratio. If the intervention costs $5 million/QALY, the patient will realize it is of negligible value over the alternative, whether it be another treatment or no treatment. The patient then has the option to seek another opinion, select another intervention, or decide whether to let the disease run its natural course.

Value-based medicine for the reference case can discern an overall negative or neutral outcome for a healthcare intervention when these outcomes are very difficult to differentiate from evidence-based data alone. It can also illustrate the underestimation of the value conferred by an intervention when only a primary evidence-based outcome is available. The quality-of-life variables addressed by VBM can dramatically improve the value of an intervention, decrease the value of an intervention, or place the intervention into the potentially harmful category. But most important, the value conferred will be the most accurate and reproducible since it is obtained using the preferences of other patients with the same disease or health state. Put another way, since VBM better evaluates the worth of a healthcare intervention to patients than evidence-based medicine (EBM), VBM allows patients to receive higher quality of care than EBM alone.

For the Provider

Providers will also benefit from VBM because they will have a better perception of the actual value their interventions to convey to patients. In addition, all physicians become patients at some point, and they will be able to utilize the information personally. We believe when all the benefits and the adverse effects associated with some interventions are included in the overall equation, providers will be surprised that the overall value conferred is either greater or less than they had previously believed.

Does a very high cost utility mean a provider should not offer an intervention? No, but it certainly should make both the patient and the provider examine other possible options.

For the Public Welfare

As the costs of healthcare continue to outpace general inflation, difficult resource allocations must be made for healthcare services. Value-based medicine will allow the most efficacious use of resources to help the most people receive the highest quality of healthcare possible for the resources expended. Considering the enormity of the healthcare expenditure in the United States ($1.773 billion, or 4.7 times that of the $380 billion defense budget in 2004; see Chapter 3), the most efficient use of healthcare resources is a critical factor for the country to remain in a globally influential position.

Identification of interventions that are not cost-effective will allow the public to have input with policymakers and healthcare professionals as to the future of the interventions. An intervention should not necessarily be discontinued because it is not cost-effective. Nonetheless, if an intervention is identified as not cost-effective, options that can bring a treatment into the range of cost-effectiveness should be considered. These include improving the effectiveness, and/or decreasing the associated costs, and/or altering the adverse effects with additional modifying interventions.

While no one can guarantee that savings from VBM will be utilized to insure the more than 40 million people in the United States who currently lack healthcare insurance, VBM will at least make money available for this purpose. We can only hope legislators have the foresight to direct the savings so all citizens might receive appropriate healthcare.

Select policy decision makers do realize the great value of healthcare economic analyses.[4] Nonetheless, in a study in the United Kingdom they also realized some of the same problems we have addressed in this book, more specifically that the lack of methodological rigor, the lack of reliability, and the poor generalizability of results preclude current widespread usage. These are all issues the readers of this text can now, at least in theory, remedy.

FINAL THOUGHTS

No matter what plan is offered for healthcare reform, there will always be naysayers. This is not a new phenomenon, but if the naysayers always had their way, we would still be toasting the Queen's birthday in the United States. There will undoubtedly be naysayers for VBM, but their 15 minutes of fame will be short as all stakeholders in healthcare realize the enormity of what VBM has to offer.

As the costs and complexities of healthcare in the United States and other countries continue to increase faster than available budgets, assessing the value of healthcare interventions will become increasingly important. At present, cost-utility analysis in healthcare offers a method that combines available data in a logical fashion and allows decision makers to consider both the costs and benefits of different resource allocation alternatives. Resource allocation decisions in the real world will never be based solely on cost-utility analysis, but as the methodologies used in economic evaluations become better known, they will play a more significant role as aids in making difficult funding decisions in healthcare.

The importance of VBM and cost-utility analysis transcends even the healthcare system. Cost-utility analysis can compare expenditures used for virtually any safety programs (speed limits, helmet use for motorcyclists, environmental protection standards, work safety standards, equipment to protect soldiers, and so on), permitting society to use its resources for the highest return for its citizens. Spending for the highest return, whether it be in healthcare or for other safety and quality-of-life endeavors, will undoubtedly improve the standard of living for society as a whole. It will also focus society on the real problem in healthcare today in the United States—not that too much is spent on healthcare services, but that it is spent inefficiently and unwisely.

> The spending of resources for the highest return, whether on healthcare services or other safety and quality-of-life endeavors, will undoubtedly improve the standard of living for society as a whole.

Articles concerning healthcare costs in the United States appear daily in the media. When the lead articles in both the *Wall Street Journal*[5] and the *New York Times*[6] on the same day are concerned with the rise in medical costs, and the cost of drugs for seniors is rising at three times the rate of inflation,[7] the issue of healthcare costs will move higher on the public policy agenda. As policymakers and the public learn about the advantages offered by VBM, changes will surely come about that are positive for all patients, our healthcare system, and the overall economic welfare of the country.

Final Thought

Value-based medicine
=
Improved quality of care
+
Efficient use of healthcare resources

CORE CONCEPTS

- Healthcare economic analyses have been increasingly used to evaluate healthcare interventions over the past decade.
- Since VBM better evaluates the worth of a healthcare intervention to a patient than EBM, VBM allows patients to receive higher-quality care than EBM does alone.

■ Value-based medicine can provide the money to make healthcare insurance available to the more than 40 million who currently lack it and make drugs available to the seniors and others in need.

REFERENCES

1. Henry D, Lopert R. Pharmacoeconomics and policy decisions: the Australian health care system. *Clin Ther.* 1999;21:909-915.

2. Meads C, Salas C, Roberts T, et al. *Clinical Effectiveness and Cost Utility of Photodynamic Therapy for Wet Age-Related Macular Degeneration.* Birmingham, West Midlands: Health Technology Assessment Group, University of Birmingham; 2002. Available at: www.nice.org.uk/Docref.asp?d=30223.

3. Chapman RH, Stone PW, Sandberg EA, Bell C, Neumann PJ. A comprehensive league table of cost-utility ratios and a sub-table of "panel-worthy" studies. *Med Decis Making.* 2000;20:451–467.

4. Hoffmann C, Stoykova BA, Nixon J, Glanville JM, Misso K, Drummond MF. Do health-care decision makers find economic evaluations useful? The findings of focus group research in UK health authorities. *Value Health.* 2002;5:71-78.

5. Martinez B. Wall Street Journal analyzes health care cost shifting. Employers cannot afford to shield employees from rising costs. *Wall Street Journal.* June 16, 2003:A1.

6. Perez-Pena R. 22 states limiting doctors' latitude in Medicaid drugs. *New York Times.* June 16, 2003:A1.

7. Abelson R. Study finds drug costs are soaring for elderly. *New York Times.* June 10, 2003.

INDEX

Page numbers in italics preceded by *f* indicate references to figures, and page numbers in italics preceded by *t* indicate references to tables.

A

Activities of daily living
 EuroQol 5D health measurement dimensions, t141
 large utility value decreases associated with functional losses, 191
 visual acuity and (questionnaire), *t114–116*
Activities of Daily Living Scale, 85, 101
ADL. *See* Activities of daily living
Adolescent obesity, 59–60
African-Americans, life expectancy, 199
Age and aging
 community underestimation of loss of quality of life (macular degeneration) 168–170, *t168, 169*
 discrimination, 198
 Medicare program, 33–37
 nursing home expenditures, 31, 33
 reference cases in cost-utility analysis, 19
Age Discrimination in Employment Act, 198
Allied health practitioners, Medicare allowed charges, *f37*
Alpha error, 58, 59
Alternative hypothesis, 58
Ambulatory surgery centers
 cost basis for cost-utility analysis, *t244*
 costs, reimbursement, 245
 recommended standards for cost-utility variables, 277
American College of Rheumatology Classification of Global Function Status in Rheumatoid Arthritis, 80, 85, 88, 159, *t89*
 categorical scales, 104
 description of, 105–106
American Heart Association Functional Capacity Classification, 85, 86, 88, *t89*
 angina associated with coronary artery disease, 187–188, *t187*
 categorical scales, 104
 description of, 104–105
Americans With Disabilities Act, 19, 164, 165
Analog scales. *See* Rating scales
Anchors. *See* Utility values
Angina
 associated with coronary artery disease, 187–188, *t187*
 multiple utility values, 159

Angina—*Cont.*
 utility values, 105
Annual discount rate, 209
Antibiotic costs, 285
Anticoagulants, cost-utility analysis, 267–270
Anxiety, 5D health measurement dimensions, *t141*
Aortic valve replacement, 196
Arterial hypertension. *See* Hypertension
Arthritis
 community underestimation of loss of quality of life, *t168*
 decision analysis with no-drug and drug-treatment options, *f174*
 rheumatoid, 80, 85, 105–106
 rheumatoid, time-tradeoff utility values, 159
 use of SF-12 and SF-36, 99
Articles, scientific. *See* Literature, scientific
Asbestos, 256
Aspirin therapy, 220
Asthma
 child utility values, 175
 community underestimation of loss of quality of life, *t168*
Atorvastatin, 303
Average wholesale price. *See* Drugs
AWP (average wholesale price). *See* Drugs

B

Bacterial pneumonia
 decision tree, 221–223, *f222*
 example of cost-utility analysis reference case study, 281–289
Beaver Dam Health Outcomes Study, 155, 159, 161–162, *t157*
 community underestimation of loss of quality of life 168–169, *t168*
Beta error, 58, 59
Bias, publication, 60
Blinding (research principle), 54, 55, 61
Breast cancer chemotherapy (example), 201
Brown, Gary C., author profile, xiii
Brown, Melissa M., author profile, xiii

C

Cancer. *See also* Eastern Cooperative Oncology Group Performance Status Scale
 chemotherapy value (example of overestimation), 200–202, *t201*

Stroke—*Cont.*
  community overestimation of loss of quality of
    life, *t170*
  time-tradeoff utility values, 159
  use of SF-36, 99
Supply and demand, 27
Surgery
  adverse effects calculated in quality-adjusted life-years
    (example), *t197*
  postoperative pain, 197
  quality-adjusted life-years, *t175*
  time-tradeoff utility value, 174, *t175*
Survival. *See* Time-tradeoff utility analysis
Systolic hypertension, 4

T

Terminal nodes, *f131, 135, 221, f222*
Test-retest reliability. *See* Reliability
The Theory of Games and Economic Behavior, 128
Therapies. *See* Interventions
"Thermometer" of feeling. *See* Feeling thermometer
Third-party insurer perspective
  cost-utility analysis, 18
  healthcare costs, 239–240
  Medicare-approved charges and, 244–245
  performing cost-utility analyses, 277, 281
  societal perspective and, 240
  types of healthcare economic analysis costs, *t238*
  use in cost-utility analysis, 240, 243
36-Item Short Form Health Survey. *See* SF-36
Time
  defining the question in cost-utility analysis, 267, 268,
    282–283
  discounting (time value of money), 207–217
  duration of treatment benefit, 270
  effect of, on disease, 173
Time-tradeoff utility analysis, 16, 85, 135–137, 146,
    151–181, *t89*
  advantages, 152, *t137*
  advantages when there are multiple diseases, 160–161
  applicability (universality) of utility values, 171
  assigning utility values to outcomes, 273–274, 283
  choosing best method for cost-utility analysis,
    145, 147
  comorbidities and, 161–166
  construct validity, 183–184
  demographic variables affecting utility values, 161
  disadvantages, *t137*
  disease severity and, 158–161
  drug adverse effects (example), *t310*
  forms of utility analysis, 129, *t126*
  guaranteed cures and, 158
  interviewer-administered as preferred method
    for, 158
  long- and short-term utility values, 173–175

Time-tradeoff utility analysis—*Cont.*
  multiple utility values, 159–160
  options, *f136*
  patient-based values as gold standard, 170–171, 176
  preferable to EuroQol 5D, 143
  preferred quality-of-life instrument, 151–152
  sample question, 136
  test-retest reliability, *t140*
  utility analysis instruments, 125
  utility value anchors (range) from death to perfect
    health, 129–131, 146, 171–173
  utility values, 129
  utility values compared to SF-36, 99
  utility values for angina associated with coronary
    artery disease, 187–188, *t187*
  utility values for irritable bowel syndrome, *t185*
  utility values for peripheral neuropathy, *t186*
  utility values, good construct validity and high
    correlation with symptom severity, 191
  utility values, quality of life studies, 75–76, *t76*
  utility values under, 154–157, *t155–157*
  utility values, visual acuity, *t188*
Tobacco. *See* Smoking
Tomography, computed. *See* Computed tomography
Torrance, G.W., 135
Total quality management, 53–70
Toxin control, 256, *t256*
Treatment event rate, 63, 64, 66, 68
Treatments. *See* Interventions
TreeAge Data 4.0, 223, 274
12-Item Short Form Health Survey. *See* SF-12

U

Uncertainty
  decision analysis demonstrates preferred strategy, 221
  decision making and, 128
  performing sensitivity analysis, 276, 286–288,
    f286, t287
Uninsured, 12, 46
United States government. *See* US government
US government healthcare spending, 33–38, *f34*
Utility analysis, 5, 6, 127–137. *See also* Cost-utility
    analysis; Time-tradeoff utility analysis; Willingness-
    to-pay utility analysis
  advantages when there are multiple diseases, 160–161
  comprehensiveness of, 128–129
  description, background, 127–128
  guaranteed cures and trading time, 158
  health parameters (diagnosis, severity, treatment,
    comorbidities), 133
  methods of, 129
  multiattribute, groups of preference-based quality-of-
    life instruments, 125, 126, 138–144
  non-interchangeable utility values between different
    forms of, 136